Standard Haematology Practice/3

Standard Haematology Practice/3
Edited by Keith Wood
on behalf of the British Committee
for Standards in Haematology

FOREWORD BY ADRIAN NEWLAND
President, British Society for Haematology

**Blackwell
Science**

© 2000 by
Blackwell Science Ltd
Editorial Offices:
Osney Mead, Oxford OX2 0EL
25 John Street, London WC1N 2BL
23 Ainslie Place, Edinburgh EH3 6AJ
350 Main Street, Malden
   MA 02148 5018, USA
54 University Street, Carlton
   Victoria 3053, Australia
10, rue Casimir Delavigne
   75006 Paris, France

Other Editorial Offices:
Blackwell Wissenschafts-Verlag GmbH
Kurfürstendamm 57
10707 Berlin, Germany

Blackwell Science KK
MG Kodenmacho Building
7–10 Kodenmacho Nihombashi
Chuo-ku, Tokyo 104, Japan

First published 2000

Set by Graphicraft Limited, Hong Kong
Printed and bound in Great Britain at
MPG Books Ltd, Bodmin, Cornwall

The right of the Author to be
identified as the Author of this Work
has been asserted in accordance
with the Copyright, Designs and
Patents Act 1988.

The Blackwell Science logo is a
trade mark of Blackwell Science Ltd,
registered at the United Kingdom
Trade Marks Registry

A catalogue record for this title
is available from the British Library

ISBN 0–632–05322–4

Library of Congress
Cataloging-in-publication Data

Standard haematology practice/3 /
   edited by Keith Wood on behalf of
   the British Committee for Standards in
   Haematology; foreword by Adrian
   Newland.
        p.   cm.
     ISBN 0–632–05322–4
     1. Haematology—Standards—
Great Britain.   I. Wood, Keith (J.
Keith)   II. British Committee for
Standards in Haematology.   III.
Title: Standard haematology practice
three.
     [DNLM: 1. Hematology—
standards.   2. Hematologic
Tests—standards.   3. Laboratory
Techniques and Procedures—
standards.   WH 100 S785   1999]
RB45.S752   1999
616.07′561′021841—dc21
DNLM/DLC
for Library of Congress   99–25479
                              CIP

DISTRIBUTORS

Marston Book Services Ltd
PO Box 269
Abingdon, Oxon OX14 4YN
(Orders: Tel: 01235 465500
         Fax: 01235 465555)

USA
Blackwell Science, Inc.
Commerce Place
350 Main Street
Malden, MA 02148 5018
(Orders: Tel: 800 759 6102
              781 388 8250
         Fax: 781 388 8255)

Canada
Login Brothers Book Company
324 Saulteaux Crescent
Winnipeg, Manitoba R3J 3T2
(Orders: Tel: 204 837–2987)

Australia
Blackwell Science Pty Ltd
54 University Street
Carlton, Victoria 3053
(Orders: Tel: 3 9347 0300
         Fax: 3 9347 5001)

For further information on
Blackwell Science, visit our website:
www.blackwell-science.com

Contents

Contents

Prepared by the Blood Transfusion Task Force

Prepared by the Clinical Haematology Task Force

List of Contributors

British Committee for Standards in Haematology

J.K. Wood (*Chairman*); I. Cavill (*Secretary*); A.K. Burnett; I.M. Franklyn; J.A.F. Napier; J.T. Reilly; J.G. Smith; I.D. Walker.

Past Members
T.W. Barrowcliffe; D. Catovsky; J.F. Davidson; J.K.M. Duguid; J.M. England (deceased); P. Garwood; J.C. Giddings; E.C. Gordon-Smith; D.A. Kennedy; M.F. Murphy; F.E. Preston; A.S.J. Rejman; R.M. Rowan.

General Haematology Task Force

J.T. Reilly (*Chairman*); B.J. Bain (*Secretary*); R. Amos; I. Cavill; C.S. Chapman; K. Hyde; E.M. Matutes; J. Parker-Williams; A. Stephens; J.K. Wood.

Past Members and Contributors
J.W. Bailey; D. Bareford; D. Barnett; G. Bird; P.L. Chiodini; S. Davies; J.M. England (deceased); E. Hodges; S.M. Lewis; D.C. Linch; I.J. Mackie; D.H. Molineux; M.F. Murphy; A.C. Newland; J. Old; R.M. Rowan; L. Secker-Walker; K. Shinton; J.G. Smith; D. Swirsky; B. Wild.

Haemostasis and Thrombosis Task Force

I.D. Walker (*Chairman*); S.J. Machin (*Secretary*); T. Baglin; T.W. Barrowcliffe; I. Cavill; B.T. Colvin; M. Greaves; C.A. Ludlam; I.J. Mackie; F.E. Preston; P.E. Rose; J.K. Wood.

Past Members and Contributors
B. Bennett; K.A.A. Fox; B.E.S. Gibson; E. Letsky; G.D.O. Lowe; M.F. Murphy; A. Reid. R. Rivers; R. Stevens; J.J Walker.

Blood Transfusion Task Force

J.A.F. Napier (*Chairman*); P.R. Kelsey (*Secretary*); M. Bruce; I. Cavill; J.F. Chapman; J.K.M. Duguid; S.M. Knowles; M.F. Murphy; L.M. Williamson; J.K. Wood.

Past Members and Contributors
J. Apperley; P. Armstrong; T. Baglin; S. Bates; P. Bowell; D. Brazier; B. Brozovic; M. Bruce; J. Butler; M. Contreras; A. Copplestone; N. Cross; P. Dendy; M. De Silva; M.J. Desmond; L. Dodson; R.D. Finney; K. Forman; M. Gesinde; B.E.S. Gibson; J. Gillon; R. Green; G. Hedley; S.E. Kinsey; R. Knight; A. Lardy; D. Lee; E. Letsky; C.E. Milkins; R. Mitchell; G. Morgan; W. Murphy; D. Norfolk; D.G. Oscier; D. Pamphilon; J. Parker-Williams; P. Phillips; G. Poole; D. Potock; A. Richards; T. Richards; S. Robson; N. Russell; M. Scott; K. Shwe; J.J. Smith; N. Tandy; A. Todd; D. Voak; R. Warwick; A.H. Waters; D. Webb; M. Whittle; F.G. Williams.

Clinical Haematology Task Force

J.G. Smith (*Chairman*); J.M. Davies (*Secretary*); J.F. Apperley; I. Cavill; P.S. Ganley; D. Gozzard; S.E. Kinsey; D.G. Oscier; J.K. Wood.

Past Members and Contributors
A. Adam; P.G. Baddeley; R.A. Barnes; A. Bristow; J.V. Clough; A.H.R. Finn; K. Forman; I.M. Franklyn; B.E.S. Gibson; D.W. Gorst; I.M. Hann; J.M.S. Johnstone; S.J. Kelly; C. Kibbler; J. Leese; J.E. Lortan; M.F. Murphy; H. Outhwaite; A.S.J. Rejman; J. Sarangi; J. Spencer; G.P. Summerfield; J.S. Thomas; J.A. Whittaker.

Foreword

The third volume of *Standard Haematology Practice* continues the tradition developed in the first two volumes, presenting the hard work that the British Committee for Standards in Haematology (BCSH), a subcommittee of the British Society for Haematology, has put in over the last 4 years.

Volume 3 not only fills a number of gaps that were not covered in the first two volumes, but is also able to update some of the guidelines seen in the first volume, reflecting the changes in current practice.

This collective volume reaffirms the commitment of the British Society for Haematology to support good practice in our speciality and the four BCSH Task Forces have put in considerable effort to fulfil this objective. In order to make sure the guidelines are as comprehensive and acceptable to other groups as possible, we have been able to include representatives from other societies and organizations that have a major interest in good haematological practice, including the British Blood Transfusion Society, the British Society for Haemostasis and Thrombosis and the Institute of Biomedical Science. We have also had considerable help from anaesthetists, paediatricians, surgeons, the Department of Health and others. In the current climate of good clinical practice, I am pleased to be able to present this compendium as an example of the Society's long-standing commitment to clinical excellence.

Adrian Newland
President
British Society for Haematology

Editor's Comments

Since 1984, the British Committee for Standards in Haematology (BCSH) of the British Society for Haematology has produced more than 50 guidelines to good haematological practice, 20 in the last 3 years. These latest form the basis of this volume, *Standard Haematology Practice*/3. Those haematologists and contributors involved in this work, more than 140 in all, are listed and I sincerely hope I have not overlooked anyone. I thank them all for their hard work. The compiling of *Standard Haematology Practice*/3 has been relatively straightforward from previously published guidelines and I thank the editors of the journals in which they appeared for the relaxation of copyright.

Keith Wood
Royal Infirmary, Leicester

Disclaimer
While the advice and information contained in this book is believed to be true and accurate at the time of going to press, neither the editor, the authors nor the publisher can accept any legal responsibility or liability for any errors or omissions that may be made.

1 Guidelines for Near-patient Testing: Haematology

Prepared by the General Haematology Task Force

1. Near-patient testing

1.1 Introduction

The purpose of these guidelines is to provide a framework for the provision of appropriate local arrangements for near-patient testing (NPT). This chapter embodies the philosophy agreed by the Joint Working Group (JWG) on External Quality Assessment (EQA) in Pathology (1992) and the national standards required for clinical pathology accreditation (Clinical Pathology Accreditation, 1993).

The need for local agreements about NPT is evident from a number of reports from the international scientific community (Marks, 1988, 1990; Nanji *et al.*, 1988; Elliot *et al.*, 1990; Farr, 1990; Hailey & Lea, 1990; Madsen *et al.*, 1990; Rachel & Plapp, 1990; Dybkaer *et al.*, 1992; Health Services Research Unit, 1992; Kennedy, 1992; Association of Clinical Biochemists, 1993; Rink *et al.*, 1993).

An example of the inherent problems of NPT is highlighted in a project to assess the reliability of measuring haemoglobin in health centres, which was coordinated by the Health Services Research Unit of the University of Warwick (1992). In this instance, the EQA results were unsatisfactory, confirming the need to monitor extra-laboratory testing. More recently, a major clinical trial has been undertaken into the value of NPT in several general practices (Health Services Research Unit, 1992; Rink *et al.*, 1993). Other important factors are the efficacy of the procedures being undertaken (Goldie & Kemp, 1993) and medico-legal and safety aspects (Department of Health, 1987a, b; Goldie & Kemp, 1993).

1.2 Scope

The scope of these guidelines relates to the management philosophy of NPT, the venues where NPT may be undertaken, the range of tests, the qualifications of the personnel involved and the timeliness of the service. Other aspects discussed are initiation of the service, training, equipment, results, monitoring of quality, accreditation, safety and cost.

The chapter focuses on the delivery of an on-site service within a hospital environment, e.g. an intensive-care unit. The guidelines do not specifically encompass general

Reprinted with permission from *Clinical and Laboratory Haematology*, 1995, **17**, 301–310.

practitioners' surgeries or other venues, e.g. pharmacies. However, much of the information could be applied to these other NPT sites and a section on key points for general practitioners considering NPT in their surgeries is included. Sites for NPT could include:

- intensive care units;
- accident and emergency departments;
- renal dialysis units;
- theatres;
- neonatal units;
- occupational health departments;
- research laboratories (undertaking clinical tests);
- general practitioners' surgeries and health centres;
- pharmacies.

Other non-accredited commercial institutions may also wish to avail themselves of the professional expertise available in central clinical laboratories.

The range of services should be clearly defined and includes blood counts (haemoglobin) and coagulation testing (prothrombin time (PT), activated partial thromboplastin time (APTT), thrombin time (TT) and activated clotting time (ACT)).

1.3 Range of equipment

The type of equipment used ranges from simple haemoglobinometers for the measurement of haemoglobin to small analysers that can produce a full blood count. Coagulation equipment ranges from simple instruments providing ACT or PT estimation to minianalysers producing PTs, TTs and APTTs. These are generally used for monitoring heparin or oral anticoagulant therapy. For blood counts, it is strongly recommended that near-patient investigators use only instrumentation that employs primary sampling (automated systems) and do not use instrumentation that involves dilution of whole blood in the preanalytical phase (semi-automated systems).

1.4 Examples of users

The types of personnel involved may include:

- medical practitioners;
- nurses;
- healthcare assistants;
- physiological measurement technicians;
- medical technical officers (MTOs);
- other non-laboratory personnel.

1.5 Philosophy

The principal philosophy is that NPT sites must work in partnership with the central laboratory. The cornerstone of this joint service should be the embodiment of the philosophy in a service-level agreement, which defines the range of services, operational details and responsibilities of both central haematology laboratory staff and on-site staff. The agreement should also define the times when the service is available, for example, 9 a.m.–5 p.m. or a 24-h service and full weekend service. Ownership of the results should belong jointly to the central haematology laboratory and the senior clinical staff of the department that is delivering the on-site service. In this way, a high level of quality will be maintained.

1.6 Management

While the on-site staff may understand the day-to-day operation and provision of results, the professional head of the central laboratory must take responsibility for all aspects of this service, after discussion with the clinicians concerned. This will include selection and procurement of the most appropriate equipment for the task in hand and assessment of the infrastructure of the on-site environment, which must meet basic laboratory standards.

Standard operating procedures (SOPs) must be written and signed by an appropriate senior member of the central laboratory staff. These SOPs will include details of procedures relating to service performance, delivery and safety regulations (HMSO, 1988; Health Services Advisory Committee, 1990). Protocols must also be produced for training of staff, monitoring performance of equipment and handling of results.

A directorate of laboratory medicine may wish to nominate or employ a peripatetic medical laboratory scientific officer (MLSO) who takes responsibility for monitoring the quality of the on-site service, perhaps in several locations.

The management arrangements should be clearly documented, together with appropriate lines of accountability. Job descriptions should contain appropriate sections on NPT.

1.7 Training

Training protocols must be established and all potential operators must achieve an adequate level of competence. This should include the basic principles of measurement, appropriate use of the equipment and consequences of inappropriate use, knowledge of normal and abnormal results, the importance of record keeping, the importance of internal quality control (IQC) and EQA and safety procedures (Kennedy, 1992). Trainees should also be awarded a certificate of competence by the central laboratory and a list of authorized users must be drawn up and approved by the head of the central laboratory. It would also be useful to make trainees aware of the recent code of conduct for NPT (Council for Professions Supplementary to Medicine, 1994). Arrangements must also be in hand for continuing professional development of the staff delivering the service, with regular training updates. Secondment of on-site staff to the central laboratories may be an appropriate method of training and continuing staff development.

1.8 Equipment

Equipment selected for on-site investigations will usually have been evaluated by the Medical Devices Agency (MDA) at the Department of Health. Potential users must ensure that equipment is safe and that results are comparable with results from instruments in the central laboratory. Central laboratory staff must take responsibility for the initial installation, setting up and calibration of equipment. It is also essential that equipment has a preventive maintenance schedule and a service contract, together with a logbook documenting operational details, faults, repairs or other corrective action. Appropriate backup arrangements for equipment must be made.

Reagents should be procured by the central laboratory and supplied in a cost-effective manner to the clinical unit concerned. A logbook of the shelf-life of reagents and batch numbers used must be maintained by on-site staff.

1.9 Safety

Standard operating procedures must be available for the collection, transportation, processing and disposal of specimens. Other protocols should be available for containment of spillages and a clearly identified policy for containment of 'high-risk' samples must be defined. All procedures must conform to the policy for *Safe Working and the Prevention of Infection in Clinical Laboratories* (Health Services Advisory Committee, 1990). Ideally, specimen analysis should be by closed-vial sampling. Dilution of whole blood in the pre-analytical phase is not recommended for the NPT environment.

Protocols must also be available for the disinfection and decontamination of equipment and laboratories. Each procedure must have undergone a full control of substances hazardous to health (COSHH) assessment – for example, if cyanide reagents are used in the determination of haemoglobin. All procedures should conform to the appropriate legislation (HMSO, 1974, 1988; Department of Health, 1987c; Health Services Advisory Committee, 1990).

1.10 Results

It is essential that results of tests are documented. For most investigations – for example, blood counts – some type of request form would be appropriate and these requests should include full patient identity details (name, hospital number, data of birth, location, date, time). In the absence of appropriate computer systems, results must be documented in a logbook, which also identifies reagent batch numbers and the name of the operator; results must be returned to the clinician in a written format, with appropriate biological reference ranges. A system must be in place to ensure that results are comparable with central laboratory results and integrated with these in the case notes of the patient. When computers are available – for example, order communications systems – NPT results must be integrated with central laboratory results in the clinical computer and their origin appropriately identified. The units used for reporting results must be the same as those in the central laboratory.

A system must also be defined where results are validated by satisfactory performance in IQC and EQA schemes. Abnormal results must be appropriately flagged. Moreover, mechanisms must be agreed for appropriate referral to the central laboratory of out-of-limits results for further investigation. Advice on interpretation and clinical matters is readily available from consultant staff in the central haematology laboratory.

1.11 Quality

The principles of total quality management (TQM) must be adhered to, beginning with sample collection and ending with the integration of results into the patient's case notes.

All aspects of quality must be considered, including personnel, equipment, reagents and appropriateness and timeliness of the service.

1.11.1 Internal quality control

Responsibility for initial calibration and all future calibration of any instrumentation must rest with the central haematology laboratory. Equally, the provision of calibration and control materials, together with clearly defined operating rules for the regular use and interpretation of IQC materials and a policy for involvement in EQA, is the responsibility of the central laboratory.

1.11.2 External quality assessment

In principle, all providers of laboratory services have access to a range of EQA schemes and it is expected that both NPT and centralized laboratory sites should be subject to EQA by a scheme recognized by the JWG (1992). In this regard, NPT should not be seen as a secondary type of testing service and subjected to less rigorous EQA. Local haematologists should involve general practitioners and other NPT users in the central laboratory's EQA scheme. Near-patient testing results are used for clinical purposes in just the same way as those from centralized laboratories. Indeed, it is possible to imagine that certain NPT sites, e.g. out-patient departments of cancer centres, might have higher throughputs than, and require just as high-quality standards as, centralized laboratories.

1.11.3 General haematology

Given the fact that NPT results are used for clinical purposes and that it is inappropriate to distinguish data produced by NPT from those of centralized laboratory services, there can be no case for avoiding full participation in EQA by NPT sites. In general haematological practice, NPT is likely to be confined to the blood count, for which, at present, only the UK National External Quality Assessment Scheme (NEQAS) is recognized by the JWG.

1.11.4 Coagulation testing

Similar EQA schemes and samples to those used in hospital laboratories for traditional tests may be used on NPT instruments utilizing citrated plasma. True like-with-like EQA of instruments using non-anticoagulated whole blood is impossible; the performance of these instruments must therefore by monitored by comparable tests in the central laboratory, using a citrated venous sample collected simultaneously. A proportion of the daily or weekly workload must be compared with results from the central laboratory. For some instruments, commercial lyophilized blood preparations with normal and abnormal clotting times are available. These mimic fresh whole blood and can be used for EQA, as well as precision studies. An additional way of providing EQA may be the use of stabilized red cells (van Dijk-Wierda *et al.*, 1978), which can be recombined with stabilized or lyophilized normal or abnormal plasmas.

1.12 Accreditation

The NPT service must be considered for national accreditation (Clinical Pathology

Accreditation, 1993) as part of the central laboratory's accreditation submission. All appropriate accreditation standards must be adhered to.

1.13 Finance

In some circumstances a cost–benefit analysis may need to be undertaken. This must include amortization of the equipment and transport costs and should also take account of the cost, quality, timeliness and appropriateness of the service.

1.14 General practitioners' surgeries

*1.14.1 Key points**

General practitioners should do the following.

1 Seek the advice and involvement of their local haematologist if they are considering NPT, in order to achieve optimum quality and cost-effectiveness.

2 Decide whether they wish to undertake procedures for diagnosis, for screening for occult disease or to monitor disease or the effect of treatment, before embarking on NPT. For example, haemoglobinometry does not serve any particular function as a single measurement for diagnosis; some patients with serious illnesses, such as leukaemia, may have a normal haemoglobin (Rejman, 1992).

3 Decide which investigations they wish to perform, bearing in mind the turn-round time of their local laboratory and patient convenience.

4 Consider the recent study, which offered a clear message that there is only a weak case for equipping general practices with the means of doing a wide range of investigations in-house (Health Services Research Unit, 1992; Rink *et al.*, 1993).

5 Be aware that investigative rates and costs may rise (Health Services Research Unit, 1992; Rink *et al.*, 1993).

6 Be aware of the full costs of NPT, including purchase price, consumables, maintenance contracts, equipment replacement costs and the cost of staff time.

7 Evaluate the safety of the testing procedures in their surgeries, including the evident risks of human immunodeficiency virus (HIV) and hepatitis from specimens during analysis.

8 Recognize the possibilities of litigation ensuing from erroneous results.

9 Recognize the need to use only trained operators.

10 Recognize the need for training programmes (including ongoing training) for their staff and ensure an appropriate match between the equipment and the skills available.

11 Ensure comparability of results with the local haematology laboratory service.

12 Take into account the need for good IQC and EQA programmes.

13 Be aware of the technical difficulties that may be encountered from NPT, such as specimen mixing, carry-over and specimen storage and disposal problems.

14 Ensure that their staff will be available for on-demand analyses.

15 Ensure that the analytical system is robust.

16 Recognize the need for backup arrangements.

---

* Others considering NPT in a non-hospital setting, e.g. pharmacists, may also find these key points useful.

17   Be aware of the high quality and close operational control of laboratory testing already available in their local central laboratory.

18   Be aware that many local haematology services will have undergone peer review for the national accreditation scheme.

The problems arising from NPT are not inconsiderable, but many of them can be overcome by involving the local haematologist in the initial decisions and ongoing provision of NPT.

2 Operational evaluation

2.1 Introduction

Near-patient testing equipment requires evaluation at three levels.

1   A full national evaluation by the MDA at one of the national evaluation centres. Such evaluations usually assess performance under optimal conditions (optimal conditions variance). This will continue to be necessary, even after the date when (for marketing in European Community (EC) countries) all medical devices will have to carry a CE mark indicating that the performance claims have been validated by the manufacturer.

2   A second operational evaluation by the MDA, which assesses the equipment in a manner commensurate with the intended operational use under routine conditions (routine conditions variance). This assesses the system's suitability for its intended use.

3   If an MDA operational evaluation has not been undertaken, the local purchaser should perform an evaluation to the same standard. If an MDA operational evaluation has been carried out, the local purchaser may wish to perform a briefer local assessment, which appraises certain aspects of the equipment in its intended location that are of particular importance to the site in question.

The national evaluation is carried out in accordance with the protocol for blood counters produced by the International Council for Standardization in Haematology (ICSH 1994) or in accordance with the protocols for coagulation instruments (Giddings *et al.*, 1989; I. Mackie, 1994, University College London, pers. comm.). Reports of these evaluations are readily available (from the MDA) and they assess the following: general operational aspects, the effects of dilution, precision, carry-over, accuracy, comparability (relative accuracy), linearity, sensitivity, specificity and reliability.

The operational evaluation would normally be undertaken by the MDA after the full national evaluation, using competent staff. The evaluation would be performed in a location equivalent to the intended operational site. The following guidelines are designed for the MDA operational evaluation to assess the clinical utility of the equipment in the near-patient location, but could also be adapted for use in the local purchaser assessment. These guidelines are designed as the minimum criteria for the operational evaluation, and a more detailed evaluation may be necessary in certain circumstances.

2.2 Principles of the Medical Devices Agency operational evaluation

1   The conditions of the evaluation should be closely allied to the users' working environment, using staff (e.g. nurses) with skills similar to those of potential users under routine conditions in the intended location of the equipment. Henceforth, these staff will be referred to as user-evaluators.

2   The operational evaluation should be designed to highlight possible sources of error or calibration drift. Moreover, the evaluation should be tailored to the type of equipment and materials under assessment. For example, the evaluation of an automated blood counter would be different from that of a simple haemoglobinometer. A capillary PT analyser, for oral anticoagulant control, would be evaluated in a different environment from an instrument using venous or arterial blood for heparin control during, for example, cardiac bypass surgery.

2.3 Before the evaluation

2.3.1 Documentation
Ensure that there is appropriate documentation and a record is kept of the following.
1   Down time and reason for breakdown.
2   Maintenance schedules.
3   Reagent usage (batch number, expiry dates, storage conditions, etc.).
4   Use of appropriate control materials.

2.3.2 Training
The training should be provided by the central haematology laboratory organizing the evaluation and/or the equipment supplier.

Trainee user-evaluators should be nurses or junior doctors, etc., of similar experience to those staff who could potentially use the equipment if approved and introduced following the evaluation.

The training should centre around the principle that user-evaluators are given basic tuition about the equipment, followed by a period of familiarization with the equipment. These staff should then be given SOPs and be allowed to follow these procedures through to the production of patient results. Training should also be planned on the assumption that operators have little or no knowledge of sources of systematic and random errors, such as the effects of high cell counts and background counts and the possibility of clots reducing platelet counts.

Trainees should be awarded a certificate of competence by the central laboratory, after appropriate training and prior to the commencement of the evaluation. An assessment of the adequacy and effectiveness of training should be made during the evaluation. A register of competent staff should be kept by the organizing laboratory.

2.4 What the evaluation should assess

2.4.1 Equipment location
Physical requirements (equipment dimensions, weight, free-standing/bench top, size of bench, flat surface, stability of bench, floor area, ease of access, power supply, noise and heat generation, air conditioning, waste disposal).

2.4.2 Safety

A COSHH, microbiological, electrical and mechanical assessment will normally have been undertaken during the national MDA evaluation.

It is important to ensure that staff using the equipment can adhere to appropriate control of infection standards. An assessment should be made of microbiological risks arising from, for example, contamination of equipment/surfaces by patient specimens, together with an assessment of appropriate decontamination and waste-disposal procedures.

A risk assessment of any potential mechanical and fire hazards (e.g. is the equipment continuously powered?) should also be made.

2.4.3 Operational aspects

These aspects should be assessed by completion of questionnaires. One questionnaire should be compiled for user-evaluators and a separate questionnaire for central laboratory staff (MLSOs, etc.).

Sample questionnaires are detailed in Appendices 1.1 and 1.2.

2.5 Random and systematic errors

Imprecision, inaccuracy and drift, etc. will have been assessed during the national MDA evaluation. The purpose of this section is to assess imprecision under routine conditions. These performance characteristics should be assessed in accordance with 'Protocol for evaluation of automated blood cell counters' (ICSH, 1994).

2.5.1 Blood-count analysers

Comparison of imprecision

Twenty to thirty patients' specimens, covering the expected clinical range (normal, high, low), should be analysed in triplicate by a user-evaluator and by a competent MLSO. These experiments will provide estimates of optimal (MLSO) and achievable (NPT user) levels of precision (mean, standard deviation (SD) and (CV). If these data are not significantly (clinically) different, the equipment should be judged appropriate for use in the operational evaluation (ICSH, 1994).

Between-batch imprecision

During the trial period (over a period of days), several user-evaluators should analyse patients' samples in triplicate, from different batches, to achieve a total of 20–30 patients' samples. The samples must cover the expected clinical range (normal, high, low). This must be undertaken under routine conditions to provide an estimate of routine between-batch variance (ICSH, 1994).

Assessment of comparability

During the trial period, a minimum of 40 samples (ICSH, 1978) should be analysed both by the NPT instrument and by the central laboratory instrument in the hospital laboratory and comparisons made in accordance with the protocol from the ICSH (1994). This should be repeated, comparing a user-evaluator and MLSO on the NPT equipment alone, to provide an estimate of achievable levels of comparability in a near-patient location.

Carry-over/interfering substances

These aspects will have been fully assessed during the national MDA evaluation. During this operational evaluation, the assessment should be limited to determining whether staff are aware of carry-over from, for example, high white-cell counts and the effects of interfering substances, such as lipids or cold agglutinins. During the course of the evaluation, a few samples of these types should be included in each evaluator's assessment and their ability to take appropriate action should be assessed.

Dilution procedures

Modern analysers sample whole blood and NPT should not involve dilutions – hence this aspect is not included.

2.5.2 Coagulation analysers

Comparison of imprecision

At least 12 samples from patients, with a range of clotting times, from normal values to just above the therapeutic range for anticoagulant control, should be analysed by a user-evaluator and by a qualified MLSO. This will provide an estimate of the achievable level of precision (median, SD and CV). If these data are not significantly different, the equipment should be judged appropriate for clinical use. If there are statistically significant differences between the data obtained by the MLSO and the user-evaluator, then it must be considered whether these differences would alter the clinical management of the patient before the instrument is judged appropriate for clinical use.

Within-batch imprecision

For instruments using anticoagulated blood or plasma, imprecision should be checked by performing 10 replicate tests from the same blood sample. Blood should be collected from a healthy normal subject, a patient with a mildly prolonged coagulation time (at the lower end of the therapeutic range for warfarin or heparin) and a patient with a moderately prolonged coagulation time (middle of the therapeutic range).

For instruments requiring finger-prick samples, precision should be checked by sampling from six separate finger pricks from the same volunteer, within a period of 2 h. This should be carried out with at least one healthy normal subject and at least one patient with a moderately prolonged coagulation time (e.g. for PT and APTT, at the mid-point of the therapeutic range for warfarin and heparin, respectively).

Some manufacturers provide lyophilized whole-blood quality-control samples for their instruments and, where available, these should also be used for precision exercises.

Between-batch imprecision

With instruments that can use anticoagulated blood or plasma, lyophilized or frozen plasma with normal and prolonged clotting times should be run twice daily throughout the trial period. Where a lyophilized commercial whole-blood sample is available, this should be used as an additional quality-control/precision sample.

For instruments that will only use non-anticoagulated whole blood, true between-batch precision cannot be tested. Useful information may be obtained by comparing the median, SD and CV obtained with each batch of NPT samples with the data obtained in the reference method in the hospital laboratory.

Assessment of comparability

A minimum of 50 blood samples should be tested and citrated blood specimens sent to the hospital laboratory for comparative analysis.

Where an instrument is evaluated for use in oral anticoagulant control, at least 40 samples with international normalized ratios (INRs) spread evenly over the therapeutic range (INR 2.5–4.0), as well as at least 10 samples from over-anticoagulated patients (INR >4.5) and 10 from healthy normal subjects, should be tested. The hospital laboratory should test the citrated plasma with their routine PT method. Some reagents do not give comparable results with individual NPT instruments. If this is the case, the hospital laboratory may wish to use a more appropriate PT method and reagent. It is recommended that the additional reagent is selected from those in common use in the UK, with an international sensitivity index (ISI) assigned by the manufacturer for the particular method used. If there is any discrepancy over the therapeutic range, it may be necessary to perform larger numbers of tests.

Where an instrument is evaluated for use in an operating theatre, intensive-care unit or renal dialysis unit for control of heparin, the 50 samples should cover the full range of heparin levels encountered in normal use. The NPT instrument APTT should be compared with an APTT and, if possible, an anti-Xa assay for heparin in the hospital laboratory, using citrated plasma. The local routine reagent and method for APTT should be used, provided that it is suitable for heparin monitoring. The APTT ratio must be calculated using the mid-point of the locally derived reference range or the geometric mean-normal APTT, derived from at least 20 fresh samples from healthy normal subjects. The anti-Xa assay for heparin may act as a useful reference point for comparing heparin levels, since the APTT is influenced by numerous variables and there is wide variation in heparin sensitivity between reagents. If an MDA operational evaluation has been performed, the above protocol must be used to ensure good precision and comparability before the introduction of the NPT instrument into clinical practice.

There is no routinely used counterpart for the ACT in the hospital coagulation laboratory. The only meaningful comparison may therefore be with the anti-Xa assay for heparin.

Some NPT instruments perform a TT, with and without protamine sulphate, for the detection of haemostatic abnormalities and heparin control. A comparison should be made with a TT on citrated plasma, with the thrombin reagent diluted appropriately to be sufficiently sensitive for the purpose for which the TT is being performed.

Appendix 1.1: Sample questionnaire: user-evaluators

Instrument name (model):
Manufacturer:
Evaluator's name:
Start date of evaluation:
End date of evaluation:
Number of patient samples analysed:
Grades
0   Poor   1   Unsatisfactory   2   Acceptable
3   Good   4   Excellent   n/a   Not applicable

GRADING

Were the SOPs easy to follow?	[ ]
Was the instruction manual/documentation easy to follow?	[ ]
Was the equipment easy to start up?	[ ]
Was the start-up rapid?	Yes/No
Was the equipment easy to shut down?	[ ]
Was the shut-down rapid?	Yes/No
Was the equipment easy to use?	[ ]
Was the equipment easy to maintain?	[ ]
Did you understand the training?	[ ]
Are there too many steps in the analysis?	Yes/No
Was the instrument generally reliable?	[ ]
Did too many faults occur with the instrument?	Yes/No
Were faults easily rectified?	Yes/No
How did you find the presentation of results?	[ ]
How would you grade the total analysis time?	[ ]
Were reagents easy to use?	[ ]
Was reagent packaging satisfactory?	[ ]

Comments

Appendix 1.2: Sample questionnaire: haematology staff assessment

Instrument name (model):
Manufacturer:
Evaluator's name:
Start date of evaluation:
End date of evaluation:
Number of patient samples analysed:
Grades
0   Poor   1   Unsatisfactory   2   Acceptable
3   Good   4   Excellent   n/a   Not applicable

	GRADING
Is the equipment in a secure environment?	Yes/No
Is the instrument tamper-proof?	Yes/No
Were patient results treated with appropriate confidentiality?	[ ]
Were the SOPs used appropriately?	[ ]
Was the rate of sample throughput satisfactory?	[ ]
Were manufacturers' manuals satisfactory?	[ ]
Were reagents used appropriately?	[ ]
Were reagents stable during the evaluation?	[ ]
Were reagents stored appropriately?	[ ]
Were failure alarms noted?	[ ]
Were out-of-control alarms noted?	[ ]
How would you grade user maintenance?	[ ]
How would you grade equipment cleaning by users?	[ ]
How would you grade the use of quality control samples?	[ ]
Was internal quality control (IQC) appropriate?	[ ]
Did IQC samples cover the appropriate clinical range?	[ ]
Was quality maintained in small batches of patient samples?	[ ]
Is there an appropriate external quality assessment (EQA) scheme available?	Yes/No
Would users register with an appropriate EQA scheme?	Yes/No/n/a
Were specimens collected properly?	[ ]
Were specimens in the correct container?	Yes/No
Were samples identified properly?	[ ]
Were samples of appropriate quality?	[ ]
Was the volume of blood appropriate (90–110% of nominal volume)?	[ ]
Were specimens stored properly?	[ ]
Were sample-mixing conditions appropriate?	[ ]
Were any samples analysed that contained clots?	Yes/No
Were any haemolysed samples analysed?	Yes/No
Were request forms appropriate?	[ ]
Were request forms stored appropriately?	[ ]
Was the method of reporting results appropriate?	[ ]
Were result reports integrated into the hospital case notes?	[ ]
Were historical results stored properly?	[ ]
Were samples disposed of properly?	Yes/No

Comments

References

Association of Clinical Biochemists (1993) *Guidelines for Implementation of Near-patient Testing.* Available from Royal Society of Chemistry, Burlington House, Piccadilly, London W1V 0BN.

Clinical Pathology Accreditation (UK) Ltd. (1993) *Accreditation Handbook, Version 6.0.* Available from CPA (UK) Ltd, 45 Rutland Park, Botanical Gardens, Sheffield SI0 2PB.

Council for Professions Supplementary to Medicine (1994) *Statement of Conduct: Near Patient Testing*. Available from the Registrar, Park House, 184 Kennington Park Road, London SE11 4BU.

Department of Health (1987a) *Blood Glucose Measurements: Reliability of Results Produced in Extra-laboratory Areas*. Hazard Notice (HN) 13, Department of Health, London.

Department of Health (1987b) *Blood Gas Measurements: the Need for Reliability of Results Produced in Extra-laboratory Areas*. Hazard Notice (HN) 31, Department of Health, London.

Department of Health (1987c) *Health Departments – Decontamination of Health Care Equipment Prior to Inspection, Service, or Repair*. Note (87) 22 DGM letter, SHHD 1987/66 WHC (87) 41.

Dybkaer R., Martin D.V. & Rowan R.M. (eds) (1992) Good practice in decentralized analytical clinical measurements. European Committee for Clinical Laboratory Standards, International Federation of Clinical Chemistry and World Health Organisation. *Scandinavian Journal of Clinical and Laboratory Investigation* (Suppl. 209).

Elliot K., Watson I.D., Tsintis P. *et al.* (1990) The impact of near-patient testing on the organisation and costs of an anticonvulsant clinic. *Therapeutic Drug Monitoring* **12**, 434–437.

Farr A.D. (1990) Near-patient 'laboratory' testing [editorial]. *Medical Laboratory Sciences* **47**, 249–250.

Giddings J.C., Hall P., Basterfield P. *et al.* (1989) Protocol for the evaluation of automated blood coagulation instruments (coagulometers) for determination of the international normalised ratio. *Medical Laboratory Sciences* **46**, 39–44.

Goldie D.J. & Kemp H. (1993) Near patient testing: the challenge for clinical pathology. *Journal of Clinical Pathology* **46**, 689–690.

Hailey D.M. & Lea A.R. (1990) Developments in near-patient testing. *Medical Laboratory Sciences* **47**, 319–325.

Health Services Advisory Committee (1990) *Safe Working and the Prevention of Infection in Clinical Laboratories*. Health and Safety Executive. HSE Books, PO Box 1999, Sudbury, Suffolk CO10 6FS.

Health Services Research Unit (1992) *New Technology in Health-care – Near Patient Testing in General Practice*. A summary of research carried out by the Health Services Research Unit, Warwick Business School, University of Warwick, and the Division of General Practice and Primary Care, St George's Hospital Medical School, London. Available from the Health Services Research Unit, Warwick Business School, University of Warwick, Coventry CV4 7AL.

HMSO (1974) *Health and Safety at Work Act*. PO Box 276, London SW8 5DT.

HMSO (1988) *Control of Substances Hazardous to Health*. PO Box 276, London SW8 5DT.

ICSH (1978) Protocol for type testing equipment and apparatus used for haematological analysis. *Journal of Clinical Pathology* **31**, 275–279.

ICSH (1994) Guidelines for evaluation of blood cell analysers including those used for differential leucocyte and reticulocyte counting and cell marker applications. *Clinical and Laboratory Haematology* **16**, 157–174.

Joint Working Group (JWG) on External Quality Assessment (EQA) in Pathology (1992) *Guide-lines on the Control of Near-patient Tests (NPT) and Procedures Performed on Patients by Non-pathology Staff*. Available from D. Kilshaw, Secretary, JWGEQA, c/o Mast House, Derby Road, Liverpool L20 1EA.

Kennedy D.A. (1992) *In vitro* diagnostics: matching available skills and equipment. *IMLS Gazette* **296**, 296–298.

Madsen H.H., Antonsen S. & Nielsen H.K. (1990) Near-patient potassium and sodium measurements: evaluation of ion-selective electrodes (Ionometer EF2) in a dialysis department. *Blood Purification* **8**, 171–176.

Marks V. (1988) Essential considerations in the provision of near-patient testing facilities. *Annals of Clinical Biochemistry* **25**, 220–225.

Marks V. (1990) Near-patient testing: implications for laboratory-based professions. *Medical Laboratory Sciences* **47**, 326–329.

Nanji A.A., Poon R. & Hinberg I. (1988) Near-patient testing. Quality of laboratory test results obtained by non-technical personnel in a decentralized setting. *American Journal of Clinical Pathology* **89**, 797–801.

Rachel J.M. & Plapp F.V. (1990) Bedside blood grouping. *Medical Laboratory Sciences* **47**, 330–336.

Rejman A. (1992) Measuring haemoglobin in the surgery: working for change. *RCGP Connection* [the membership magazine of the Royal College of General Practitioners].

Rink R., Hilton S., Szczepura A. *et al.* (1993) Impact of introducing near-patient testing for standard investigations in general practice. *British Medical Journal* **307**, 775–778.

van Dijk-Wierda C.A., van Halem-Visser L.P., van der Hoaff-van Halem R. & Loeliger E.A. (1978) The preparation of control blood for external quality assessment programmes in oral anticoagulant control. *Thrombosis and Haemostasis* **39**, 210–214.

2 The Role of Cytology, Cytochemistry, Immunophenotyping and Cytogenetic Analysis in the Diagnosis of Haematological Neoplasms
Prepared by the General Haematology Task Force

1 Introduction

In recent years, immunophenotyping and cytogenetic analysis have become increasingly important in characterizing haematological neoplasms, while the role of cytochemistry has diminished. This guideline discusses the place of these three methods of investigation and outlines the essential tests needed for clinically meaningful diagnosis. Details of recommended techniques are given elsewhere (ICSH, 1985, 1993; Rooney & Czepulkowski, 1992; BCSH, 1994a, b). The terminology and classifications used in this guideline are those recommended by the French–American–British Cooperative Group. Our recommendations are summarized in Tables 2.1–2.3 and are discussed in more detail in the following text.

Table 2.1 Essential and useful techniques

Essential techniques
Cytology
Cytochemistry
    Either Sudan black B or myeloperoxidase reaction
    Either α-naphthyl acetate esterase or a combined reaction,
    such as α-naphthyl acetate esterase plus naphthol
    AS-D chloroacetate esterase
    Perls' stain for haemosiderin
Immunophenotyping
    Use of primary and secondary panels of antibodies for
    diagnosis of the acute leukaemias and the chronic
    lymphoproliferative disorders, as recommended in previous
    guidelines (BCSH, 1994a, b)

Useful techniques
Cytochemistry
    Neutrophil alkaline phosphatase reaction
    Tartrate-resistant acid phosphatase reaction
Immunophenotyping
    Use of panels of selected antibodies for the diagnosis of large
    granular lymphocyte leukaemia and hairy-cell leukaemia

Reprinted with permission from *Clinical and Laboratory Haematology*, 1996, **18**, 231–236.

Table 2.2 Role of specific tests

Test	Role
Cytology	Examination of Romanowsky-stained films is essential in the diagnosis of all haematological neoplasms
Cytochemistry	
MPO/SBB	Essential in acute leukaemia unless myeloid differentiation is obvious; essential in MDS unless the diagnosis of RAEB-t has been established from the Romanowsky-stained film; useful in acute transformation of CGL
NSE/CE	Essential in acute leukaemia if M2, M4 or M5 AML is suspected
NAP	Useful in chronic myeloid leukaemias if cytogenetic and DNA analysis are not available; sometimes useful in the diagnosis of other MPD; useful in the diagnosis of PNH developing in aplastic anaemia
TRAP	Useful in the diagnosis of hairy-cell leukaemia but not essential if detailed immunophenotyping is available and/or trephine biopsy is characteristic
Immunophenotyping	Essential in acute leukaemias unless obviously myeloid; useful in acute transformation of CGL unless blast cells are clearly myeloid; can be used in the diagnosis of PNH; essential in lymphoproliferative disorders
Cytogenetic analysis	Strongly recommended in all cases of acute leukaemia; important if the diagnosis of MDS is suspected; useful in MDS in indicating prognosis; strongly recommended in CGL but not generally useful in other MPD; useful in confirming the diagnosis of specific lymphoproliferative disorders

MPO, myeloperoxidase; SBB, Sudan black B; NSE, non-specific esterase; CE, combined esterase; NAP, neutrophil alkaline phosphatase; TRAP, tartrate-resistant acid phosphatase; MDS, myelodysplastic syndromes; CGL, chronic granulocytic leukaemia; AML, acute myeloid leukaemia; DNA, deoxyribonucleic acid; MPD, myeloproliferative disorders; PNH, paroxysmal nocturnal haemoglobinuria; RAEB-t, refractory anaemia with excess of blasts in transformation.

Table 2.3 Role of cytogenetic analysis

Condition	Diagnostic value	Prognostic value	Affects choice of treatment	Indicated to monitor disease
AML	Yes	Yes	Yes	Yes
ALL/BL	Yes	Yes	Yes	Yes
MDS	Yes	Yes	Yes	Rarely
AA	No	Rarely	Rarely	Not relevant*
CGL	Yes (95%)	Yes	Yes	Yes
MPD	Rarely	Rarely	Rarely	Not relevant
NHL	Yes	Yes, but only in context of histology	No	Yes

* Unless dysplastic features appear.
AML, Acute myeloid leukaemia; ALL/BL acute lymphoblastic leukaemia/Burkitt's lymphoma; MDS, myelodysplastic syndromes; AA, aplastic anaemia; CGL, chronic granulocytic leukaemia; MPD, myeloproliferative disorders; NHL, non-Hodgkin's lymphoma.

2 Cytology

Despite advances in other areas, careful microscopical examination of Romanowsky-stained peripheral blood (PB) and bone-marrow (BM) films remains fundamental in haematological diagnosis. Microscopy alone may provide a definitive diagnosis of acute myeloid leukaemia (AML) and the myelodysplastic syndromes (MDS) and a provisional cytological diagnosis of acute lymphoblastic leukaemia (ALL) (which requires immunophenotypic confirmation). Microscopy is also crucial in the diagnosis of chronic myeloid leukaemias and is necessary in the diagnosis of other myeloproliferative disorders (MPD). In the lymphoproliferative disorders (LPD), microscopy is important but may be unreliable if not supplemented by immunophenotyping.

Cytology can fail in a number of situations. For example, splenic lymphoma with villous lymphocytes, follicular lymphoma and the small-cell variant of T-prolymphocytic leukaemia can all be misdiagnosed as chronic lymphocytic leukaemia. Similarly, not all cases of mature B-cell ALL (B-ALL) have an L3 morphology and rare cases with L3 morphology are not B-ALL.

Although cytology is usually reliable in the diagnosis of both Philadelphia (Ph)-positive and Ph-negative (*BCR-ABL*-positive) chronic granulocytic leukaemia (CGL), consistent diagnosis of the other chronic myeloid leukaemias is not always achieved. Nevertheless, at present, cytology is the best technique available for diagnosing and classifying the Ph-negative chronic myeloid leukaemias.

Certain PB characteristics are useful in distinguishing between atypical chronic myeloid leukaemia (aCML) and chronic myelomonocytic leukaemia (CMML) (Galton, 1992; Bennett *et al.*, 1994). Anaemia, thrombocytosis and monocytosis are more common in aCML than in CGL, eosinophilia and basophilia are less consistently present and granulocytic dysplasia is common. Atypical chronic myeloid leukaemia differs from CMML in that there are significant numbers of immature granulocytes in the PB, often more than 15% and almost always more than 5%. Eosinophilia and basophilia are uncommon in CMML. The monocyte count does not, by itself, confirm a diagnosis of CMML, since it exceeds $1 \times 10^9/l$ not only in CMML but also in many cases of aCML.

Erroneous interpretation of specialized investigations often results from neglect of basic microscopy. Such investigations should therefore only be interpreted in the context of clinical, haematological and cytological features. Before proceeding to more specialized tests, it is important to have a preliminary assignment of the particular case to the broad groups of acute leukaemia, MDS, MPD or LPD.

3 Cytochemistry

Essential cytochemical tests are: (i) myeloperoxidase (MPO) or Sudan black B (SBB); (ii) non-specific esterase (NSE) (e.g. α-naphthyl acetate esterase) or combined esterase (CE) (e.g. α-naphthyl acetate esterase plus naphthol AS-D chloroacetate esterase); and (c) Perls' stain.

Some cases of AML M1 can be identified cytologically (e.g. if Auer rods are present), but SBB/MPO cytochemistry is necessary to identify the remainder. Non-specific esterase/CE identifies most cases of AML M5, but, in a minority of cases of AML M5a, SBB/MPO and NSE/CE reactions are negative and the diagnosis is based on cytology combined with immunophenotyping. Acute myeloid leukaemia M0 is not detected by SBB/MPO and cytochemistry is not generally useful in the diagnosis of M7 AML. Sudan black B/MPO may also detect Auer rods in cases of MDS in which none are detectable on a Romanowsky stain. Finally, SBB/MPO and NSE/CE sometimes demonstrate myeloid differentiation in blast transformation of CGL and other MPD.

The Perls' stain for iron is indicated in all cases of suspected MDS, since it may provide evidence to support the diagnosis and is necessary for the further categorization of cases of refractory anaemia or refractory anaemia with ring sideroblasts. Occasionally, a haemoglobin H preparation is indicated to investigate suspected acquired haemoglobin H disease, and a Kleihauer test can be used to demonstrate the presence of cells containing haemoglobin F.

The neutrophil alkaline phosphatase (NAP) and tartrate-resistant acid phosphatase (TRAP) reactions are less useful cytochemical reactions. A low NAP score supports a diagnosis of CGL (Ph-positive or negative) but is redundant if cytogenetic or molecular genetic analysis is available. The NAP score is normal in about 5% of cases of uncomplicated chronic-phase CGL and this can lead to unnecessary uncertainty about the diagnosis in otherwise typical cases. The NAP score can also be reduced in aCML, paroxysmal nocturnal haemoglobinuria (PNH) and 30–50% of cases of MDS. Thus a patient with CMML may have a normal or low NAP score. Tartrate-resistant acid phosphatase positivity is present in the great majority of cases of hairy-cell leukaemia and in some cases of the variant form. Positive reactions are, however, also seen in a minority of cases of B-prolymphocytic leukaemia and splenic lymphoma with villous lymphocytes. Whether a laboratory needs to perform NAP and TRAP reactions is therefore dependent on whether it has access to techniques yielding more specific results.

With the advent of immunophenotyping, the periodic acid–Schiff and acid phosphatase reactions are no longer necessary in haematological diagnosis.

4 Immunophenotyping

Immunophenotyping is essential in the diagnosis of ALL and M0 and M7 AML. It is therefore indicated in all cases of acute leukaemia that are not demonstrated to be myeloid with a Romanowsky stain and cytochemistry. Although immunophenotyping is not yet of importance in determining choice of treatment in AML, the results may indicate groups with poor prognosis, such as those with CD7 positivity (Urbano-Ispizua *et al.*, 1992; Kita *et al.*, 1993) or CD34 positivity (Geller *et al.*, 1990; Solary *et al.*, 1992).

Immunophenotyping is useful in determining blast-cell lineage in transformation of CGL, since about one-third of transformations are lymphoblastic. (Lymphoid and myeloid transformations cannot be reliably distinguished by cytochemistry, since the last cells in myeloid transformation are often either megakaryoblasts or very undifferentiated myeloblasts, resembling those of M0 AML.) Immunophenotyping is of little importance in investigating transformation of other MPD, since transformation is almost always myeloid.

Immunophenotyping is essential in LPD. The demonstration of clonality is important when the diagnosis of a lymphoid neoplasm is in doubt and when it is uncertain if a plasma-cell infiltrate is reactive or neoplastic. When there is an established diagnosis of LPD, immunophenotyping is very important in establishing lineage and making a specific diagnosis (BCSH, 1994b).

An unusual application of immunophenotyping is its ability to support a diagnosis of PNH. Immunophenotyping of PB neutrophils and erythrocytes by flow cytometry, to detect reduced expression of CD59 and CD58, respectively, may be more sensitive than Ham's test in detecting the emerging PNH clone in cases of aplastic anaemia (Hillmen *et al.*, 1992). (Suitable antibodies, BRIC 5 (CD58) and BRIC 229 (CD59), are available from the International Blood Group Reference Laboratory, Blood Products Laboratory, Elstree, Herts., UK.)

5 Cytogenetic analysis

Cytogenetic analysis of the BM should normally be performed at diagnosis in all cases of acute leukaemia. The karyotype is used to stratify patients into good, poor and intermediate prognostic groups (Table 2.4). The chromosomal abnormality provides a totally leukaemia-specific clonal marker, which indicates the choice of chromosomal or breakpoint-specific probes which can be used, with sensitive molecular techniques, to monitor remission. Cytogenetic analysis can also be useful when the diagnosis of AML is in doubt. Since the role of all-*trans*-retinoic acid in M3 and M3 variant AML has been defined, cytogenetic analysis (to detect t(15;17)(q22;q11–12)) has become relevant not only to prognosis but also to the choice of therapy.

Prognostic groups in ALL are shown in Table 2.4. The worst prognostic groups, Ph-positive cases and those with t(4;11)(q21;q23), need the most intensive protocols or BM transplantation. Survival of t(1;19)(q23;p13) patients is greatly improved by intensive therapy (Rivera *et al.*, 1991), while hyperdiploidy with 51–68 chromosomes and dic(9;12)(p11;p12) are indications for sparing the patient the more intensive treatment regimes at any age. Because of the more successful outcome with alternative intensive chemotherapy (Murphy *et al.*, 1986; Hann *et al.*, 1990), the confirmation of Burkitt's lymphoma-related ALL by karyotypic analysis is an important priority.

Karyotypic analysis is important in neonates with apparent congenital leukaemia in order to distinguish transient abnormal myelopoiesis in Down's syndrome (including mosaic Down's syndrome, which may not be phenotypically readily apparent) from other cases of congenital leukaemia, which are often associated with the very adverse t(4;11)(q21;q23) karyotype. Although it is likely that transient abnormal myelopoiesis in Down's syndrome is actually spontaneously remitting AML, this diagnosis does not have the same implications as that of other forms of congenital leukaemia, since remission may occur with only supportive management.

Table 2.4 The prognostic significance of some cytogenetic abnormalities*

Disease	Prognosis		
	Good	Intermediate	Poor
AML	t(8;21)(q22;q22)	+8	t(9;22)(q34;q11)
	t(15;17)(q22;q12)	11q23†	t(6;9)(p23;q34)
	inv(16)(p13q22)		inv(3)(q21q26)
			12p-
			complex (often including abnormality of chromosome 5, 7 or both)
ALL	Hyperdiploidy with		t(8;14)(q24;q32)‡
	51–68 chromosomes		t(2;8)(p11.2;q24)‡
	dic(9;12)(p11;p12)		t(8;22)(q24;q11)‡
			t(9;22)(q34;q11)
			t(4;11)(q21;q23)
			t(1;19)(q23;p13)§
MDS	Normal	+8	-5
	Isolated 5q-		-7
	Isolated 20q-		7q-
			inv(3)(q21q26)
			t(6;9)(p23;q34)
			complex

* This list is not exhaustive.
† Except t(4;11)(q21;q23).
‡ Prognosis is greatly improved with alternative chemotherapy (Murphy *et al.*, 1986; Hann *et al.*, 1990).
§ Prognosis is greatly improved with intensive chemotherapy (Rivera *et al.*, 1991).
AML, acute myeloid leukaemia; ALL, acute lymphoblastic leukaemia; MDS, myelodysplastic syndromes.

Cytogenetic analysis is not recommended for patients with acute leukaemia in remission, since it is not sufficiently sensitive to detect low levels of the clone. If monitoring of the leukaemic clone is needed, molecular techniques are required. The karyotype of a relapse BM will distinguish between return of the original leukaemia and induction of a new neoplasm.

In suspected MDS, demonstration of a clonal cytogenetic abnormality confirms the diagnosis, although it must be borne in mind that a normal karyotype does not exclude the diagnosis. Karyotypic abnormalities which in AML are associated with a poor prognosis are, when found in MDS, predictive of early leukaemic transformation or death from complications of cytopenia. The prognostic significance of specific cytogenetic abnormalities is shown in Table 2.4. It will be noted that in MDS only a normal karyotype and 5q- or 20q- occurring as single abnormalities are indicative of a relatively good prognosis. Karyotype may influence choice of therapy, e.g. iron chelation, therapy which could be appropriate for refractory anaemia with 5q- as the only cytogenetic abnormality, would have little relevance in a patient with inv(3)(q21q26) or t(6;9)(p23;q34), in whom early blast transformation and death would be likely. In childhood myelodysplastic disorders/MPD, cytogenetic analysis will help to distinguish the infantile monosomy 7 syndrome from juvenile chronic myeloid leukaemia.

In aplastic anaemia, cytogenetic analysis is not indicated if resources are short. It is rarely successful and the detection of a clonal cytogenetic abnormality is rare. Nevertheless, a chromosomal abnormality found in an otherwise typical aplastic anaemia is indicative of a neoplastic clone and is of importance for prognosis and choice of therapy. The development of dysplastic features in aplastic anaemia suggests that a neoplastic clone is present and is thus an indication for cytogenetic analysis.

Among chronic myeloid leukaemias, it is important to identify the Ph-positive cases, including those with variant translocations. Although there is little evidence that the variants differ from the classical 9;22 translocation in their prognostic significance, their detection provides an important baseline from which to monitor the course of the disease. The presence of additional karyotypic abnormalities at diagnosis or their development during the course of the illness is indicative of clonal evolution and may herald an accelerated phase or blast transformation. Cytogenetic response to treatment (interferon or BM transplantation) is a valuable and prognostically important investigation in CGL. However, deoxyribonucleic acid (DNA) or ribonucleic acid (RNA) analysis, to detect the *BCR-ABL* chimeric gene, is more sensitive in monitoring the leukaemic clone and, in Ph-negative CGL, it replaces cytogenetic analysis for this purpose.

Cytogenetic analysis is not generally useful in other MPD. However, in patients presenting as essential thrombocythaemia, it is important to detect the poor-risk groups, e.g. Ph-positive cases and those with inv(3)(q21q26). Cytogenetic analysis is therefore indicated in patients with atypical features, e.g. marked basophilia or blast cells in the PB.

In LPD, cytogenetic analysis may confirm a provisional diagnosis, e.g. when t(14;18)(q32;q11) is detected in suspected follicular lymphoma, t(11;14)(q13;q32) in suspected mantle-cell lymphoma or t(2;5)(p23;q35) in suspected T-lineage anaplastic large-cell lymphoma. However, most translocations are not totally specific for a histological category, so karyotype must be interpreted in the light of the cytological features. For example, t(11;14) is detected not only in mantle-cell lymphoma but also in a significant proportion of patients with splenic lymphoma with villous lymphocytes and in some patients with B-prolymphocytic leukaemia. Cytogenetic analysis can be important in demonstrating clonality and thus confirming a diagnosis of large granular lymphocyte leukaemia, particularly in CD3-negative cases in which there is no rearrangement of T-cell receptor genes. In LPD, cytogenetic abnormalities have prognostic significance, but only when the precise diagnosis and the karyotype are considered together. For example, when detected in a large-cell lymphoma, t(14;18) does not have the same significance as when detected in a centroblastic/centrocytic lymphoma. In general, when resources are scarce, cytogenetic analysis is not indicated in lymphoma unless it is likely to give important prognostic information or influence choice of therapy.

The role of cytogenetic analysis in haematological neoplasms is summarized in Table 2.3.

6 Practical points

When blood samples for immunophenotyping and cytogenetic analysis are sent to specialist centres, certain procedures must be followed if optimal results are to be achieved and waste of valuable resources is to be avoided. All samples should be accompanied by full clinical details, the provisional diagnosis, the results of a full blood count and, in the case of immunophenotyping, a film of PB, BM or both. It may be necessary to despatch samples to the specialist centre before full information is available, but in this eventuality a follow-up telephone call is essential. It is important to stress, for example, that, in LPD, immunophenotyping and karyotypic analysis of the BM are only relevant when there is infiltration by neoplastic cells. A BM film should be examined promptly and, if there is no infiltration, the specialist laboratories should be notified immediately so that processing of the sample does not proceed. This is particularly important for cytogenetics laboratories, where most of the labour-intensive work remains to be done.

For immunophenotyping, heparinized or ethylenediaminetetra-acetic acid (EDTA)-anticoagulated samples are suitable. Samples should reach the referral laboratory within 24 h. They should not be refrigerated and should be transported at ambient temperature. Either PB or BM is suitable, as long as neoplastic cells are present. Even samples containing a low proportion of neoplastic cells may give useful information. However, if the percentage of neoplastic cells is low, a larger volume of blood should be sent, e.g. 40–50 ml, whereas, if the count is very high, 8–12 ml will suffice.

Samples for cytogenetic analysis should be taken into 5 ml of tissue culture medium containing 100 international units (iu) of preservative-free heparin. Samples should not be refrigerated and should be transported at ambient temperature to reach the specialist laboratory within the same working day. Either PB or BM may be suitable. For acute leukaemia, a BM specimen is preferred, but PB is an alternative if the white-cell count is high (e.g. $>20 \times 10^9$/l) and if the blast count is significant (e.g. >30%). In CGL, BM is preferred, but, in cases with a high white-cell count in whom no BM specimen is available, PB may be satisfactory. In MDS, a BM specimen is needed.

7 Conclusion

A precise diagnosis is necessary in haematological neoplasms in order to determine prognosis and guide the choice of treatment. A specific diagnosis always requires cytology and often also requires cytochemistry, immunophenotyping and cytogenetic analysis. The relative importance of each of these methods of investigation varies according to the differential diagnosis in an individual patient. Whether specific investigations are required in an individual laboratory depends on the frequency with which patients with haematological neoplasms are encountered and on the ease of access to regional or supraregional diagnostic services.

References

BCSH, General Haematology Task Force (1994a) Immunophenotyping in the diagnosis of acute leukaemia. *Journal of Clinical Pathology* **47**, 777–781.

BCSH, General Haematology Task Force (1994b) Immunophenotyping in the diagnosis of chronic lymphoproliferative disorders. *Journal of Clinical Pathology* **47**, 871–875.

Bennett J.M., Catovsky D., Daniel M.-T. *et al.* (1994) The chronic myeloid leukaemias: guidelines for distinguishing chronic granulocytic leukaemia, atypical chronic myeloid leukaemia and chronic myelomonocytic leukaemia. Proposals of the French–American–British Cooperative Leukaemia Group. *British Journal of Haematology* **87**, 746–754.

Galton D.A.G. (1992) Haematological differences between chronic granulocytic leukaemia, atypical chronic myeloid leukaemia and chronic myelomonocytic leukaemia. *Leukaemia and Lymphoma* **7**, 343–350.

Geller R.B., Zahurak M., Hurwitz C.A. *et al.* (1990) Prognostic importance of immunophenotyping in adults with acute monocytic leukaemia: the significance of stem cell glycoprotein CD34 (My 10). *British Journal of Haematology* **76**, 340–347.

Hann I.M., Eden O.B., Barnes J. & Pinkerton C.R. (1990) 'MACHO' chemotherapy for stage IV B lymphoma and B cell acute lymphoblastic leukaemia. *British Journal of Haematology* **76**, 359–364.

Hillmen P., Hows J.M. & Luzzatto L. (1992) Two distinct patterns of glycosylphosphatidylinositol (GPI) linked protein deficiency in the red cells of patients with paroxysmal nocturnal haemoglobinuria. *British Journal of Haematology* **80**, 399–405.

ICSH (1985) Recommended procedures for cytological procedures in haematology. *Clinical and Laboratory Haematology* **7**, 55–74.

ICSH (1993) Recommended procedures for the classification of acute leukaemias. *Leukemia and Lymphoma* **11**, 37–49.

Kita K., Miwa H., Nakase K. *et al.* (1993) Clinical importance of CD7 expression in acute myelocytic leukemia. *Blood* **81**, 2399–2405.

Murphy S.B., Bowman W.P., Abramowitch M. *et al.* (1986) Results of treatment of advanced stage Burkitt's lymphoma and B cell (SIg+) acute lymphoblastic leukemia with high-dose fractionated cyclophosphamide and coordinated high-dose methotrexate and cytarabine. *Journal of Clinical Oncology* **4**, 1732–1739.

Rivera G.K., Raimondi S.C., Hancock M.L. *et al.* (1991) Improved outcome in the childhood acute lymphoblastic leukaemia with reinforced early treatment and rotational combination chemotherapy. *Lancet* **337**, 61–66.

Rooney D.E. & Czepulkowski B.H. (eds) (1992) *Human Cytogenetics: A Practical Approach*, Vol. II, *Malignancy and Acquired Abnormalities*, 2nd edn. Oxford University Press, Oxford.

Sokal J.E., Gomez G.A., Baccarani M. *et al.* (1988) Prognostic significance of additional cytogenetic abnormalities at diagnosis of Philadelphia chromosome positive-chronic granulocytic leukaemia. *Blood* **72**, 294–298.

Solary E., Casasnovas R.-O., Campos L. *et al.* & the Groupe d'Etude Immunologique des Leucémies (1992) Surface markers in adult acute myeloblastic leukemia: correlation of CD19+, CD34+ and CD14+/DR-phenotypes with shorter survival. *Leukaemia* **5**, 393–399.

Urbano-Ispizua A., Matutes E., Villamor N. *et al.* (1992) The value of detecting surface and cytoplasmic antigens in acute myeloid leukaemia, *British Journal of Haematology* **81**, 178–183.

3 Use and Evaluation of Leucocyte Monoclonal Antibodies in the Diagnostic Laboratory: a Review

Prepared by the General Haematology Task Force

1 Introduction

Hybridoma technology, developed in the mid-1970s by Köhler and Milstein (1975), made it possible to produce virtually limitless quantities of highly specific monoclonal antibodies (mAbs) that recognize distinct epitopes of cellular antigens. There is currently available a large number of such reagents (greater than 1100), which detect different molecules on both normal and neoplastic cells from the various lineages. In 1982, at the First International Workshop on Leucocyte Differentiation Antigens, the term 'cluster of differentiation' (CD) was introduced to help classify antibodies detecting antigens with similar tissue distribution. Five workshops have now been held and 130 CD groups established, a number that is likely to increase in the future. Only a minority of these reagents, however, are of value for the routine diagnosis of leukaemic disorders. It should be stressed that, to date, no leukaemia-specific antibodies have been produced and that all antibodies in diagnostic use recognize antigens that are also present on normal cells. It is for this reason that panels of antibodies, including both monoclonal and polyclonal reagents, are needed to obtain diagnostic information. In addition, determination of peripheral-blood lymphocyte subsets, by immunological techniques, has been shown to be useful in the evaluation of immune deficiencies and autoimmune disorders and for monitoring transplant rejection therapy.

Antibodies may be of different immunoglobulin class (e.g. immunoglobulin G (IgG)/ IgM), subclass (e.g. IgG_1/IgG_2) and isotype (e.g. IgG_{2a}/IgG_{2b}). They can also be unconjugated or conjugated to different fluorochromes (e.g. fluorescein isothiocyanate (FITC), tetramethylrhodamine isothiocyanate (TRITC), phycoerythrin (PE), peridinin chlorophyll protein (Per-CP), PE-Cy5 and PE Texas red), enabling multicolour analysis. Newer and more sensitive fluorochromes are currently being developed. In addition to the wide variety of antibodies and fluorochromes, there are a number of different techniques available for the detection of cellular antigens, including direct and indirect immunofluorescence, using either flow cytometry or microscopy, on whole blood or separated cells. In most laboratories, immunocytochemical techniques are used for cytoplasmic antigen detection, although the recent availability of permeabilizing agents (e.g. PermeaFix-Ortho) will increase the use

Reprinted with permission from *Clinical and Laboratory Haematology*, 1996, **18**, 1–5.

of flow cytometry in this area. In view of this variety of methodology, it is vital that each antibody is correctly evaluated, for each individual technique, prior to its routine clinical use. The British Committee for Standards in Haematology has drafted guidelines for the minimum antibody panels required for the immunophenotyping of both acute and chronic leukaemias (British Committee for Standards in Haematology, 1994a, b). These documents do not give details on the selection and evaluation of antibodies and give only brief technical details on the use of antibodies.

The following review, incorporating results from the UK National External Quality Assessment Scheme (NEQAS) in leucocyte immunofluorescence and immunocytochemistry, highlights the practical procedures that should be considered in a laboratory's evaluation and use of antibody reagents.

2 Designation

The introduction of the CD system for categorizing mAb reactivity provides a consistent method for evaluating and comparing antibodies. All antibodies designated as reacting against a CD antigen should have been evaluated in one of the five international workshops on human leucocyte differentiation antigens (Bernard *et al.*, 1984; Reinherz, 1986; McMichael, 1987; Knapp, 1989; Schlossman *et al.*, 1994). However, discrepant data in the literature may, in part, be attributed to the use of different commercial sources and hence different clones of a particular mAb (Reilly *et al.*, 1995). Unevaluated research and/or locally produced antibodies, i.e. those which have not been officially recognized as reacting against a CD, should generally be avoided in clinical diagnostic work. This does not apply to antibodies such as FMC7, antimyeloperoxidase and anti-terminal deoxynucleotidyl transferase (TdT), which bind to antigens that have yet to be assigned a CD number.

3 Antibody labelling

Cells directly labelled with FITC-conjugated antibodies will not be as bright as those stained using indirect FITC methods. Shapiro (1988) reported that the decreased sensitivity may be as much as five- to sixfold. This is of practical importance when the antigen expression is low. Phycoerythrin and the newer fluorochromes (e.g. tandem colour fluorochromes) have a much higher quantum yield than FITC, thus increasing sensitivity. The UK NEQAS in leucocyte immunofluorescence has consistently shown statistically significant differences between samples analysed with FITC- and PE-conjugated antibodies for the following antigens: CD3, CD5, CD13, CD14, CD33. For example, in a survey investigating CD13 detection, eight of 24 laboratories who used FITC-conjugated antibodies obtained values of less than 50% (overall mean 58%), of which three were negative results, defined as less than 20% (British Committee for Standards in Haematology, 1994a). In contrast, all 12 laboratories using PE-conjugated reagents obtained results greater than 50% (mean 77%). Therefore, when available, PE conjugates or tandem colour fluorochromes should be used for single-colour analysis. In the case of two-colour analysis (see below), the more sensitive fluorochrome-conjugated antibody should be used for the mAb detecting the weaker antigen.

4 Multicolour analysis

Two-colour immunofluorescence has become widely accepted as the method of choice for analysing normal and leukaemic cells (Shapiro, 1988; Uckun *et al.*, 1989). It is an ideal method for demonstrating the coexpression of antigens in cases of biphenotypic leukaemias, particularly when the sample contains a mixture of normal and leukaemic cells. In addition, two-colour analysis is the recommended technique for immune monitoring, i.e. for quantitation of $CD3^+CD4^+$ and $CD3^+CD8^+$ cells (Centers for Disease Control, 1992). Single-colour analysis will consistently overestimate both populations by up to 5% and significantly more in cases with a high $CD3^-CD8^+$ natural killer (NK) population. Care is also required in the selection of antibody combinations to ensure the availability of appropriate (i.e. class, subclass, isotype) negative-control reagents. It is possible that in certain two-colour combinations one antibody may prevent the binding of the second. This occurs when both antibodies (one of which has a higher avidity) compete for spatially adjacent sites (e.g. CD3 and the T-cell antigen receptor complex). Finally, the development of fluorochromes, in addition to PE and FITC, which can be detected with a single laser, and the availability of computer software capable of rapid data analysis have enabled the incorporation of triple-colour analysis in routine leukaemia diagnosis and detection of minimal residual disease (Campana *et al.*, 1990). However, this may lead to further technical problems, including more complicated spectral compensation, as well as the need for added expertise for instrument set-up, data collection and analysis.

5 Reagent selection

There are a number of factors that require consideration in the choice of reagents. The nuclear enzyme TdT is best detected by immunofluorescence or immunocytochemical techniques, using immunoadsorbed, purified polyclonal antibodies. Monoclonal anti-TdT antibodies are not always as sensitive as polyclonal reagents (Lanham *et al.*, 1986) and are best used as cocktails. In addition, antibodies may only work with one technique; for example, IgM antibodies may be suitable for immunofluorescence but not for immunocytochemistry, as is the case for FMC7 and anti-CD57. It should be appreciated, however, that different antibodies directed against a CD may identify the same or different epitopes on a specific molecule. Various anti-CD34 antibodies, for example, react with different sites on CD34 and, as a result, have different binding properties (Lansdorp *et al.*, 1989). This may account for variation in results when the same sample has been analysed by different laboratories.

6 Antibody controls

Appropriate antibody controls must always be included in the investigative panel. It is not appropriate to use mouse immunoglobulin containing all the immunoglobulin classes, as increased binding may be due to one subclass only. Therefore, both antibody class (including subclass and isotype) and fluorochrome-matched immunoglobulins should be used to determine the degree of non-specific binding. This is particularly important for setting positive/negative fluorescence thresholds on the flow cytometer or, if using ultraviolet microscopy or immunocytochemistry techniques, to provide a visual background staining level. For small-volume samples, it may be necessary to use a single control reagent (composed of a cocktail of relevant antibodies). Such reagents, however, do not allow the identification of the antibody in the event of non-specific binding. It is important to stress that the control antibody should be appropriately matched to the concentration and fluorochrome : protein (F : P) ratio of the test antibody.

7 Antibody concentration

Antibodies from the same manufacturer can exhibit batch-to-batch variation. In addition, some control antibodies are not marketed at the same concentration as the test antibody. Ideally, the F : P ratio should be 1 : 1. Many available reagents have high F : P ratios and are better avoided if alternatives exist (overconjugation can produce highly charged acidic species, which tend to stick non-specifically to cells, especially if they are fixed). It is important to establish the correct working dilutions for every new antibody, including those from different batches, for each detection system. Data from the UK NEQAS show that laboratories use a wide variety of antibody dilutions, even when antibodies are obtained from the same source. Ideally, the titre value should be determined for every antibody, and this is of particular value in the investigation of suspected non-specific binding. Titre value is defined as the amount of antibody that is required to saturate the maximum number of antigen-binding sites on a selected cell population. This is measured by the median positive fluorescence channel for the different antibody dilutions. The saturation or titre value is obtained by plotting the median peak channel fluorescence (MPCF) against antibody concentration and is the point at which the MPCF plateaus (see below). The saturation value should be constant over at least two dilutions, and curves that fail to plateau are usually the result of non-specific binding. When using indirect techniques, it is important that each antibody is diluted to a predetermined level, so as to obtain maximum sensitivity and specificity. Under such circumstances, a 'chequer-board' titration is the recommended procedure (see below). Clone and batch numbers of all reagents must be documented.

8 Storage

Storage conditions and expiry dates must be followed. Repeated freezing and thawing of purified or conjugated antibodies should be avoided, as this can lead both to antibody aggregation, resulting in non-specific binding, and to fluorochrome degradation and loss of antibody activity. In addition, repeated freeze/thawing results in loss of antibody and fluorochrome activity. A common error is the failure to mix reagents adequately following thawing, leading to increased concentration of antibody at the bottom of the tube or vial. Phycoerythrin-conjugated antibodies should not be frozen.

9 Fixatives

The UK NEQAS in leucocyte immunocytochemistry has highlighted the effect that different fixatives may have on antigen detection (Forrest & Barnett, 1989). Recent trials have repeatedly demonstrated that CD3, CD5, CD13 and CD33 antigens are best preserved by using cold, pure, acetone fixation. Laboratories using formalin-containing fixatives (especially greater than 0.5%) may miss these diagnostically important antigens. Cold, pure, acetone fixation, therefore, is recommended for all antigen detection.

10 Cell concentration

Cell-separation techniques should involve standardization of final cell counts (10^6 cells/ml, in phosphate-buffered saline).

11 Fc blocking

Blocking of Fc receptors is important, particularly when analysing leukaemias with a significant monocytic component (Lawlor *et al.*, 1986). Such samples require preincubation with either rabbit or human serum prior to analysis. In general, Fc receptor affinity varies according to antibody class, with IgM antibodies exhibiting the least binding (degree of Fc binding increases as follows: IgM, IgG_1, IgG_{2a} and IgG_{2b}). In practice, the preferential use of IgG_1 mAbs is to be recommended. Care is required during the washing stages in indirect methods, as traces of the first antibody in the supernatant can form complexes with the second antibody and bind to Fc receptors on irrelevant cells. An additional precaution that can be taken during indirect immunofluorescence analysis is the use of fluorescent $(Fab)^2$ fragments of xenogenic antimouse immunoglobulin (i.e. Fc-cleaved).

12 Quality control

Both internal and external quality controls (QCs) should be undertaken when performing leukaemia or lymphocyte subset analysis. Internal QC procedures can include immunophenotyping fresh or frozen known positive and negative cells. In addition, control cells and calibration beads are now available for evaluation of mAb by flow cytometry, although primarily for lymphocytic antigens (e.g. Absolute Control (Ortho Diagnostic), CD-Chex (Streck Laboratories), Cyto-Trol (Coulter) and Sphero Beads (Dako)). Flow-cytometer users should also undertake QC of the linearity of fluorochrome amplification, as well as fluorescence intensity, by means of commercial calibrants (e.g. Calbrite (Becton-Dickinson), Immuno-Brite (Coulter)). All calibration results should be documented to give an indication of machine performance and drift. A detailed discussion of analyser QC is, however, outside the scope of this guideline and is adequately covered elsewhere (Lawry & Lowdell, 1994). The above procedures do not replace the need for external quality assessment. This is essential, especially in laboratories in which techniques are run on an *ad hoc* or infrequent basis. This may involve participation in locally organized quality assurance schemes, in which small discussion groups and helpful advice can be generated, as well as participation in the UK NEQAS for leucocyte immunophenotyping.

13 Antibody selection

Despite the experience of a number of QC schemes worldwide, there is no consensus as to the best antibody within a CD for diagnostic use. Such evaluations would require multisite studies and the development of reference materials that express the antigens of clinical importance. Research in this area is currently under way, although the problem should not be underestimated.

Appendix 3.1: Protocol for antibody evaluation

Ideally, every antibody should be titrated against each sample requiring analysis. This is impracticable, in terms of both time and resources. In practice, the following procedures should be undertaken.

Flow cytometry

Direct technique

Determine the optimum antibody dilution, using a sample (normal or leukaemic) known to express the relevant antigen, ideally at the same density. In the case of the whole-blood technique, different volumes of directly conjugated antibody are added to a fixed volume of blood, to give rise to doubling dilutions of antibody. The sample is then analysed and two graphs plotted.

1 Median peak channel fluorescence (MPCF) against antibody dilution (linear/log).
2 Percentage cell positivity against antibody dilution (linear/log).

   The optimum antibody dilution is that which lies on the plateau area of both plots, i.e. a dilution that results in maximal fluorescence and cell positivity (Fig. 3.1). Failure to achieve a plateau effect in either plot suggests non-specific binding.

Indirect technique

To determine the optimum dilution of both the primary and secondary antibodies, use a chequer-board analysis. The final working concentrations are the conditions that give satisfactory maximum fluorescence and cell-positivity counts when plotted as above.

Microscopy: immunoenzymatic/fluorescence techniques

1 Optimum antibody dilution is dependent on observer subjectivity, since it depends on

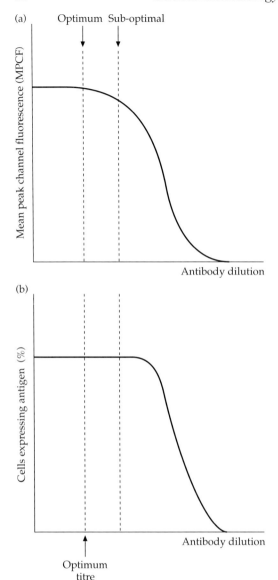

Fig. 3.1 Determination of optimum antibody dilution.

the visual comparison of positivity against the background levels of negative controls. Ensure accurate pH of buffers, as the fluorescence signal can be quenched with a pH above and below 7.2. Controls for specificity of anti-TdT reagents should include cytospin preparations from known cases of acute lymphoblastic leukaemia (positive control) and acute myeloid leukaemia (negative control).

2 Known positive and negative controls are required. The dilution of the first-layer antibody should be determined by serial dilutions. The working dilutions of the second- and third-layer antibodies should be those recommended by the manufacturer.

References

Bernard A., Boumsell L., Dausset J., Milstein C. & Schlossman S.F. (eds) (1984) *Leukocyte Typing I*. Springer-Verlag, Berlin.

British Committee for Standards in Haematology (1994a) Immunophenotyping in acute leukaemias. *Journal of Clinical Pathology* **47**, 777–781.

British Committee for Standards in Haematology (1994b) Immunophenotyping in chronic (mature) lymphoproliferative disorders. *Journal of Clinical Pathology* **47**, 871–875.

Campana D., Coustan-Smith E. & Janossy G. (1990) The immunological detection of minimal residual disease in acute leukaemia. *Blood* **76**, 163–171.

Centers for Disease Control (1992) Guidelines for the performance of CD4+ T-cell determination in persons with human immunodeficiency virus infection. *Morbidity and Mortality Weekly Report* **41** (RR 8), 1–17.

Forrest M.J. & Barnett D. (1989) Laboratory control of immunocytochemistry. *European Journal of Haematology* **42**, 67–71.

Knapp, W. (ed.) (1989) *Leucocyte Typing IV*. Oxford University Press, Oxford.

Köhler G. & Milstein C. (1975) Continuous cultures of fused cells secreting antibody of predetermined specificity. *Nature* **256**, 495–497.

Lanham G.R., Bollum F.J. & Stass S.A. (1986) Detection of terminal deoxynucleotidyl transferase using monoclonal antibodies directed against native and denatured sites. *American Journal of Clinical Pathology* **86**, 88–91.

Lansdorp P.M., Dougherty G.J. & Humphries R.K. (1989) CD34 epitopes. In Knapp W. *et al.* (eds) *Leucocyte Typing IV*, pp. 826–827. Oxford University Press, Oxford.

Lawlor E., Finn T., Temperley I.J. & McCann S.R. (1986) Monocytic differentiation in acute myeloid leukaemia: a cause of Fc binding of monoclonal antibodies. *British Journal of Haematology* **64**, 339–346.

Lawry J. & Lowdell M. (1994) Quality control in clinical flow cytometry. In Massey M. (ed.) *Flow Cytometry: Clinical Applications*, pp. 45–66. Blackwell Science, Oxford.

McMichael A.J. (ed.) (1987) *Leukocyte Typing III*. Oxford University Press, Oxford.

Polliak A., Rabinowitz R., Leizerowitz R., Keren-Zur Y. & Schlesinger M. (1993) Myelomonocytic antigens are rarely expressed on B-lymphocytic leukaemia cells. *Leukaemia and Lymphoma* **9**, 125–131.

Reilly J.T., Granger V. & Barnett D. (1995) Leukaemia immunophenotyping: effect of antibody source and fluorochrome on antigen detection. *Journal of Clinical Pathology* **48**, 186.

Reinherz B.F. (ed.) (1986) *Leukocyte Typing II*. Springer-Verlag, New York.

Schlossman S., Boumsell L., Gilks W. *et al.* (1994) *Leukocyte Typing V: White Cell Differentiation Antigens*. Oxford University Press, Oxford.

Shapiro H.M. (ed.) (1988) *Parameters and Probes: Practical Flow Cytometry*, 2nd edn, pp. 150–152. Alan R. Liss, New York.

Uckun F.M., Muraguchi A., Ledbetter J.A. *et al.* (1989) Biphenotypic leukemic lymphocyte precursors in CD2+ CD19+ acute lymphoblastic leukemia and their putative normal counterpart in human fetal hematopoietic tissues. *Blood* **73**, 1000–1015.

4 The Laboratory Diagnosis of Malaria
Prepared by the General Haematology Task Force

1 Introduction

A published audit, National External Quality Assessment Scheme (NEQAS) data and the observations of reference centres on slides submitted to them for confirmation of diagnosis have revealed shortcomings in the diagnosis of malaria in the UK. In the published audit (Milne *et al.*, 1994), malaria parasites were detected in 233 of 267 cases submitted to two reference centres. A diagnosis of malaria had been made in the referring laboratory in seven cases in which the reference centre detected no parasites. There was also significant misdiagnosis with regard to species. This was most often misdiagnosis of *Plasmodium ovale* as another species, but in 24 single infections and in one double infection *Plasmodium falciparum* was not specifically identified (20 cases) or was misidentified as another species. A high frequency of technical errors (e.g. wrong pH or a poor-quality film) was also noted. Similar observations have been made in NEQAS surveys (NEQAS data quoted by permission of the NEQAS organizer, the late Dr J.M. England). In one survey, 12% of participants detected a variety of parasites in a normal film and there was also a problem with species identification. Twenty-eight per cent of participants failed to identify *Plasmodium vivax* correctly, the most frequent error being misidentification as *P. falciparum*. Rapid and accurate diagnosis is important if malaria is to be treated expeditiously and appropriately. Since technical errors may lead to delay in diagnosis and inappropriate treatment or lack of treatment, it is important for adequate laboratory procedures to be defined. This is the aim of this guideline.

2 Recommended procedures

2.1 Microscopy in the detection of malaria parasites and in the identification of species

2.1.1 Basic procedures
Thick and thin films (Dacie & Lewis, 1995; Bain, 1996) should be prepared and examined

Reprinted with permission from *Clinical and Laboratory Haematology*, 1997, **19**, 165–170.

in all cases of suspected malaria. The thick film should be used for detection of malaria parasites and the thin film for identification of species. It is useful to prepare four thin films and four thick films, so that two of each can be stained, leaving spare films for sending to a reference centre (see Appendix 4.1) and for further study if there is diagnostic difficulty. Thin films should be fixed and stained with a Giemsa stain or a Leishman stain at a pH of 7.2 (see Appendices 4.2 and 4.3). Thick films should be stained unfixed after drying at 37°C for 15 min; a Giemsa stain can be used, but a modified Field's stain (see Appendices 4.2 and 4.3) is preferred, because it is more rapid. Routine May–Grünwald–Giemsa (MGG) and Giemsa stains, including those used in automated staining machines, are unlikely to be satisfactory, because of an inappropriate pH. In the case of a gravely ill patient, it is useful to stain an extra fixed thin film with a modified Field's stain, since this permits very speedy diagnosis of *P. falciparum*. A Giemsa or Leishman stain is still required for precise identification of other species. Films should be made without delay, since morphological alteration of parasites occurs with storage of ethylenediaminetetra-acetic acid (EDTA)-anticoagulated blood.

A minimum of 200 oil-immersion fields (×100 objective) should be examined in the thick film; this will take about 5–10 min for an experienced observer but longer for less experienced observers or for those who do not often examine films containing malaria parasites. If an observer is uncertain as to whether or not malaria parasites are present in the thick film, an entire thin film should be examined. This is likely to take 20–40 min. Following the detection of malaria parasites in a thick film, the thin film should be examined to determine the species. It should be noted that detection of *P. falciparum* gametocytes in the absence of other stages of the life cycle may be clinically significant in an untreated symptomatic patient, since it may indicate a suppressed active infection (Warhurst & Williams, 1996).

2.1.2 Quantification of parasites

Whenever *P. falciparum* is detected, the percentage of parasitized cells should be quantified, cells containing only gametocytes being excluded from the count. Quantification should be performed using a thin film, 1000 red cells being examined. The use of graticule, e.g. a Miller ocular micrometer, facilitates quantification. In the case of a double infection, the quantification applies only to *P. falciparum*. If the parasite count is less than 1 in 1000 cells, it is useful to quantify on a thick film, since this will be sufficient to give some idea of response to treatment. One method is shown in Table 4.1. Alternatively, parasite numbers per microlitre can be calculated in relation to the number of white cells (Warhurst & Williams, 1996) or from the percentage parasitaemia and the red-cell count. Quantification is important, since exchange transfusion should be considered in patients with more than 10% of parasitized red cells and severe complications (Wilkinson *et al.*, 1994). Quantification of parasites should be repeated daily until no parasites (other than gametocytes) remain.

Table 4.1 Estimation of parasitaemia from thick films, using a × 100 oil-immersion objective

Parasites observed	Percentage of red cells parasitized
10–20 per field	1
1–2 per field	0.1
1–2 per 10 fields	0.01
1–2 per 100 fields	0.001
1–2 per 1000 fields	0.0001

Table 4.2 The 95% and 99% confidence limits of parasite counts if 1000 red cells are counted

Observed percentage	95% confidence limits	99% confidence limits
0	0.00–0.37	0.00–0.53
1	0.48–1.84	0.35–2.11
2	1.2–3.1	1.0–3.4
3	2.0–4.3	1.8–4.7
4	2.9–5.4	2.6–5.9
5	3.7–6.5	3.4–7.0
6	4.6–7.7	4.2–8.2
7	5.5–8.8	5.1–9.3
8	6.4–9.9	5.9–10.45
9	7.3–10.95	6.8–11.6
10	8.2–12.0	7.7–12.7
15·	12.8–17.4	12.2–18.1·

The above table is derived from Diem & Lentner (1970) *Documents Geigy*, 7th edn. As an approximation, the confidence intervals can be calculated from the formula $p \pm (z.\text{SE}(p))$ when $\text{SE}(p)$ is the standard error of p and z is 1.95996 for 95% confidence intervals and 2.5758 for 99% confidence intervals. $\text{SE}(p)$ is calculated as $[p(1-p)/n]^{1/2}$ when p is the observed proportion and n is the total number of cells counted. The figures are predicted from probability theory and show the minimum variability without taking account of technical or observational errors.

2.1.3 Confirmation of diagnosis and species

All malaria films should be examined by two trained observers. The second observer may examine the films simultaneously or subsequently (e.g. next morning when the films have been examined on call). The second observer should have significant experience in the diagnosis of malaria and should keep his/her skills updated. The observer confirming the presence and species of malaria parasites should also confirm that the parasite count is of the correct order. However, it is not to be expected that a second parasite count will be exactly the same as the first, since the confidence limits of low counts are fairly wide (Table 4.2) and an amended count should only be issued if the first count was wrong.

2.1.4 Identification of the species when the thick film is positive and the thin film is negative

There are three possible ways to deal with identification of species when the thin film is negative. All may be satisfactory, depending on the circumstances.

1   It is often possible for an experienced observer to determine the species on a thick film.

2   If only one or two ring forms are seen and it is not possible to determine the species with certainty, it is prudent for the patient to be treated as for *P. falciparum* infection.

3   A test for malaria antigen can be used to confirm the presence of *P. falciparum* (see Section 2.2). This can be useful out of hours.

2.1.5 Negative films despite a strong clinical suspicion of malaria

When the parasite count is very low, examining 1000 rather than 200 high-power fields on a thick film will increase the yield of positive results. When there is a strong clinical suspicion of malaria but initial films are negative, a repeat should be suggested. Laboratories should consider including a statement in every report that negative films do not exclude a diagnosis of malaria and that repeat films should be requested if clinically indicated. Relevant haematological abnormalities, such as thrombocytopenia, may strengthen a clinical suspicion of malaria and be a further indication for a repeat blood sample and films.

2.1.6 Notification

When malaria parasites are detected clinical staff should be reminded that malaria is a notifiable disease. Laboratories that wish to notify cases themselves are free to do so since this will ensure that a higher percentage of cases are actually notified and duplicate reporting will be detected.

2.2 Supplementary tests

2.2.1 ParaSight F

ParaSight F (Gamidor Ltd.), which tests for the presence of soluble *P. falciparum* antigen in the blood, has been the subject of a Department of Health evaluation (Chiodini *et al.*, 1996) and, although both false positives and false negatives occur, it has been found to have a high degree of sensitivity and specificity. It is useful as follows.

1   To confirm *P. falciparum* diagnosed on a blood film, particularly when there is a relatively inexperienced observer (e.g. if on-call tests are being performed by a medical laboratory scientific officer (MLSO) who does not often examine films for malaria parasites) or in hospitals that examine films for malaria parasites infrequently.

2   To detect *P. falciparum* infection when an inexperienced observer is uncertain whether or not parasites are present (e.g. on call). A more experienced observer should subsequently confirm the diagnosis on thick and thin films and quantitate the parasitaemia.

3   To help determine species when there is a positive thick film but a negative thin film.

4   To help determine species when there is a mixed infection.

2.2.2 *Quantitative buffy-coat blood parasite detection method*

The quantitative buffy-coat (QBC) blood parasite detection method (Gamidor Ltd.) permits detection of parasites by fluorescence microscopy following exposure of the blood to acridine orange (Moody *et al.*, 1990). This test can be regarded as an optional backup to thick and thin films. Some laboratories use this method as the initial screening test backed up by thick and thin films on QBC-positive samples.

Disadvantages are as follows.

1   The costs of the equipment and of each test are high.

2   Howell–Jolly bodies also fluoresce with acridine orange.

3   Identification of species is not usually possible, a blood film being required for this purpose.

2.2.3 *Other tests*

Other tests are under development, e.g. assay of parasite lactate dehydrogenase (LDH).

3 Quality control

1   As part of internal quality control:

    (a)   All malaria films should be examined by two observers.

    (b)   All new batches of Giemsa or Leishman stain should be tested with a known *P. vivax* or *P. ovale* infection to ensure that Schuffner's dots are stained and that parasitized cells are decolourized. Blood films for this purpose can be wrapped in Parafilm or aluminium foil and frozen. Frozen films must be brought to room temperature before unwrapping to prevent condensation and red-cell lysis.

2   All laboratories doing tests for malaria parasites should participate in one or both of the available NEQAS schemes.

3   Films on all positive cases should be sent to a reference centre (see Appendix 4.1) for confirmation. An unstained thick film and an unstained thin film should be sent and, if possible, a blood sample. Postal regulations relevant to the transport of biological materials should be adhered to. Slides of equivocal or negative cases may also be sent if there are particular reasons to do so, e.g. a positive test for malaria antigen or a strong clinical suspicion of malaria.

4   Continuing education and maintenance of expertise

All laboratories have a need to ensure that new staff are adequately trained and laboratories which do not often examine blood for malaria parasites need, in addition, to ensure that staff maintain their skills. The following steps are useful.

1   Sets of mixed positive and negative thick and thin films should be available for examination during training and for periodic practice; suitable films include NEQAS films and films that have had the species verified by a reference centre. In addition, reference centres can often supply spare films for this purpose.

2 High-quality photographs of malaria parasites should be available for reference (see Appendix 4.4).

3 Films from NEQAS can be examined by all MLSOs and medical staff who carry out microscopy for malaria diagnosis. It is useful to do this as a training exercise after the correct answer is known, so that relevant features can be demonstrated immediately to any staff who fail to make a correct diagnosis.

4 Training courses are available (see Appendix 4.5).

Appendix 4.1: Reference centres

Diagnostic Laboratory
Liverpool School of Tropical Medicine
Pembroke Place
Liverpool L3 5QA

Department of Clinical Parasitology
Hospital for Tropical Diseases
Mortimer Market Centre
Capper Street
London WC1E 6AU

PHLS Malaria Reference Laboratory
London School of Hygiene and Tropical Medicine
Keppel Street
London WC1E 7HT

Scottish Parasite Diagnostic Laboratory
Stobhill Hospital
Balornock Road
Glasgow G21 3UW

Appendix 4.2: Suppliers of reagents and kits

Supplier	Approximate cost (1999, excluding VAT) and code for ordering
1 Modified Field's stain HD Supplies 44 Rabans Close Rabbans Lane Industrial Estate Aylesbury HP19 3RS	HD 1410 (A), HD 1415 (B), £4.60 for 25G A or B, i.e. £9.20 for both reagents to provide 1 l of stain
Merck Ltd. (formerly BDH) Hunter Boulevard Magna Park Lutterworth LE17 4XN	Field stain A 'Gurr', No. 34121 2G, 25 g, £20.68, Field stain B, 'Gurr' No. 34122 2Y, 25 g, £20.68

Continued p. 38

Appendix 4.2 (*Contd.*)

Supplier	Approximate cost (1999, excluding VAT) and code for ordering
2 Giemsa stain Merck Ltd. (as above)	BDH improved R66 Giemsa stain, 'Gurr', 35086 5P, £16.95 for 1 l
3 Leishman stain HD Supplies (as above) Merck Ltd. (as above)	HS 400, £3.65 for 500 ml 35022 4L, £10.30 for 500 ml 35022 6N, £29.05 for 2.5 l
4 Buffer tablets Merck Ltd. (as above)	Buffer tablets 'Gurr' pH approximately 7.2, 33201 2W, 50 tablets, £17.82 (1 tablet produces 100 ml of buffer solution)
5 ParaSight F Gamidor Ltd. (UK Supplier) Biomedical Services 67 Milton Park Abingdon OX14 4RX	£202.35 for 50-test kit
6 QBC Blood Parasite Detection Gamidor Ltd. (as above)	£206.19 for 100-test kit
7 ICT Diagnostics MalaPac test Launch Diagnostics Ltd. Ash House Ash Road New Ash Green Longfield Kent DA3 8JD	£116.00 for 25-card kit £28 for 5-card kit

Appendix 4.3: Methods

Leishman stain

1   Make a thin film and air-dry rapidly.

2   Place film in a staining rack, flood film with Leishman stain and leave for 30 s to 1 min to fix.

3   Add twice as much buffered distilled water (preferably from a plastic wash-bottle, as this allows better mixing of the solutions), pH 7.2.

4   Leave to stain for 10 min.

5   Wash off stain with tap water.

6   Dry film upright.

Stain recipe

1 Add glass beads to 500 ml of methanol.
2 Add 1.5 g of Leishman's powder.
3 Shake well, leave on a rotary shaker during the day and then incubate at 37°C overnight. There is no need to filter.

or

Use commercially prepared stain, product number HS 400, HD Supplies (see Appendix 4.2).

Field's stain

1 Make a thick film and leave to air-dry or dry in a 37°C incubator for 15 min.
2 Stain in 'A' for 5 s and then drain.
3 Rinse gently in tap water for 5 s and then drain.
4 Stain in 'B' for 3 s and then drain.
5 Rinse gently in tap water for 5 s and then drain.
6 Air-dry upright.
7 Examine the area where the white-cell nuclei are stained metachromatically.

Giemsa stain

Thin films

1 Fix thin film in methanol for 1 min and then air-dry.
2 Add stain and leave for 10–40 min, depending on the specific stain used (e.g. 40 min for Merck R66 stain). Stain upside down in a staining plate or place in a trough.
3 Pour off the stain and wash slide with tap water for a few minutes.
4 Dry upright.

Thick films

1 Heat film in incubator at 37°C for 15 min.
2 Proceed as for thin films (see above).

Stain recipe

Giemsa powder   3.8 g
Methyl alcohol   250 ml
Glycerol   250 ml

Add stain and glass beads to bottle. Add glycerol and alcohol, shake vigorously and place at 37°C for 24 h with further frequent shaking. Remove from the incubator and shake again over 24 h. The stain is then ready for use. Filter small amounts as required.

Appendix 4.4: Photographs of malarial parasites

Supplier	Product
Tropical Health Technology 14 Belville Close Doddington March PE15 0TT	Learning Bench Aid No. 1 Microscopical Diagnosis of Malaria
World Health Organization, Geneva, or HMSO	*Basic Laboratory Methods in Medical Parasitology*, (1992) WHO, Geneva

Appendix 4.5: Training courses

Training courses are provided at three reference centres. Up-to-date prices are available from the relevant centres.

1 The Liverpool School of Tropical Medicine runs an annual 4-day course dealing with blood parasites, which is suitable for MLSOs and haematologists/pathologists and is approved for continuing medical education (CME) and for continuing professional development (CPD).

2 The UK NEQAS Blood Parasitology Teaching Scheme, based at the Hospital for Tropical Diseases, includes the attendance of one person a year at a 1-day regional training course. The course is suitable for MLSOs and haematologists/pathologists and is approved for CME and CPD. Participation in this teaching scheme is open to laboratories enrolled in either UK NEQAS (H) or UK NEQAS Blood Parasitology.

3 The Public Health Laboratory Service, Malaria Reference Laboratory runs a 3-day course dealing with the laboratory diagnosis of malaria, which includes a self-assessed practical test. This course is suitable for haematologists and others involved in the laboratory diagnosis of malaria and is approved for CPD.

References

ACDP (1995) *Categorization of Biological Agents According to Hazard and Categories of Containment*, 4th edn. HSE Books, London.

Bain B.J. (1996) *Blood Cells: a Practical Guide*. Blackwell Science, Oxford.

Chiodini P.L., Hunte Cooke A., Moody A.H. *et al.* (1996) *MDA Evaluation of the Becton Dickinson Parasight F test for the Diagnosis of* Plasmodium falciparum. Medical Devices Agency, Department of Health.

Dacie J.V. & Lewis S.M. (1995) *Practical Haematology*, 8th edn. Churchill Livingstone, Edinburgh.

Diem K. & Lentner G. (1970) *Documents Geigy. Scientific Tables*, 7th edn. Geigy Pharmaceuticals, Macclesfield.

Health Services Advisory Committee, Health and Safety Commission (1992) *Safety in Health Service Laboratories: Safe Working and the Prevention of Infection in Clinical Laboratories*. HSE Books, London.

Milne L.M., Kyi M.S., Chiodini P.L. & Warhurst D.C. (1994) Accuracy of routine laboratory diagnosis of malaria in the United Kingdom. *Journal of Clinical Pathology* **47**, 740–742.

Moody A.H., Hunt-Cooke A. & Chiodini P.L. (1990) Experience with the Becton–Dickinson QBCII® centrifugal haematology analyser for haemoparasites. *Transactions of the Royal Society of Tropical Medicine and Hygiene* **84**, 782.

Warhurst D.C. & Williams J.E. (1996) ACP Broadsheets No. 148. Laboratory diagnosis of malaria. *Journal of Clinical Pathology* **49**, 533–538.

Wilkinson R.J., Brown J.L., Pasvol G., Chiodini P.L. & Davidson R.N. (1994) Severe falciparum malaria: predicting the effect of exchange transfusion. *Quarterly Journal of Medicine* **87**, 553–557.

5 Guidelines for the Enumeration of CD4⁺ T Lymphocytes in Immunosuppressed Individuals

Prepared by the General Haematology Task Force

1 Introduction

The acquired immune deficiency syndrome (AIDS) results from a severe and progressive functional loss of CD4$^+$ T lymphocytes. The aetiological agent is the human immunodeficiency virus (HIV), which causes a progressive depletion of CD4$^+$ T lymphocytes, together with activation and dysfunction of many other cells involved in the immune response. The resulting clinical immunodeficiency is manifest by the occurrence of opportunistic infections, selective increase in specific tumours, frequent association with wasting and potential involvement of the central nervous system. Because of the association of disease progression with the decline in CD4$^+$ T lymphocytes, the management of HIV-infected individuals requires the precise and accurate measurement of this lymphocyte subset (Centers for Disease Control, 1992; Nicholson, 1994). Quantitation of CD4$^+$ T lymphocytes is determined by flow-cytometric immunophenotyping of peripheral whole blood and is essentially based upon a product of three laboratory variables: the white blood cell count (WBC), the lymphocyte count and the percentage of lymphocytes that express the CD4 antigen. Flow-cytometric immunophenotyping facilitates the identification of individual cells according to size, granularity and antigen expression. The reliance of analysis of these parameters and the move of flow cytometry from research to routine clinical practice have increased the need for standardization. To ensure the accuracy and reliability of CD4$^+$ T-lymphocyte counting, on both an intra- and interlaboratory basis, standard methods, as well as guidelines for quality assurance and quality control, are required. This guideline provides information on: (i) frequency of CD4 testing; (ii) laboratory safety; (iii) specimen collection, transport and storage; (iv) specimen processing and controls; (v) instrument quality control; (vi) sample analysis; (vii) data analysis, storage and reporting; and (viii) quality assurance.

2 Frequency of CD4 testing

The frequency of monitoring a patient's CD4 count will depend upon a number of factors,

Reprinted with permission from *Clinical and Laboratory Haematology*, 1997, **19**, 231–241.

including the treatment and the rate of disease progression. All HIV+ patients should have at least one baseline CD4 measurement at the time of diagnosis and then monthly for 3 months following HIV diagnosis. Following this, asymptomatic patients will require CD4 counts every 6 months, while symptomatic patients require analysis at 3-monthly intervals. Individuals with rapidly decreasing levels, as detected on the first three measurements, should have a CD4+ T-lymphocyte count checked monthly. The CD4+ T-lymphocyte count should be used as a guide for the administration of antiretroviral therapy, *Mycobacterium avium-intracellulare* (MAI) prophylaxis and *Pneumocystis carinii* pneumonia (PCP) prophylaxis in adults. The threshold for antiviral/MAI therapy is a CD4 count $<0.5 \times 10^9/l$ and for PCP prophylaxis a CD4 count $<0.2 \times 10^9/l$.

3 Laboratory safety

Each individual laboratory must have local guidelines describing the procedures involved in the laboratory handling of pathological specimens. The Advisory Committee on Dangerous Pathogens (1995) has recently reviewed and published workplace guidelines, which provide information on the categorization of and protection against blood-borne infections, such as HIV and hepatitis. All laboratory workers must be familiar with these guidelines before undertaking such work.

The decontamination of the flow cytometer, following the analysis of HIV specimens, must be performed in accordance with the manufacturer's recommended instructions. Stream-in-air flow cytometers should not be used for CD4+ T-lymphocyte counting on HIV-infected material. If this is not possible, measures to avoid aerosols or droplets of sample material must be undertaken (if in doubt, contact the manufacturer of the instrument). The use of a flow cytometer equipped with an autosample loader/biosampler to minimize sample handling is recommended.

Sample preparation should be performed in a designated area, which should be thoroughly decontaminated after use. Test-tubes should be individually capped in order to prevent spillage and to retain aerosols that may be created during mixing. Spillages of HIV-infected material should be dealt with immediately by using an appropriate decontaminating solution in accordance with health and safety guidelines. After staining, lysing and washing, buffered paraformaldehyde (pH 7.0–7.4, 2% solution) or a proprietary cell-fixing reagent should be added to the samples in order to minimize the infection risk. All samples must remain in fixative after analysis. Flow-cytometer systems that employ a sample loader/biosampler may use a 'lyse-no-wash' procedure in order to minimize handling. In these instances, fixation of the specimen may not be required prior to analysis, providing the loader is sealed when in use. However, following analysis, all samples should be inactivated prior to disposal, using either a 10% solution of sodium hypochlorite, a viral-inactivating reagent or, ideally, a combined viral inactivating and mycobactericidal reagent. The sample loader/biosampler should be thoroughly decontaminated after use, in accordance with the manufacturer's guidelines. Specimens should be disposed of by appropriate methods.

4 Specimen collection

All specimens from individual patients should, wherever possible, be collected by venepuncture at the same time of day to minimize diurnal variation, which can produce significant changes in absolute CD4 counts. It is important that the correct anticoagulant is used,
with 0.34 M di- or tripotassium ethylenediaminetetra-acetic acid (K_2EDTA or K_3EDTA)
being preferred. Haematological analysis must be completed within 6 h of venepuncture.
If a specimen is to be referred to a central laboratory for analysis, resulting in a delay of
over 6 h, then a total WBC must accompany the sample (it is preferable that the total WBC
and flow-cytometric differential, rather than a haematological analyser-derived absolute
lymphocyte count, be used to calculate the absolute CD4 lymphocyte count). All samples
must be labelled with a unique patient identifier and data and time of collection and be fully
processed within 18 h to minimize anticoagulant effect. The use of Soundex or hospital
reference numbers to ensure confidentiality is preferred. The possible risk of infection
should be clearly indicated on sample(s) and laboratory request form(s).

Storage and transportation must be between 10°C and 30°C and samples should not be
subjected to temperatures below 10°C (Ekong *et al.*, 1992). Packaging and transportation
of HIV-infected material should be in accordance with the regulations of the postal and/or
courier service used. Specimen integrity must be examined upon receipt and repeat specimens requested if there is evidence of gross haemolysis or clots or if the specimen is
received >18 h from time of venepuncture.

5 Specimen processing and controls

There are several methods of specimen processing and determination of absolute T-
lymphocyte subsets, all of which involve the staining of lymphocytes in whole blood with
monoclonal antibodies directly conjugated with fluorochromes. The lymphocyte population is analysed by flow cytometry and the absolute lymphocyte subset values are calculated
accordingly.

5.1 Two-colour flow cytometry and ultraviolet microscopy

In the early 1980s, determination of CD4[+] T lymphocytes was usually undertaken using
Ficoll density-separated lymphocytes and ultraviolet (UV) microscopy. It must be stressed
that enumeration of CD4[+] T lymphocytes should no longer be undertaken by either UV
microscopy or single-colour analysis. There have been a number of technological advances
that have enabled the routine use of whole-blood lysis with multicolour parametric analysis.
In the mid- to late 1980s, changes in software and conjugation of new fluorochromes to
monoclonal antibodies facilitated identification of lymphocytes, using either light-scatter
gating procedures or differential staining with CD45 and CD14 (Loken *et al.*, 1990). These
approaches, however, have several disadvantages. Firstly, a forward angle/side scatter
(FSC) gate approach does not enable the identification of gate contaminants and may result
in falsely low percentage values, while the requirement for larger panels (up to six tubes

Table 5.1 Monoclonal antibody panels required for T-gating, lineage gating and CD45/SSC gating (these are examples only; exact combinations and/or fluorochrome assignment will depend upon instrument configuration and software analysis/gating procedure used)

T-gating fluorochrome order, e.g. (FITC/PE/PE-Cy5)	Lineage gating fluorochrome order, e.g. (FITC/PE/PE-Cy5)	CD45/SSC gating fluorochrome order, e.g. (FITC/PE/PE-Cy5)	Tube
CD3/CD4/CD8	Isotype controls e.g. ($IgG_1/IgG_{2a}/IgG_1$)	IgG_1/IgG_1/CD45 (this tube is optional)	No. 1
	CD3/CD4/CD8	CD3/CD19/CD45	No. 2
	CD16 and/or CD56/CD19/CD3	CD3/CD4/CD45	No. 3
		CD3/CD8/CD45	No. 4
		CD3/CD16 and/or CD56/CD45	No. 5

in a panel) increases analysis time, specimen handling and, ultimately, cost. Secondly, it is impossible to detect tube-to-tube variation when using a light-scatter gate derived from CD45/CD14 'back-gating'. In addition, the isotype control tube does not provide a control for CD45/CD14 staining, while the light-scatter gate may contain granulocytes and/or red-cell debris, necessitating result correction (basophils cannot be resolved from the lymphocyte population based upon a light-scatter gate using CD45/CD14).

In view of the above limitations, the optimal method for T-lymphocyte evaluation is now multiparametric or three-colour lymphocyte immunophenotyping. This approach has substantial advantages, as it enables analysis of high-purity lymphocyte gates with low levels of debris and/or contaminating cells. Thus it is recommended that CD4⁺ T-lymphocyte determination is performed using a minimum of three-colour lymphocyte immunophenotyping, employing one of the following three gating strategies: (i) T-gating; (ii) lineage gating; and (iii) CD45/side scatter (SSC) gating. Each of these approaches will be described in more detail below.

5.2 T-gate method

This approach, using whole-blood lysis, is best suited to flow cytometers capable of generating absolute lymphocyte counts (Mandy *et al.*, 1992). The technique can be used on instruments without such facilities but will complicate the reporting of both absolute lymphocyte counts and percentages. (Note that the light-scatter profile (FSC vs. right-angle SSC) is not used as the primary gate.) The absolute numbers of T-lymphocyte subsets can be derived from a single tube containing a mixture of anti-CD3, anti-CD4 and anti-CD8, conjugated to fluorescein isothiocyanate (FITC), phycoerythrin (PE) and a third fluorochrome (e.g. peridin chlorophyll protein (PerCP)), respectively (Table 5.1). Isotype controls are not necessary. Following staining, lysis and washing, the specimen is analysed using a combination of right-angle light scatter and the CD3 fluorescence channel. This allows identification of the T-lymphocyte cluster and the setting of the relevant gate (Fig. 5.1). Events are collected and then analysed using the remaining fluorescence channels, i.e. FL2 VFL3

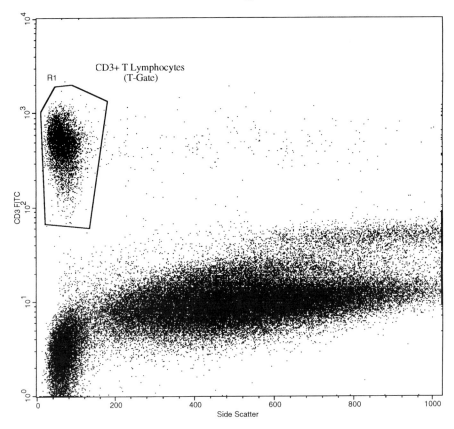

Fig. 5.1 T-gate method (CD3/SSC) dot plot of a whole-blood lysis specimen. R1 denotes the CD3$^+$ T-lymphocyte analysis region.

(Fig. 5.2). The events collected through this gate are, by definition, T lymphocytes (i.e. expressing CD3), allowing the identification of CD4$^+$ and CD8$^+$ populations. This method of analysis excludes B lymphocytes, CD8$^+$ natural killer (NK) cells, monocytes and debris. The CD4$^+$ and CD8$^+$ lymphocytes, therefore, are expressed as a percentage of the total CD3$^+$ lymphocytes and not the total lymphocyte population. The advantages and disadvantages of the T-gating method are listed in Table 5.2. Advantages include the following: (i) a large T-gate may be used to maximize recovery without sacrificing purity; (ii) the identification of dual positive populations (CD3$^+$CD4$^+$ and CD3$^+$CD8$^+$) are determined in a single tube; (iii) immature and γδ T cells are not included in the CD4$^+$ and CD8$^+$ determinations; and (iv) an isotype control is not required. However, these advantages should be considered along with the disadvantages, which include the following: (i) the exclusion of B lymphocytes and NK cells results in the lack of a full lymphocyte immunophenotypic profile; (ii) CD4$^+$ and CD8$^+$ lymphocyte populations are expressed as a percentage of CD3$^+$ lymphocytes and not of the total lymphocyte population; (iii) use of a single-tube assay does not enable the calculation of the lymphosum (total T cells (CD3%) + B cells (CD19%) + NK cells (CD3$^-$CD16 and/or CD56^{+0}%) = 100% ± 5%) nor does it enable replicate comparisons of CD3$^+$ cells,

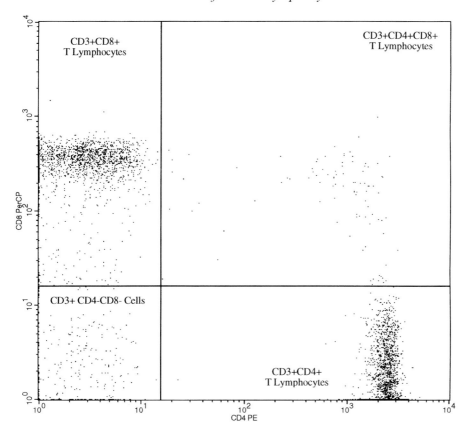

Fig. 5.2 Analysis of CD3⁺ T lymphocytes identified in Fig. 5.1 (R1) for expression of CD4 and CD8.

Table 5.2 Advantages and disadvantages of using T-lineage gating procedures

T-gate method advantages	T-gate method disadvantages
A large T-gate can be used to maximize recovery	B and NK lymphocytes, vital for lymphosum, are excluded
A pure T-gate is obtained, thus avoiding result correction	
Identification of dual CD4⁺ and CD8⁺ populations is possible	CD4⁺ and CD8⁺ populations are expressed as a percentage of CD3⁺ lymphocytes
Immature and γδ T cells are not included	Use of a single tube does not provide lymphosum or allow comparative CD3 determinations for internal QA
Isotype controls are not required	
A one-tube panel is used	
Cost is lower than a conventional, larger, two-colour panel	Absolute values for CD4 and CD8 cannot be determined without using a flow cytometer with absolute counting capability
There are fewer tubes to handle and process than with a two-colour panel	
It is suitable for both paediatric and adult specimens	The T sum (CD4 + CD8 = CD3) may not be helpful in cases when CD3⁺CD4⁻CD8⁻ cells present
There is an increased number of evaluable samples when compared with the use of FSC/SSC gating strategies	Is best suited to instruments with absolute count capability

QA, quality assessment.

which are required for quality-control purposes; (iv) absolute values of CD4$^+$ and CD8$^+$ cells cannot be determined if the flow cytometer has no direct counting facility; and (v) the T sum (CD4 + CD8 = CD3) may not necessarily be helpful in HIV cases where CD3$^+$CD4$^-$CD8$^-$ cells are present. The role of this technique, therefore, is best suited to instruments or reagent systems that provide direct absolute counts, using either beads or precision delivery.

5.3 Lineage gating

A logical development of the T-gating method is the inclusion of B lymphocytes and NK cells. This was first proposed by Mercolino *et al.* (1995) and is referred to as 'lineage gating'. The procedure encompasses T-lineage as well as B-lineage gating strategies, so as to include all the lymphocyte subsets. As a result, using three tubes (including isotype controls), it is possible to analyse T, B and NK lymphocytes, as well as obtaining duplicate T-lymphocyte analysis and lymphosum enumeration. The latter two procedures are required for internal quality-control purposes. The panel of tubes for lineage gating are detailed in Table 5.1.

Lineage-gating analysis incorporates the whole-blood lysis technique. An isotype control tube is used to set a light-scatter gate (FSC vs. SSC) on the lymphocyte population. Events collected within this gate are then used to determine the negative and positive regions on the three fluorescence channels. The use of the control tube also enables the identification of non-specific staining in the SSC vs. fluorescence gates used in the analysis of specific cell populations. The second tube, containing the fluorochrome-conjugated CD3, CD4 and CD8 antibodies, is used to analyse T lymphocytes in the manner described for T-gating. The third tube, containing an NK marker (i.e. anti-CD16), a B-lymphocyte marker (i.e. anti-CD19) and the T-lymphocyte marker anti-CD3, enables the calculation of the lymphosum, as well as allowing a duplicate check of CD3$^+$ T lymphocytes. Several gates are used to achieve these values, including light-scatter gates, T, B and NK gates (for an in-depth description of the procedure, see Mercolino *et al.*, 1995). In addition to the advantages of T-gating, the technique enables: (i) the exclusion of debris and non-lymphoid cells from analysis, thus increasing the recovery, without compromising on purity, and negating the requirement for flow-cytometric values to be corrected for non-lymphocyte contamination; (ii) a complete lymphocyte profile from three tubes (including controls) to be obtained, making it suitable for small-volume samples; (iii) a lymphosum to be obtained, thus providing an internal quality-control check; (iv) the T-lymphocyte subsets to be reported as a percentage of the total lymphocytes; and (v) the resolution of the basophils from the lymphocyte population. The disadvantages of this approach are: (i) that it can only be used on flow cytometers with absolute count facilities; (ii) that it is dependent on advanced software and gating techniques; (iii) that the use of SSC is the primary method of discriminating lymphocytes from granulocytes; and (iv) that difficulties may be encountered in NK-cell gating if a single marker is used for their identification, due to the heterogeneity of antigen expression by NK cells. The advantages and disadvantages of the linear-gating method are listed in Table 5.3.

Table 5.3 Advantages and disadvantages of lineage-gating approach

Lineage-gating advantages	Lineage-gating disadvantages
Any debris and non-lymphocyte cells are excluded from analysis	It is best suited to instruments with absolute counting capabilities
A complete profile is obtained from three tubes (including isotype controls)	Advanced software and gating techniques are required
A lymphosum is obtained, thus providing an internal QA check	The approach utilizes SSC as the primary method of discriminating lymphocytes from granulocytes
It is suitable for both paediatric and adult specimens	
The T-lymphocyte subsets are reported as a percentage of total lymphocytes	The use of a single NK marker may present difficulties in NK identification
It resolves basophils from the lymphocyte population	
The cost may be lower than the conventional, larger, two-colour panel	
There are fewer tubes to handle and process than with a larger two-colour panel	
It increases the number of evaluable samples compared with the use of FSC/SSC-gating strategies	

QA, quality assurance.

5.4 CD45/side-scatter gating

It is well recognized that relying solely upon light-scatter gating may lead to problems with contamination. As a result, methods have been devised to optimize the placement of light-scatter gates and, at the same time, provide information of gate contamination by non-lymphocytes and debris. The use of a tube containing both anti-CD45 and anti-CD14 was initially proposed by Loken *et al.* (1990) to overcome such problems and is the basis of the Centers for Disease Control (CDC) recommendations for CD4⁺ T-lymphocyte immuno-phenotyping (Centers for Disease Control, 1992, 1993).

However, several problems still exist with this approach. Firstly, the tube containing anti-CD45 and anti-CD14 is not subjected to isotype-control monitoring. Secondly, the gate set using this combination is assumed to be constant throughout the panel used. Finally, the remaining panel uses a light-scatter gate, making discrimination between debris and lymphocytes difficult and discrimination between basophils and lymphocytes imposs-ible. Nicholson *et al.* (1996) therefore proposed the use of a three-colour procedure, incor-porating anti-CD45, which is used to provide an immunological tube-to-tube check of the lymphocyte analysis region. The approach requires that anti-CD45 is incorporated into each combination of antibodies (see Table 5.1). As with T- and lineage gating, the approach uses fluorescence vs. side scatter. The CD45 expression is used to identify the lymphocyte population (CD45^bright, low-linear SSC) (Fig. 5.3). The lymphocyte gate thus defined is relatively free from contaminating cells and debris. The remaining two or more fluores-cence channels are then analysed through this region (Fig. 5.4). Because there are very few contaminating events, the need to correct for non-lymphocyte contamination is reduced and the accuracy of lymphocyte determination increased. For a more in-depth descrip-tion of this procedure, see Nicholson *et al.* (1996). As with the T-gating method, isotype controls are not required and the remaining unstained cells are used to determine the

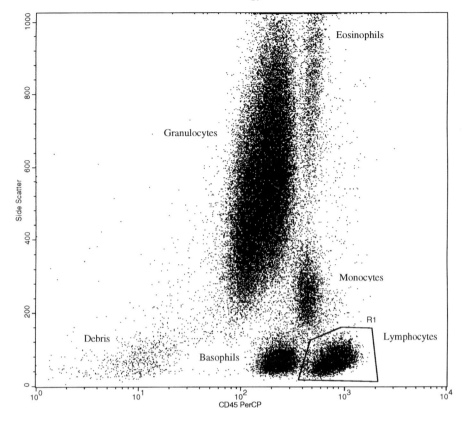

Fig. 5.3 CD45/side-scatter (SSC) dot plot of a whole-blood lysis specimen. The relative position of each leucocyte population is shown. R1 denotes the lymphocyte analysis region. (Data collected on a Becton Dickinson FACScan using Cell Quest software™.)

negative and positive fluorescence boundaries. Table 5.1 details the antibody combinations which should be used to enable immunophenotyping of HIV-infected individuals by this method.

There are several advantages to using CD45 gating: (i) it can be used with instruments and reagent systems that do not provide absolute counts; (ii) the use of anti-CD45 in each tube allows consistent gating checks on an intertube basis; (iii) no debris is collected in the analysis gate; (iv) non-lymphocyte contamination is minimal; (v) it discriminates basophils from lymphocytes (not possible by CD45/CD14 gating); (vi) high-purity lymphocyte data are collected, which avoids the need for result correction; (vii) replicate CD3 determinations are obtained, while the CD3⁺CD4⁺ and CD3⁺CD8⁺ populations are determined in only two tubes; (viii) cost may be lower than with a larger, two-colour panel; (ix) no isotype controls are required; (x) there are fewer tubes to handle and process; and (xi) there are increased numbers of evaluable samples compared with FSC/SSC gating strategies. However, there are also several disadvantages which need to be considered: (i) added expertise is

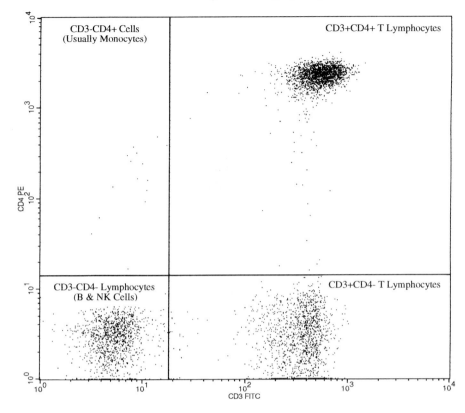

Fig. 5.4 Analysis of CD4+ T lymphocytes, using the R1 region designated in Fig. 5.3.

required for machine set-up (including spectral compensation), data collection and data analysis; (ii) the third fluorochrome may not be detected by older flow cytometers; (iii) CD4 and CD8 determination is performed in separate tubes; (iv) some lymphocytes may be lost from analysis, due to weak CD45 expression; and (v) discrimination of lymphocytes from smaller monocytes may be difficult in some cases. The advantages and disadvantages of the CD45/SSC-gating method are listed in Table 5.4.

To overcome the limitations of three-colour immunophenotyping, four-colour technology is now becoming available, incorporating CD45/SSC or lineage gating. These approaches, although in their infancy, have the ability to simultaneously detect CD3+CD4+ and CD3+CD8+ T lymphocytes. There are few data available at present comparing its performance with the above three strategies. Thus, any laboratory intending to use four-colour analysis should undertake statistical comparisons with their current method (i.e. lineage gating or CD45/SSC) before its introduction, to demonstrate that there are no significant differences. Furthermore, it can only be used with flow cytometers suitably equipped with either an extra laser and/or electronic hardware/software capable of detecting and analysing the fourth fluorochrome.

Table 5.4 Advantages and disadvantages of CD45/SSC gating

CD45/SSC-gating advantages	CD45/SSC-gating disadvantages
It can be used with instruments that do not provide absolute counts	Added technical expertise is required
The use of anti-CD45 in each tube allows a consistent tube-to-tube gating check	for machine set-up, data collection and data analysis
No debris is collected in the analysis gate	The third and fourth fluorochromes may not be detected by older flow cytometers
The inclusion of non-lymphocyte contamination in the gate is minimal	Some lymphocytes may have weak expression of CD45 and thus be
It resolves basophils from lymphocytes	excluded from the analysis
The use of a high-purity lymphocyte gate avoids the need for result correction	Discrimination of lymphocytes from small monocytes may be difficult
Replicate CD3 determinations are obtained	
CD3$^+$CD4$^+$ and CD3$^+$CD8$^+$ populations are obtained from two tubes	
The cost may be lower than the conventional, larger, two-colour panel	
No isotype controls are required	
There are fewer tubes to handle and process than with the two-colour panel	
It increases the number of evaluable samples compared with the use of FSC/SSC gating strategies	
It is suitable for both paediatric and adult specimens	

6 Recommended gating strategy

The choice of the above gating procedures will ultimately determine the panel used for CD4$^+$ T-lymphocyte determination. The panels recommended within these guidelines facilitate the use of internal quality-control checks (with the exception of T-gating). Any abbreviated panel, therefore, will result in the loss of these checks. It is important that careful review of the results is undertaken to ensure consistency with previously obtained results. The use of replicate CD3 evaluations can be used to indicate variability in lysis (there should be less than 3% variation between CD3 percentages when using a panel that contains four replicates of CD3). The recommended gating strategy, for most laboratories, is either CD45/SSC (using three or more separate fluorochromes) or lineage gating.

7 Sample preparation

The whole-blood lymphocyte-staining method is well described. Briefly, peripheral blood is collected in the manner stated earlier and a volume of blood added to premixed three-colour monoclonal antibodies at the concentrations recommended by the manufacturer. If premixed monoclonal antibodies are not commercially available, the user will have to determine the optimum concentrations to use. Each antibody should be titred against each of the others and compared with those results obtained when using single staining (Reilly, 1996). Following incubation (in the dark), the red cells are lysed (using a proprietary lysing reagent) and washed in accordance with the manufacturer's recommendations. Several commercial systems are now available which employ the 'lyse-no-wash' technique, thereby reducing specimen handling, cell disruption and loss due to centrifugation and washing. If a wash step is included, it is advisable to vortex the cells prior to analysis to break up cell aggregates. Cell specimens should be fixed as described earlier.

Several control steps should be employed in the analysis of CD4⁺ lymphocytes, including the use of isotype controls, process controls (both reagent and process) and flow-cytometer controls (beads) (the quality control of the flow cytometer will be covered in Section 8). The use of isotype controls has several advantages, and their use needs to be evaluated in each individual laboratory. They provide assistance, for example, in determining photomultiplier tube (PMT) settings, cursor placement and the identification of positive/negative boundaries where continuous antigen expression is present. Disadvantages are that: (i) the antibody concentration may not have the same characteristics as the test antibodies; (ii) the fluorochrome conjugation may be different and may bind differently to individual cell populations; (iii) isotype controls are not required when antigen expression is discontinuous; (iv) isotype controls differ between manufacturers and negative peaks must match the test negative peak; and (v) there is an extra cost burden for the analysis. In view of these considerations, multicolour (three or more fluorochromes) immunophenotyping can be performed in the absence of isotype controls, the cursor placement being set using the unlabelled (negative) cell population. The cursor placement from the initial analysis tube can be used for all other tubes for a given patient's panel.

The use of a process control is recommended to enable the monitoring of reagent performance, staining, lysis and analysis. Such controls must be run at least once a week (prior to any of the week's work being processed) and preferably on a daily basis. They must also be run: (i) if there has been a change in reagent and/or laboratory personnel; (ii) after instrument service and/or instrument calibration; and (iii) in any situation where the validity of the technique may be suspect. Process controls should be used to test the labelling procedure and, if possible, to test the lysing step. They should also be stable over time (for a minimum of 30 days). Target values should have been assigned to these specimens by the manufacturer. Results obtained from these reagents must be plotted on a Levy–Jennings-type plot, thus providing a visual indication of drift or bias over time. A fresh normal specimen must not be used as a process control, due to variability between individuals. However, such material can be used for instrument set-up and correcting for spectral overlap.

8 Instrument quality control

A stream-in-cuvette flow cytometer must be used to process HIV-infected material. Daily calibration of the instrument must be carried out to ensure optimal performance. This procedure is undertaken using commercial beads in order to: (i) monitor the light scatter and fluorescence peak channel coefficients of variation; (ii) monitor light and fluorescence peak channel drift; (iii) monitor instrument sensitivity; and (iv) facilitate compensation set-up to adjust for spectral overlap. All values should be logged daily, together with instrument settings. All settings should be re-established following a change in bead batch or after an instrument service. Beads, however, only provide guidance for the final flow-cytometer set-up and optimization of settings is achieved using a fresh normal specimen.

9 Sample analysis

The choice of gating strategy will influence the method of analysis. If computer-assisted analysis is not used, manual gating strategies must be employed. It is preferable for data to be acquired ungated and for a minimum of 2500 lymphocyte events to be collected. If the data are acquired gated – for example, using CD45/SSC – then the gate placement should be checked for each tube, in order to adjust for tube-to-tube variation. Marked differences between tubes usually indicate sample-preparation error and the tube (or panel) should be repeated. In addition, if a monocyte contamination of >5% is observed within the gate, the tube should be repeated. If this problem recurs, a new specimen should be requested. To facilitate evaluation of problem samples, a tube containing CD14, CD45 and CD3 may be added to determine the extent of monocyte contamination within the CD45/SSC gate. This approach, however, is rarely required when using CD45/SSC gating. The individual operator should define, in his or her own working environment, the specimen acceptance and rejection criteria when using such software. If in doubt, repeat staining or analysis of a repeat specimen should be performed.

10 Data analysis

The procedure for gating strategies has been detailed earlier and data analysis, therefore, will clearly depend on the strategy chosen. If the lineage gating strategy is employed, computer-assisted analysis software is available that defines the analysis region and sets the positive and negative quadrant boundaries for fluorescence staining, based upon the isotype control used, and subsequently calculates the lymphocyte subset values for each of the tests. If T-gating or CD45/SSC gating strategies are employed, the use of isotype controls can be eliminated by using the unlabelled (negative) populations in each tube to set the positive/negative quadrant boundaries. Cursor settings are determined by using the fluorescence patterns from CD3, CD4 and CD8. Since cells expressing both CD3 and CD4 stain brightly, the discrimination between negative and positive populations allows easy placement of the quadrant boundaries. Furthermore, the cursor placement from this tube can be used for subsequent tubes. As stated earlier, there is no need to correct for non-lymphocyte contamination when using the three described gating strategies.

11 Data storage

All primary files, worksheets and copy report forms should be kept for a minimum of 6 months. It is preferable to store data electronically. The flow-cytometry data should be stored as list-mode files. All electronically stored data should be retained for at least 2 years following the death of the patient. Deletion of the data or destruction of paper records should be in accordance with the Department of Health's document HC(89)20, *Preservation, Retention and Destruction: Responsibilities of Health Authorities under Public Records Act*, and locally agreed guidelines.

12 Data reporting

Counts of CD4+ T lymphocytes should be reported as both percentage and absolute values. The use of T-lineage gating procedures, however, will only allow the reporting of T-lymphocyte subsets as a percentage of the total T lymphocytes, thereby giving rise to higher calculated CD3+CD4+ and CD3+CD8+ percentages when compared with lineage gating and CD45/SSC gating approaches. Therefore, if T-gating is employed, this should be highlighted to the clinician. Wherever possible, gating strategies should be used that allow the lymphocyte subsets to be reported as a percentage of total lymphocytes (i.e. lineage or CD45/SSC gating). Analysis techniques for the monitoring of patient CD4+ T-lymphocyte percentages must be consistent and not varied from T-lineage to other gating strategies without prior discussion with the clinical users. Calculation of absolute values of lymphocyte subsets is also subject to technical variation. The most precise method (i.e. giving the lowest CV) is that used by the new generation of flow cytometers (e.g. using either precision fluidics or bead technology), which enable absolute values to be calculated directly, thereby obviating the need for a haematology-analyser-derived total WBC. Therefore, wherever possible, the use of such instruments is preferred. If such instrumentation is not available, then haematology parameters derived as stated earlier should be used in the calculation. The haematology values should be calculated from blood drawn at the same time as that used for immunophenotyping. It is important that adequate haematology quality assurance is in place before using such parameters. Data from the relevant monoclonal antibody combinations should be reported (Table 5.1), with the corresponding reference limits obtained from a normal population and adjusted for age in young children. The reference limits should be obtained from a minimum of 70 normal individuals. These ranges should be checked on an annual basis, or following any change in instrumentation or methodology (including reagents).

13 Quality assurance

It is expected that laboratories performing CD4+ T-lymphocyte testing will be fully conversant with all procedures employed. Such laboratories should meet Clinical Pathology Accreditation (CPA) (UK) Ltd. standards and be accredited as appropriate. In addition, both internal and external quality assurance should be undertaken. Internal quality assurance has been described earlier. Satisfactory performance should be demonstrable in external proficiency testing schemes such as UK National External Quality Assessment Scheme (NEQAS) leucocyte immunophenotyping schemes. All quality-assurance activities should be documented.

14 Key points

1 All HIV patients should have at least one baseline CD4$^+$ T-lymphocyte count determined during the 3 months following diagnosis.

2 In HIV individuals CD4$^+$ T-lymphocyte counts are measured to determine the need for prophylactic antiviral ($<0.5 \times 10^9$/l) or anti-*Pneumocystis carinii* ($<0.2 \times 10^9$/l) therapy.

3 Use Soundex or hospital reference numbers to ensure confidentiality.

4 The risk of infection must be clearly identified on the sample(s) and laboratory request form(s).

5 Stream-in-air flow cytometers should not be used for CD4$^+$ T-lymphocyte determination in HIV-infected individuals.

6 Peripheral-blood specimens should be collected in EDTA and fully processed within 18 h. Haematology analysis must be performed within 6 h of collection. Specimens must be stored at between 10˚C and 30˚C.

7 Cell specimens should be fixed in 2% paraformaldehyde or proprietary cell fixative for a minimum of 30 min after staining and prior to analysis.

8 Single-colour and UV microscopy must not be used for CD4$^+$ T-lymphocyte determination.

9 Three- or four-colour lymphocyte immunophenotyping is the recommended procedure, employing either: (i) T-gating; (ii) lineage gating; or (iii) CD45/SSC gating. Wherever possible the use of lineage gating or CD45/SSC gating is preferred.

10 It is preferable for CD4 and CD8 antibodies to be PE-conjugated.

11 Isotype controls are not required for T-gating and CD45/SSC-gating methods.

12 Process controls to monitor reagent, staining and, ideally, lysis procedures should be used at least once a week and preferably daily.

13 Flow-cytometer performance should be monitored daily, using unstained and fluorescent latex beads.

14 Analysis gates should have <5% monocyte contamination.

15 CD4$^+$ T lymphocytes should be reported as both percentage and absolute values. If T-gating is used, the clinician should be notified that the T-lymphocyte subset percentage values are expressed as a percentage of the total T lymphocytes only.

16 Wherever possible, calculation of absolute CD4$^+$ T-lymphocyte numbers should be obtained, using a flow cytometer that generates these values independently of haematology-derived parameters.

17 Laboratories providing a routine CD4$^+$ T-lymphocyte enumeration service should meet CPA (UK) Ltd. standards and be accredited where appropriate.

18 Participation (together with satisfactory performance) in external proficiency-testing schemes should be demonstrable.

19 All primary files, worksheets and copy report forms should be kept for a minimum of 6 months. The data should also be stored electronically and retained for at least 2 years following the death of the patient.

References

Advisory Committee on Dangerous Pathogens (1995) *Protection Against Blood-borne Infections in the Workplace: HIV and Hepatitis*. HMSO, London.

Centers for Disease Control (1992) Guidelines for the performance of CD4+ T-cell determinations in persons with human immunodeficiency virus infection. *Morbidity and Mortality Weekly Report* **41**, 1–19.

Centers for Disease Control (1993) Revised classification system for HIV infection and expanded surveillance case definition for AIDS among adolescents and adults. *Morbidity and Mortality Weekly Report* **41**, 1–35.

Ekong T., Hill A.M., Gompels M., Brown A. & Pinching A.J. (1992) The effect of the temperature and duration of sample storage on the measurement of lymphocyte subpopulations from HIV-1-positive and control subjects. *Journal of Immunological Methods* **151**, 217–225.

Loken M.R., Brosnan J.M., Bach B.A. & Ault K.A. (1990) Quality control in flow cytometry: 1: establishing optimal lymphocyte gates for immunophenotyping by flow cytometry. *Cytometry* **11**, 453–459.

Mandy F.F., Bergeron M., Recktenwald D. & Izaguirre C.A. (1992) A simultaneous three-color T cell subset analysis with single laser flow cytometers using T cell gating protocol: comparison with conventional two-color immunophenotyping method. *Journal of Immunological Methods* **156**, 151–162.

Mercolino T.J., Connelly M.C., Meyer E.J. *et al.* (1995) Immunologic differentiation of absolute count with an integrated flow cytometric system: a new concept for absolute T cell subset determinations. *Cytometry (Communications in Clinical Cytometry)* **22**, 48–59.

Nicholson J.K.A. (1994) Immunophenotyping specimens from HIV-infected persons: laboratory guidelines from the Centers for Disease Control and Prevention. *Cytometry* **18**, 55–59.

Nicholson J.K.A., Hubbard M. & Jones B.M. (1996) Use of CD45 fluorescence and side-scatter characteristics for gating lymphocytes when using the whole blood lysis procedure and flow cytometry. *Cytometry* **26**, 16–21.

Reilly J.T. (1996) Use and evaluation of leucocyte monoclonal antibodies in the diagnostic laboratory: a review. *Clinical and Laboratory Haematology* **18**, 1–6.

6 The Laboratory Diagnosis of Haemoglobinopathies

Prepared by the General Haematology Task Force

1 Introduction

Disorders of globin-chain synthesis, both thalassaemias and structurally abnormal haemo-globins, are common in the UK and constitute a significant public-health problem. Diagnosis may be required: (i) to confirm a provisional diagnosis, such as sickle-cell disease or β-thalassaemia major; (ii) to explain a haematological abnormality, such as anaemia or microcytosis; (iii) to identify an abnormality in the presymptomatic phase, as in neonatal screening; (iv) to predict serious disorders of globin-chain synthesis in the fetus and offer the option of termination of pregnancy; (v) to permit genetic counselling of prospective parents; or (vi) as preoperative screening for the presence of sickle-cell haemoglobin. Improved fully automated systems and reagents for techniques such as high-performance liquid chromatography (HPLC) and isoelectric focusing (IEF) have led to their introduction in many laboratories. Immunological methods for the identification of variant haemoglobins have also become available. There is therefore a need for an updated guideline defining the role of new techniques in relation to traditional techniques. To save repetition, previous guidelines (Globin Gene Disorder Working Party of the BCSH General Haematology Task Force, 1994; Thalassaemia Working Party of the BCSH General Haematology Task Force, 1994) should be consulted. This guideline discusses techniques and defines their place in specific diagnostic settings. The detection of unstable haemoglobins, methaemoglobins and high-oxygen-affinity haemoglobins is not discussed, but laboratories should either have methods for detecting these variant haemoglobins or should send such samples to a reference laboratory.

It should be noted that the identification of haemoglobins is often presumptive, based on a characteristic electrophoretic mobility or other characteristics in an individual of appropriate ethnic origin. Definite identification usually requires deoxyribonucleic acid (DNA) analysis or amino acid sequencing. Family studies are also of considerable importance in elucidating the nature of disorders of haemoglobin synthesis.

Reprinted with permission from *British Journal of Haematology*, 1998, **101**, 783–792.

2 Techniques

2.1 Full blood count

A full blood count (FBC) is usually indicated in all individuals being investigated for a suspected disorder of globin-chain synthesis. The exception is in neonatal screening. Red-cell indices are of particular importance in screening for β- and α°-thalassaemia trait and in distinguishing between δβ-thalassaemia and hereditary persistence of fetal haemoglobin (HPFH).

2.1.1 When are further tests indicated?

A blood film is useful, in addition to a blood count, when an unstable haemoglobin, sickle-cell disease or thalassaemia is suspected. A reticulocyte count is indicated if haemolysis is likely, e.g. if an unstable haemoglobin, haemoglobin-H disease or sickle-cell disease is suspected. In addition, definitive tests to identify normal and variant haemoglobins are indicated in suspected haemoglobinopathies, regardless of the results of the FBC and blood film.

2.2 Haemoglobin electrophoresis on cellulose acetate at alkaline pH (pH 8.2–8.6)

Cellulose acetate electrophoresis enables the provisional identification of haemoglobins A, F, S/G/D, C/E/O-Arab, H and a number of less common variant haemoglobins. With good electrophoretic techniques, haemoglobin F levels >2% can be recognized visually; when an increased level is detected, quantification is required. Good techniques also enable a split A_2 band to be recognized. This is useful in helping to distinguish α-chain variants, e.g. haemoglobin G Philadelphia, from β-chain variants, e.g. haemoglobin D Punjab. It is also essential if β-thalassaemia trait is to be diagnosed in individuals who also have a δ-chain variant (see below).

   Haemoglobin A_2 can be quantified by cellulose acetate electrophoresis, followed by elution and spectrometry, but this is a labour-intensive technique if large numbers of samples require testing. Quantification of haemoglobin A_2 by scanning densitometry is not recommended, as the precision is not good enough for the diagnosis of β-thalassaemia trait (ICSH, 1978).

   Variant haemoglobins, including haemoglobin S, can be quantitated by scanning densitometry (Legg *et al.*, 1995). However, it is necessary to have good separation of bands and it should be noted that this method is imprecise if the concentration is low, e.g. haemoglobin F can be quantified with reasonable precision only when it is appreciably elevated. Quantification of variant haemoglobins can be diagnostically useful, e.g. in helping to distinguish haemoglobin Lepore from heterozygosity for haemoglobins S/D/G and in the differential diagnosis of sickle-cell/$β^+$ thalassaemia (S$β^+$ thal) and sickle-cell anaemia (SS).

2.2.1 When are further tests needed?

Patients who show a band with the mobility of haemoglobin S require a sickle solubility test (or alternative) to confirm the presence of haemoglobin S; if this is negative, an alternative technique to identify haemoglobins D and G is needed. Those with a single band with the mobility of haemoglobin S require not only a sickle solubility test but an alternative technique to distinguish SS from compound heterozygosity for haemoglobin S and other haemoglobins, e.g. D and G, with the same mobility as haemoglobin S. Samples which show a band with the mobility of C/E/O-Arab require electrophoresis at acid pH (using citrate agar or a commercial or other agarose gel which has been shown to give similar separation of variant haemoglobins) or investigation by an appropriate alternative technique (see below), to distinguish between these haemoglobins and, when there is a single band with this mobility, to distinguish homozygotes from compound heterozygotes; the alternative technique should also distinguish haemoglobin C from haemoglobin C-Harlem. It should be noted that DNA analysis can be used to identify D-Punjab and O-Arab. Elevated haemoglobin F should be quantitated and a Kleihauer test should be performed when δβ-thalassaemia is suspected (i.e. when red-cell indices suggest thalassaemia, an F band is visible on electrophoresis and haemoglobin A_2 is not elevated) and also when HPFH is suspected.

2.3 Haemoglobin electrophoresis on citrate agar or agarose gel at pH 6.0–6.2

Electrophoresis at acid pH on citrate agar or appropriate agarose gel is usually used as a supplement to cellulose acetate electrophoresis at alkaline pH. There are differences in the relative mobilities of variant haemoglobins between citrate agar and agarose gel. Both techniques distinguish haemoglobin S from D/G but do not distinguish between most types of D and G. They will distinguish haemoglobin C from E, C-Harlem and O-Arab.

Electrophoresis at acid pH is indicated in the investigation of suspected high-affinity haemoglobins, even when electrophoresis at alkaline pH is normal, since some high-affinity haemoglobins have abnormal mobility at acid pH but normal mobility at alkaline pH.

2.3.1 When are further tests indicated?

Further tests are needed to distinguish haemoglobins D and G from each other (see above). A sickle solubility test is indicated when mobility at acid pH suggests haemoglobin C-Harlem, a variant haemoglobin in which the sickle mutation is one of two mutations, rather than haemoglobin C. A sickle-cell solubility test is similarly indicated if electrophoretic mobility suggests the presence of one of the other variant haemoglobins in which the sickle mutation is one of two mutations. Performing a sickle solubility test when any variant haemoglobin is detected (WHO, 1994) will avoid missing any such cases.

2.4 Quantification of haemoglobin A_2 by microcolumn chromatography

This is a satisfactory method for quantification of haemoglobin A_2 for the diagnosis of β-thalassaemia trait. Special columns are required for haemoglobin-A_2 quantification in the presence of haemoglobin S, but it should be noted that this test is not essential for diagnosis, since $Sβ^+$ thal can be distinguished from sickle-cell trait (AS) on the basis of haemoglobin S comprising a higher proportion of total haemoglobin than haemoglobin A in $Sβ^+$ thal (>50%) and a lower proportion (<50%) in AS. This technique is of some value in

Table 6.1 Variant haemoglobins which can be distinguished from each other by isoelectric focusing*

Instrument/reagent system	Distinguished from each other
Isolab	A, F, S, C, D-Punjab, G-Philadelphia/Lepore, E/A$_2$/O-Arab
Helena Rapid Electrophoresis	A, F, S, C, D-Punjab, G-Philadelphia, E/A$_2$,† O-Arab
Pharmacia Phast	Information not available

* Haemoglobins that can be distinguished from each other are separated by a comma; those which cannot be distinguished from each other are separated by a solidus.
† Haemoglobin C may also show some overlap with haemoglobins E/A$_2$.

distinguishing between SS (haemoglobin A$_2$ <4%) and Sβ° thalassaemia (haemoglobin A$_2$ >4%) (Dacie, 1988; Serjeant, 1992). However, it should be noted that coexisting α-thalassaemia trait will influence these values and interpretation should be undertaken with considerable caution.

2.4.1 When are further tests indicated?
Microcolumn chromatography should be combined with haemoglobin electrophoresis at alkaline pH in order to detect any variant haemoglobins. High and low haemoglobin-A$_2$ percentages can be distinguished visually on an electrophoretic strip and this can sometimes be a useful check on microcolumn chromatography results. It should be noted that unstable haemoglobins can be associated with an increased haemoglobin-A$_2$ percentage and, if the red-cell indices do not suggest a straightforward β-thalassaemia trait, a test for an unstable haemoglobin is indicated.

2.5 Isoelectric focusing
The haemoglobins that can be distinguished from each other by IEF differ between different instrument/reagent systems (Table 6.1). In addition, an increased percentage of haemoglobin A$_2$ may be observed, but this technique has not been validated for haemoglobin-A$_2$ quantification.

2.5.1 When are further tests indicated?
The presence of haemoglobin S should be confirmed by a sickle solubility test or an alternative technique. A high or borderline haemoglobin A$_2$ on IEF should be confirmed by microcolumn chromatography or an alternative technique.

2.6 High-performance liquid chromatography
The HPLC technique can be used for the quantification of haemoglobins A$_2$ and F and the detection, provisional identification and quantification of variant haemoglobins. The haemoglobins that can be distinguished from each other by HPLC vary somewhat between different instruments and reagent systems (Table 6.2). This technique provides precise quantification of haemoglobin A$_2$ and is therefore suitable for the diagnosis of β-thalassaemia trait. However, haemoglobin A$_2$ may not be accurately quantified in the presence of haemoglobin

Table 6.2 Variant haemoglobins which can be distinguished from each other by high-performance liquid chromatography,* based on published information and on the experience of the Working Party of the General Haematology Task Force of the British Committee for Standards in Haematology

Instrument/reagent system	Distinguished from each other
Primus Variant System 99	A, F, S, C, E/A$_2$, D-Punjab, G-Philadelphia, O-Arab
Kontron Instruments Haemoglobin System PV	A, F, S, C, E/A$_2$,† D-Punjab, G-Philadelphia
BioRad Variant ('β thal short program')	A, F, S, C, E/A$_2$, D-Punjab, G-Philadelphia, O-Arab
Glycomat 765 'Green' Kit	
In haemoglobin-A$_2$ mode	A, F,‡ S, C, D-Punjab/G-Philadelphia/E/A$_2$
In variant mode	A, F, S, C, D-Punjab, G-Philadelphia, E/A$_2$
Glycomat 'Gold' Kit (also Biomen Gold Kit)	
In haemoglobin-A$_2$ mode	A, F, S, C, D-Punjab/G-Philadelphia, E/A$_2$
In variant mode	A, F, S, C, D-Punjab, G-Philadelphia, E/A$_2$
Shimadzu Industry Standard HPLC	S, D-Punjab, G-Philadelphia, C, E/A$_2$, O-Arab
Protech Scientific Ltd. HaemaChrom	Information not available

* Haemoglobins that can be distinguished from each other are separated by a comma; those which cannot be distinguished from each other are separated by a solidus.
† Haemoglobins E and A$_2$ have fairly similar retention times and some overlap might occur.
‡ Haemoglobin F and glycosylated haemoglobin A (haemoglobin A$_1$) are not distinguished.

S. In addition, haemoglobin A$_2$ cannot usually be separated from haemoglobin E, thus hindering the differential diagnosis between E/B° thalassaemia and homozygosity for haemoglobin E.

Automated HPLC systems that have been the subject of recent evaluations include the Bio-Rad Variant, Primus Variant System 99 and Kontron Haemoglobin System PV (Waters *et al.*, 1996; Bain & Phelan, 1997a, b; Wild & Stephens, 1997).

2.6.1 *When are further tests indicated?*
The nature of any variant haemoglobin detected by HPLC which is of potential clinical relevance (e.g. for genetic counselling) should be confirmed by an alternative technique.

2.7 Sickle solubility tests
The kits for sickle-cell solubility tests, which are predominantly used in the UK, will detect haemoglobin S down to a concentration of 20% (and sometimes below – in some cases, as low as 8%) (Bain & Phelan, 1997a). This method is therefore capable of detecting all cases of AS beyond the period of early infancy, even when there is coexisting α-thalassaemia trait. Kits which have been the subject of an evaluation for the Medical Devices Agency of the Department of Health and which have been found to be satisfactory are Sickledex (Ortho Diagnostics), Sickle-SOL (Baxter Diagnostics Inc.), Microgen Bioproducts S-TEST (Microgen Bioproducts Ltd.) and Sickle-Check (Lorne Laboratories Ltd.) (Bain & Phelan, 1997a). The method of Dacie & Lewis (1995), although less sensitive than commercial kits,

also detects haemoglobin S down to a concentration of 20%. Most methods require that all negative or equivocal sickle solubility tests be centrifuged before reading, to increase sensitivity and reliability.

2.7.1 When are further tests indicated?

All positive and equivocal sickle solubility tests should be confirmed by haemoglobin electrophoresis or an alternative technique, both for confirmation and to distinguish AS from SS and from compound heterozygous states. In an emergency, e.g. preanaesthetic, this distinction can be made with reasonable accuracy with a sickle solubility test combined with a blood film and a blood count. It is also recommended that all negative sickle solubility tests be confirmed by haemoglobin electrophoresis or an alternative technique.

In general, a sickle solubility test is not indicated in an infant before the age of 6 months, since a negative result may be misleading. However, a sickle solubility test can sensibly be performed in an emergency, prior to an anaesthetic, since, if it is negative, it is unlikely that anaesthesia will cause any clinical problems. The wording of the report on such a test must state that a negative test does not exclude the presence of a low percentage of haemoglobin S and that further testing is necessary and will follow.

2.8 Immunoassay for variant haemoglobins

Kits are currently available for the immunoassays of haemoglobins S, C, E and A, known respectively as HemoCard Hemoglobin S, HemoCard Hemoglobin C, HemoCard Hemoglobin E and HemoCard Hemoglobin A (Isolab Inc.). This technique is potentially useful and, when functioning properly, all HemoCards detect the relevant variant haemoglobins, at least down to 10% and sometimes down to 5% (Bain & Phelan, 1997a, b; Chapman *et al.*, 1997). However, there have been problems with intermittent failure of the method.

2.9 Quantification of haemoglobin F and Kleihauer test

Quantification of haemoglobin F is indicated if raised haemoglobin F is detected beyond early infancy, e.g. in sickle-cell disease, thalassaemia major or intermedia, suspected HPFH and suspected δβ-thalassaemia. A Kleihauer test should be performed whenever an increased percentage of haemoglobin F is detected and the differential diagnosis is between δβ-thalassaemia trait, when the distribution of haemoglobin F is usually heterocellular, and HPFH, in which the distribution of haemoglobin F is usually pancellular. A 2-min alkali denaturation test is recommended for the quantification of haemoglobin F. Techniques for the Kleihauer test will be the subject of a separate BCSH guideline. It should be noted that, in the differential diagnosis of HPFH and δβ-thalassaemia, quantification of haemoglobin F and a Kleihauer test are supplementary to the assessment of red-cell indices.

2.10 Haemoglobin H inclusions

A haemoglobin-H preparation is indicated to confirm the presence of haemoglobin H in suspected inherited or acquired haemoglobin-H disease.

Table 6.3 Disorders of globin-chain synthesis which should be predicted in a fetus and prospective parents

---

Disorders of globin-chain synthesis which should be predicted in a fetus

β-Thalassaemia major (including haemoglobin E/β°-thalassaemia)

β-Thalassaemia intermedia (including haemoglobin E/β°-thalassaemia)

Haemoglobin Barts hydrops fetalis

Sickle-cell anaemia

Compound heterozygous states causing other forms of sickle-cell disease (sickle cell/β-thalassaemia, sickle cell/haemoglobin C disease, sickle cell/haemoglobin D-Punjab, sickle cell/haemoglobin O-Arab)

Disorders of globin-chain synthesis which should be detected in prospective parents

β-Thalassaemia* heterozygosity or compound heterozygosity

Haemoglobin-E heterozygosity, homozygosity or compound heterozygosity

α°-Thalassaemia heterozygosity or haemoglobin-H disease

Sickle-cell heterozygosity, homozygosity or compound heterozygosity

Haemoglobins C, D-Punjab and O-Arab

---

* The presence of haemoglobin Lepore or of δβ-thalassaemia trait has exactly the same significance as β-thalassaemia trait and diagnosis of these traits is required whenever diagnosis of β-thalassaemia trait is required.

3 Clinical settings in which tests are required

3.1 For genetic counselling of prospective parents either before or during pregnancy

The disorders of globin-chain synthesis which should be predicted in a fetus and the abnormalities which should therefore be detected in prospective parents are given in Table 6.3. A flow chart illustrating the procedures for their detection is given in Fig. 6.1. It should be noted that it may not always be possible to predict whether a fetus will have β-thalassaemia major or β-thalassaemia intermedia. Selective testing may be considered if the percentage of patients from ethnic minorities is low (Standing Medical Advisory Committee on Sickle Cell, Thalassaemia and Other Haemoglobinopathies, 1993), but this policy is dependent on reliable information on ethnic origin being available. It should be noted that screening for haemoglobinopathies and thalassaemias is just as important when pregnancy may result from artificial insemination from a donor or from *in vitro* fertilization as when conception occurs naturally.

3.2 β-Thalassaemia trait

The detection of the great majority of cases of β-thalassaemia trait requires either: (i) that all women are screened for β-thalassaemia trait by scrutiny of the red-cell indices; or (ii) that all women are tested for β-thalassaemia trait, regardless of red-cell indices, by universal measurement of haemoglobin-A_2 percentage. Selection by ethnic origin is undesirable, since β-thalassaemia trait and haemoglobin Lepore (which has the same significance) can occur in a very wide range of ethnic groups, including Northern Europeans. If a woman is already pregnant, testing should be done regardless of apparent iron deficiency, since a diagnosis of iron deficiency does not exclude coexisting β-thalassaemia. When screening is based on red-cell indices, all women with a mean cellular haemoglobin (MCH) <27 pg

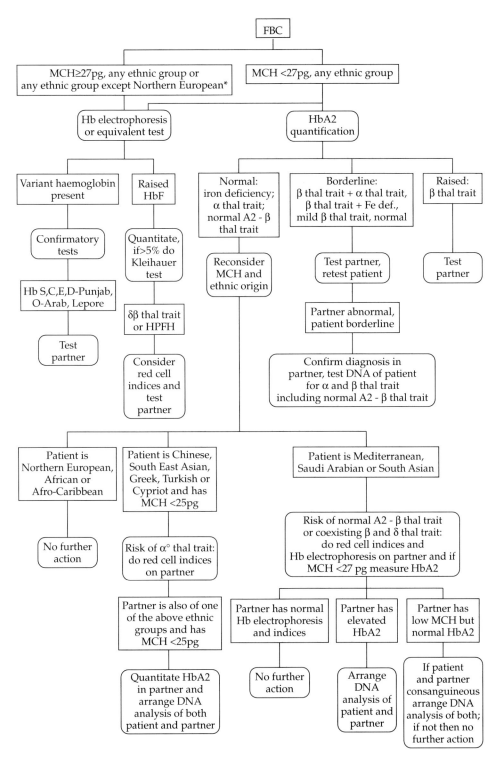

Fig. 6.1 Flow chart demonstrating procedure for diagnosis of α°-, β- and δβ-thalassaemia trait and clinically significant haemoglobin variants in pregnant women ('patients') and their partners. * Selective screening is acceptable in low-incidence areas, but only if accurate information on ethnic origin is available. Hb, haemoglobin; Fe def., iron deficiency.

(Rogers *et al.*, 1995) should have further tests performed. The screening of all women necessitates the use of a less labour-intensive technique, such as HPLC, whereas selective screening can be carried out either by cellulose acetate electrophoresis and microcolumn chromatography or by HPLC. If numbers are relatively small, electrophoresis followed by elution can be used. Important technical points which should be considered in quantifying haemoglobin A_2 have been discussed in detail in a previous British Committee for Standards in Haematology (BCSH) guideline (Thalassaemia Working Party of the BCSH General Haematology Task Force, 1994). Both δβ-thalassaemia trait and the presence of haemoglobin Lepore have the same significance as β-thalassaemia; haemoglobin electrophoresis at alkaline pH and quantification of haemoglobin F, when elevated, by an alkali denaturation test will permit their diagnosis. Both can also be diagnosed by means of IEF or HPLC. It should be noted that quantification of haemoglobin F is not essential in straightforward β-thalassaemia trait, since, although it is elevated in a significant proportion of patients, the diagnosis can be made from consideration of the red-cell indices and the proportion of haemoglobin A_2. However, an elevated level should be noted because of its relevance to a Kleihauer test performed for quantification of fetomaternal haemorrhage. Each laboratory should have procedures in place to ensure that the presence of an elevated proportion of haemoglobin F in a pregnant woman does not lead to misdiagnosis of fetomaternal haemorrhage and that an alternative technique is available for ensuring that the dose of anti-D given to Rhesus-negative women is adequate.

It should be noted that there are some problem areas in the diagnosis of β-thalassaemia trait. One is the existence of β-thalassaemia trait in which the haemoglobin A_2 level is borderline or even normal. These cases can be divided into: (i) those with both normal red-cell indices and normal haemoglobin A_2; and (ii) those with abnormal red-cell indices but a normal haemoglobin A_2. The majority of heterozygotes of the former group will be missed in the routine diagnostic laboratory. The commonest mutations responsible are -101 (C → T) and -92 (C → T). Mean values reported for individuals carrying the latter mutation are mean cellular volume (MCV) 83.9 fl, MCH 28.6 pg and haemoglobin A_2 3.4% (Pagano *et al.*, 1995). Patients in the second group, i.e. those with abnormal red-cell indices and a normal haemoglobin A_2 concentration, have an α-thalassaemia trait-like phenotype. This abnormality results from a small group of mild β-thalassaemia mutations, such as CAP + 1 (A → C) in South Asians (Indians) and, occasionally, from IVI-6 (T → C) in Mediterranean individuals. Heterozygotes for the CAP + 1 mutation have, for example, been observed to have the following mean values: MCV 79 fl, MCH 24.7 pg, haemoglobin A_2 3.4% (J. Old, pers. obs.). The phenotype of abnormal red-cell indices with a normal haemoglobin A_2 concentration can also result from the coinheritance of δ-thalassaemia (in *cis* or *trans*) and a 'high haemoglobin A_2' β^+- or β°-thalassaemia mutation. Such coinheritance of β- and δ-thalassaemia trait occurs in Sardinians and in Cypriots. The majority of such cases will be detected if the procedures we recommend for the detection of α°-thalassaemia trait are followed (Fig. 6.1).

It should also be noted that coinheritance of either α°-thalassaemia trait or homozygous α^+-thalassaemia trait and mild β-thalassaemia trait makes it more likely that the diagnosis of β-thalassaemia trait will be missed. In a small proportion of such individuals, the MCV and MCH will be raised to normal values. This modifying effect means that the diagnosis of β-thalassaemia trait may be missed in individuals with mild β^+-thalassaemia mutations, such as CAP + 1 (A → C), and coexisting α-thalassaemia trait. The coinheritance of α-thalassaemia trait and a β-thalassaemia mutation, which would usually lead to abnormal red-cell indices but a normal haemoglobin A_2 concentration, may result in the patient having normal red-cell indices as well as a normal haemoglobin A_2 concentration.

A further problem occurs if an A_2 variant is present. Failure to detect a split A_2 band may cause the diagnosis of β-thalassaemia trait to be missed, as a result of incorrect haemoglobin A_2 quantification.

3.3 α°-Thalassaemia trait

Screening for α°-thalassaemia trait (genotype $--/\alpha\alpha$) by scrutiny of the red-cell indices (supplemented by measurement of haemoglobin A_2 to exclude β-thalassaemia trait when the MCH is appropriately reduced) should be carried out in all women of the following ethnic origins: Chinese, South-East Asian, Greek, Turkish, Cypriot. The need to screen other Mediterranean populations is less well established. If the woman and her partner are consanguineous, the indications for screening are stronger. It is not necessary to screen South Asian (Indian subcontinent), African and Afro-Caribbean women for α°-thalassaemia, since a severe α-thalassaemia trait phenotype is likely to arise from the $-\alpha/-\alpha$ genotype and not the $--/\alpha\alpha$ genotype. However, it should be noted that a borderline haemoglobin A_2 in a patient with thalassaemic indices may be consequent on the coexistence of α- and β-thalassaemia (with or without iron deficiency); further investigation is necessitated by the possibility of β-thalassaemia trait, not the possibility of α-thalassaemia trait. It is considered reasonable not to test Northern European women since, although α°-thalassaemia trait does occur in white British individuals, it is very uncommon and, unless the partner was from a high-incidence ethnic group, an adverse fetal outcome would be extremely unlikely. The likelihood of detecting a significant abnormality must be set against the expense of testing and the anxiety generated.

Initial screening for α°-thalassaemia trait is by the red-cell indices (Higgs, 1993). Further testing is indicated if the MCH is <25 pg and β- and δβ-thalassaemia trait and haemoglobin Lepore have been excluded. Occasional cases of α°-thalassaemia trait have an MCH between 25 and 26 pg, but in large series such cases constitute no more than 1%. Of a total of more than 270 cases of α°-thalassaemia trait diagnosed in four British laboratories in recent years, only two patients had an MCH between 25 and 26 pg and one of these had active liver disease. Another had such a high MCH that the result was probably erroneous.

To avoid unnecessary expensive investigations and the engendering of anxiety in suspected α°-thalassaemia trait, it is useful to determine the red-cell indices of the partner and proceed to DNA analysis only if both partners have an MCH <25 pg.

It should be noted that the presence of β-thalassaemia trait does not exclude the simultaneous presence of α°-thalassaemia trait. Failure to detect both abnormalities may lead to a failure to predict haemoglobin Barts hydrops fetalis when one partner has α°-thalassaemia trait and the other has both α°- and β-thalassaemia trait. In appropriate ethnic groups (i.e. those listed above), further detailed investigation is therefore indicated if one partner has β-thalassaemia trait and the other has probable α°-thalassaemia trait (Lam *et al.*, 1997).

3.4 Variant haemoglobins

Screening for variant haemoglobins should be carried out on pregnant women of all ethnic groups, with the possible exception of Northern Europeans. Ideally, women of all ethnic groups should be screened, since clinically significant variant haemoglobins also occur, albeit at a low frequency, in Northern Europeans and since reliable information on ethnic origin is often not available. Screening can be done by cellulose acetate electrophoresis at alkaline pH, IEF or HPLC. When electrophoresis is used as the primary method, the detection of a variant haemoglobin with the mobility of haemoglobin S requires a sickle solubility test or an immunoassay for haemoglobin S for confirmation. Further testing should also be performed to identify haemoglobin D-Punjab (which is clinically significant) and to distinguish it from haemoglobin G-Philadelphia (which is not); this may be done by IEF or HPLC. Further testing should be performed to distinguish between haemoglobins C, E and O-Arab, for which IEF, HPLC or an immunoassay is suitable.

3.5 Testing of partners

The tests necessary in the partner when a variant haemoglobin or α- or β-thalassaemia trait is detected are given in Table 6.4.

3.6 Diagnosis of disorders of haemoglobin synthesis in the fetus

Diagnosis of disorders of globin-chain synthesis in the fetus is indicated when a serious disorder is predicted (see Table 6.2). Fetal DNA diagnosis should be carried out in specialized laboratories, in accordance with the previous BCSH guideline (Thalassaemia Working Party of the BCSH General Haematology Task Force, 1994). Tests most commonly used in the National Haemoglobinopathy Reference Laboratory, including tests that have been developed since the previous guideline, are given in Table 6.5.

Submission of samples for fetal diagnosis to a reference laboratory should ideally be preceded by submission of samples from both parents, together with precise details of their respective ethnic origins and a relevant clinical history.

3.7 Neonatal screening

Neonatal screening is performed to detect the presence of clinically important haemoglobin variants and the absence of haemoglobin A.

3.7.1 Blood samples

Testing can be carried out on liquid blood – either cord blood or capillary specimens – or on capillary specimens blotted on to filter-paper and allowed to dry. The latter are usually known as 'Guthrie spots'. Liquid-blood specimens are less suitable for large-scale testing programmes. Guthrie spots have the advantage that collection of specimens for

Table 6.4 Tests to be performed in the partner of a woman with a disorder of globin-chain synthesis or tests to be performed in a woman when her partner is found to have a disorder of haemoglobin synthesis

Disorder found in woman	Tests to be performed in partner to exclude clinically important interactions*
β-Thalassaemia trait†	Red-cell indices and haemoglobin A_2 quantification when indicated to exclude β-thalassaemia trait;† haemoglobin electrophoresis or alternative technique to exclude sickle-cell trait, haemoglobin E and haemoglobin O-Arab
Haemoglobin Lepore and δβ-thalassaemia trait	As for β-thalassaemia trait
α°-Thalassaemia trait	Red-cell indices, proceeding to DNA analysis in both parents if ethnic origin is appropriate and MCH is <25 pg in both
Haemoglobin S	Haemoglobin electrophoresis (or alternative technique) to exclude haemoglobins S, C, D-Punjab and O-Arab; red-cell indices and, if indicated, quantification of haemoglobin A_2 to exclude β-thalassaemia trait†
Haemoglobins C and D-Punjab	Haemoglobin electrophoresis or alternative technique to exclude haemoglobin S
Haemoglobin O-Arab	Haemoglobin electrophoresis or alternative technique to exclude haemoglobin S and, if MCH is <27 pg, haemoglobin electrophoresis or alternative technique and quantification of haemoglobin A_2 to exclude β-thalassaemia trait†
Haemoglobin E	Red-cell indices and quantification of haemoglobin A_2, if indicated, to exclude β-thalassaemia trait†

* In this table, the term 'haemoglobin electrophoresis' should be interpreted as 'haemoglobin electrophoresis or alternative technique, such as HPLC'.
† The presence of haemoglobin Lepore or of δβ-thalassaemia trait has exactly the same significance as β-thalassaemia trait and diagnosis of these traits is required whenever diagnosis of β-thalassaemia trait is required.

Table 6.5 Techniques for fetal DNA analysis for disorders of globin-chain synthesis most often used in the National Haemoglobinopathy Reference Laboratory

α°-Thalassaemia	Southern blot analysis GAP PCR
β-Thalassaemia	
Known mutations	PCR, allele-specific priming
	GAP PCR
Unknown mutations	DGGE or heteroduplex analysis
	RFLP linkage
	DNA sequencing
Hb Lepore	GAP PCR
δβ-Thalassaemia	GAP PCR
Hereditary persistence of fetal haemoglobin	GAP PCR
Hb S	PCR, DdeI digestion
Hb C	PCR, allele-specific priming
Hb E	PCR, allele-specific priming
Hb D-Punjab	PCR, EcoRI digestion
Hb O-Arab	PCR, EcoRI digestion

Hb, haemoglobin; PCR, polymerase chain reaction; RFLP, restriction fragment length polymorphism; DGGE, density gradient gel electrophoresis.

haemoglobinopathy screening can be carried out at the same time as collection of specimens for other neonatal screening programmes. When cord-blood samples are used, the risk of maternal contamination should be minimized by obtaining the specimen by needle aspiration from a cleaned site on the cord. Maternal contamination (estimated to occur in <0.5% of samples) should be suspected if haemoglobin A_2 is present or if there is a high percentage of haemoglobin A. However, it should be noted that some neonatal samples do contain haemoglobin A_2.

3.7.2 Techniques

Liquid-blood samples can be screened using cellulose acetate electrophoresis, IEF or HPLC techniques. Eluates from Guthrie-spot cards provide a more dilute sample, which may not always be suitable for analysis by cellulose acetate electrophoresis. Therefore, HPLC or IEF is more appropriate as a first-line technique. These samples are subject to increasing degradation of haemoglobins with age. Spots should therefore ideally be tested within 7 days of sampling. Ageing of the dried-blood samples leads to conversion to methaemoglobins. This, in turn, leads to variation in the baseline of chromatograms for all HPLC systems, together with an increased number of peaks in the early part of the trace, interfering, in particular, with the detection and quantification of haemoglobin H and haemoglobin Barts. This may not be deemed clinically important, as neonatal screening does not usually aim to detect haemoglobin H disease or α°-thalassaemia trait. Ageing of blood samples also leads to widening of the peaks of normal and variant haemoglobins, requiring careful interpretation. Both IEF and HPLC appear to detect all clinically significant variants and detect haemoglobin A down to concentrations of <5%.

Sickle solubility tests are not sensitive enough to detect the small quantities of haemoglobin S found in neonatal samples. HemoCard kits may be sensitive down to concentrations of 10% of haemoglobins S, C and E. However, there is some variation in sensitivity between cards and there is no HemoCard available for haemoglobin D-Punjab or haemoglobin O-Arab.

A presumptive identification of any variant haemoglobin detected can be made on the same sample using a second technique. Further confirmation and clarification of the clinical significance of abnormalities detected should be carried out at a later date, ideally around 6 weeks of age.

The International Council for Standardization in Haematology (ICSH) has published recommendations for neonatal screening for haemoglobinopathies (ICSH, 1988). Available methods have been assessed more recently for the Medical Devices Agency of the Department of Health (Chapman *et al.*, 1997).

3.8 Preoperative screening

Screening for haemoglobin S is traditionally carried out before surgery, so that anaesthetists can be aware of the potential clinical problems. However, it should be noted that, with modern anaesthetic techniques, such testing may be unnecessary. If testing is considered necessary, then all patients who are not of Northern European origin should be tested.

For routine planned surgery, an FBC, sickle solubility test and haemoglobin elec-trophoresis are usually performed in advance. For emergency surgery, an FBC and sickle solubility test are usually performed. If the sickle solubility test is positive but the blood count is normal, then SS and Sβ°-thalassaemia can be excluded. A blood film will help to exclude Sβ+ thal and sickle cell/haemoglobin C disease. Some HPLC systems can accept samples out of sequence and provide a rapid answer.

3.9 Investigation of microcytosis

If the FBC is suggestive of iron deficiency, then haemoglobin electrophoresis is not an appropriate initial investigation (except in a pregnant woman where a rapid diagnosis is required). Iron deficiency can lower the haemoglobin A_2 concentration and, although most cases of β-thalassaemia trait can be diagnosed despite iron deficiency, cases which other-wise would have only a mild elevation of the haemoglobin A_2 may be missed (Wasi *et al.*, 1968; Alperin *et al.*, 1972; Kattamis *et al.*, 1972). The patient should be investigated for iron deficiency and treated, if appropriate. If there is a persistent microcytosis after recovery from iron deficiency, further investigation should be undertaken.

If the red-cell indices are strongly suggestive of thalassaemia trait (e.g. high red blood-cell count, normal haemoglobin concentration and low MCV), then investigation for β-thalassaemia trait (and, in appropriate ethnic groups, haemoglobin-E trait) is an appropri-ate initial investigation. Any one of the methods recommended above for quantification of haemoglobin A_2 is satisfactory (HPLC, IEF or haemoglobin electrophoresis at alkaline pH plus elution or microcolumn chromatography). If iron deficiency is excluded and the haemoglobin A_2 percentage is normal, the diagnosis of α-thalassaemia trait should be con-sidered. If the patient is in the reproductive age range and of an appropriate ethnic group (see above) and the MCH is <25 pg, definitive testing for α°-thalassaemia trait should be considered. If the patient is not of an ethnic group in which α°-thalassaemia trait is likely or if the MCH is >25 pg, further testing is not indicated. The report can be worded 'haemoglobin electrophoresis (or HPLC) is normal; alpha thalassaemia trait not excluded'. In appropriate ethnic groups (e.g. Cypriots and Sardinians), the possibility should be borne in mind that thalassaemic indices with a normal haemoglobin A_2 may be due to coexisting β- and δ-thalassaemia. The diagnosis of β-thalassaemia trait can be confirmed by globin-chain synthesis or DNA studies.

In the non-urgent investigation of microcytosis, the various published formulae for discriminating between iron deficiency and thalassaemia trait (summarized in Bain, 1995) can be used to indicate which diagnosis is more likely and which test should be carried out first. However, it should be noted that such formulae should not be used in decision-making with reference to women who are already pregnant, since the question which is then being asked is not which diagnosis is more likely but whether β- and α°-thalassaemia trait can be excluded.

3.10 Investigation of other haematological abnormalities

Investigation to confirm or exclude the presence of a variant haemoglobin may be useful in the investigation of target cells, irregularly contracted cells and, occasionally, an unexplained high Hb or cyanosis, or when non-lysis of red cells in an automated haematology counter suggests the possible presence of a variant haemoglobin. Haemoglobin electrophoresis, IEF or HPLC is suitable.

4 Acknowledgements

We thank Mr Jaspal Kaeda from Hammersmith Hospital, Dr Alison May from the University of Wales College of Medicine and Mr Martin Jarvis from the North Middlesex Hospital for providing some of the data on red-cell indices in α°-thalassaemia trait; other data were provided by the National Haemoglobinopathy Reference Service. Miss Lynne Dewhurst, Manchester Royal Infirmary, helped in the preparation of Fig. 6.1.

5 Useful addresses

National Haemoglobinopathy Reference Service, Institute of Molecular Medicine, John Radcliffe Hospital, Headington, Oxford OX3 9DS. Telephone 01865 222449 or 01865 222388 (Lab); fax 01865 222500; e-mail: jold@hammer.imm.ox.ac.uk.

Further testing is also available from the following: Dr Mary Petrou, Perinatal Centre, University College London Medical School, Department of Obstetrics and Gynaecology, 86–96 Chenies Mews, London WC1E 6HX. Telephone 0171 388 9246; fax 0171 380 9864. Dr D.M. Layton, South Thames Regional Centre for Prenatal Diagnosis of Blood Disorders, Department of Haematological Medicine, King's College Hospital, Denmark Hill, London SE5 9RS. Telephone 0171 346 3242; fax 0171 346 3514.

References

Alperin J.B., Dow P.A. & Petteway M.B. (1972) Hemoglobin A2 levels in health and various hematological disorders. *American Journal of Clinical Pathology* **67**, 219–226.
Bain B.J. (1995) *Blood Cells: a Practical Guide*, 2nd edn, p. 203. Blackwell Science, Oxford.
Bain B.J. & Phelan L. (1997a) *An Evaluation of the Primus Corporation CLC 330TM Primus Variant System 99 (PVS99)*, Medical Devices Agency, London.
Bain B.J. & Phelan L. (1997b) *An Evaluation of the Kontron Instruments Haemoglobin System PV*. Medical Devices Agency, London.
Chapman C., Amos R.J., Henthorn J.S. & Chambers K. (1997) *Evaluation of Methods for Testing Neonatal Samples for Disorders of Haemoglobin Synthesis*. Medical Devices Agency, London.
Dacie J.V. (1988) *The Haemolytic Anaemias*, 3rd edn, Vol. 2, Pt 2, p. 134. Churchill Livingstone, Edinburgh.
Dacie J.V. & Lewis S.M. (1995) *Practical Haematology*, 8th edn, p. 266. Churchill Livingstone, Edinburgh.
Globin Gene Disorder Working Party of the BCSH General Haematology Task Force (1994) Guidelines for the fetal diagnosis of globin gene disorders. *Journal of Clinical Pathology* **47**, 199–204.
Higgs D.R. (1993) α-Thalassaemia. *Baillière's Clinical Haematology* **6**, 117–150.
International Committee for Standardization in Haematology (ICSH) (1978) Recommendations for selected methods for quantitative estimation of HbA2 and for HBA2 reference preparation. *British Journal of Haematology* **38**, 573–578.
International Committee for Standardization in Haematology (ICSH) (1988) Recommendations for neonatal screening for haemoglobinopathies. *Clinical and Laboratory Haematology* **10**, 335–345.

Kattamis C., Panayotis L., Metaxotou-Mavromati A. & Matsaniatis N.J. (1972) Serum iron and unsaturated iron-binding-capacity in β thalassaemia trait: their relation to the levels of haemoglobins A, A2 and F. *Medical Genetics* **9**, 154–159.

Lam T.H., Ghosh A., Tang M.H.Y. & Chan V. (1997) The risk of α-thalassaemia in offspring of β-thalassaemia carriers in Hong Kong. *Prenatal Diagnosis* **17**, 733–736.

Legg R., Sykes E., Karcher R. & Chu J. (1995) Quantitation of hemoglobin S by Bio-Rad MDMS HPLC, cellulose acetate elution, Paragon gel densitometry and Bio-Rad variant HPLC. *Clinical Chemistry* **41**, S102.

Pagano L., Desicato S., Viola A., De Rosa C. & Fioretti G. (1995) Identification of the −92 (C → T) mutation by the amplification refractory mutation system in Southern Italy. *Hemoglobin* **19**, 307–310.

Rogers M., Phelan L. & Bain B. (1995) Screening criteria for β-thalassaemia trait in pregnant women. *Journal of Clinical Pathology* **48**, 1054–1056.

Serjeant G.R. (1992) *Sickle Cell Disease*, 2nd edn, p. 44. Oxford University Press.

Standing Medical Advisory Committee on Sickle Cell, Thalassaemia and Other Haemoglobinopathies (1993) *Report of a Working Party of the Standing Medical Advisory Committee on Sickle Cell, Thalassaemia and other Haemoglobinopathies*. HMSO, London.

Thalassaemia Working Party of the BCSH General Haematology Task Force (1994) Guidelines for the investigation of the α and β thalassaemia traits. *Journal of Clinical Pathology* **47**, 289–295.

Wasi P., Disthasongchan P. & Na-Nakorn S. (1968) The effect of iron deficiency on the levels of haemoglobin A2. *Journal of Laboratory and Clinical Medicine* **71**, 85–91.

Waters H.M., Howarth J.E., Hyde K. *et al.* (1996) *Evaluation of the Bio-Rad Variant Beta Thalassaemia Short Program*. Medical Devices Agency, London.

WHO Working Group on Haemoglobinopathies (1994) *Guidelines for the Control of Hemoglobin Disorders*. World Health Organization, Geneva.

Wild B.J. & Stephens A.D. (1997) The use of automated HPLC to detect and quantitate haemoglobins. *Clinical and Laboratory Haematology* **19**, 171–176.

7 Guidelines for the Use of Thrombolytic Therapy

Prepared by the Haemostasis and Thrombosis Task Force

1 Introduction

Therapeutic fibrinolysis now has an established place in the effective treatment of occlusive thromboembolism. It reduces morbidity and mortality, as has been demonstrated by large-scale multicentre clinical trials. There is, for example, overwhelming evidence that pharmacological fibrinolysis markedly reduces mortality following myocardial infarction and there is increasing evidence of its value in the successful management of peripheral arterial occlusion. Although results of large-scale clinical trials in venous thromboembolic disease are not available, there is evidence for it having a beneficial effect, particularly in acute pulmonary embolism.

Endogenous fibrinolysis is initiated by plasminogen activators (Fig. 7.1), which include tissue plasminogen activator (tPA) and urinary-type plasminogen activator (urokinase (UK)). Their activity is inhibited by plasminogen activator inhibitors (PAIs); the predominant fast-acting one within the circulation is type I; type II may be important in regulating extravascular fibrinolysis and during pregnancy (as large amounts are produced by the placenta and released into the maternal circulation). Type III inhibitor is identical to protein C inhibitor. These, along with the second line of slow-acting inhibitors, i.e. complement C1 inhibitor, α_2-antiplasmin and α_2-macroglobulin, are all swamped by infusion of pharmacological doses of fibrinolytic activators. The plasma contains relatively large amounts of plasminogen which, along with activator, is incorporated into the developing thrombus. It is unusual for there to be free plasmin within the circulation, as it is rapidly inactivated by α_2-antiplasmin.

Of the activators, recombinant tPA (alteplase) and UK have been used extensively therapeutically and produce their pharmacological effect by directly converting plasminogen to plasmin. Streptokinase (SK) and its anisoylated derivative become activators after binding to plasminogen (see below).

1.1 Streptokinase

Upon infusion, SK (Kabikinase, Streptase) binds to plasminogen, both in the circulation

Reprinted with permission from *Blood Coagulation and Fibrinolysis*, 1995, **6**, 273–285.

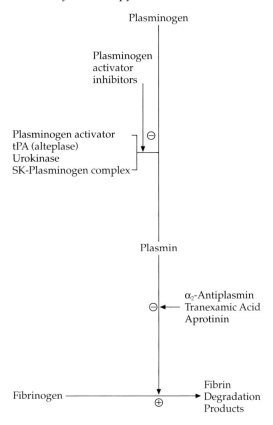

Fig. 7.1 Diagram of the fibrinolytic system.

and in thrombus, and undergoes an autocatalytic reaction to become an activator of plasminogen. Although it causes preferential dissolution of thrombus, it also results in systemic lysis, with diminution of the concentration of coagulant proteins, particularly fibrinogen and factors V and VIII. As it is a non-human protein, specific anti-SK antibodies develop and infusions can therefore be given for a maximum of 3–5 days only and there should be at least 2 years between courses of therapy (Jalihal & Morris, 1990; Lee *et al.*, 1993). A recent streptococcal infection may result in the development of anti-SK antibody; this usually only delays the development of the therapeutic effect of SK given in relatively low doses. With large doses of SK, the antibody is rapidly neutralized and early lysis results. Large doses of SK may, however, deplete circulating plasminogen such that there is insufficient remaining to promote lysis when plasma is tested *ex vivo*, but, as thrombus is preferentially enriched in plasminogen, lysis may still occur *in vivo*.

Streptokinase is available in vials of 100 000, 250 000, 600 000 and 1 500 000 international units (iu), which can be reconstituted and infused in 0.9% w/v sodium chloride or 5% w/v glucose. Details of its use for specific indications are given below. It is licensed for use in the treatment of acute myocardial infarction, deep venous thrombosis (DVT), acute major pulmonary embolism and acute arterial thromboembolism.

1.2 Anisoylated plasminogen streptokinase activator complex

Anisoylated plasminogen streptokinase activator complex (APSAC) (anistreplase) is a derivative of the SK–plasminogen activator complex in which the active site is inactivated by an anisoyl residue. After infusion, it becomes preferentially concentrated in thrombus, where gradual spontaneous deacylation occurs to reveal the active site. It is available in vials of 30 units and should be reconstituted using 5 ml of water for injection BP (*British Pharmacopoeia*) or 0.9% w/v sodium chloride. As for SK, systemic lysis is also observed. Additionally, anti-SK antibodies will arise after its use and neither it nor SK should be read-ministered within 2 years.

1.3 Alteplase

Alteplase (Actilyse) is a tissue-type plasminogen activator and, after infusion, it binds preferentially to fibrin and therefore becomes localized in thrombus. Binding to fibrin also enhances its enzymic activity to convert plasminogen to plasmin. Alteplase has also been used to treat intracardiac and aortic and venous thrombosis in neonates, who have been noted to be relatively resistant to lysis, possibly due to their low level of circulating plasminogen (see use of alteplase in peripheral arterial disease, p. 85). Although it causes preferential lysis of thrombus-bound fibrin, some systemic activation of lysis is also observed, giving rise to degradation of circulating fibrinogen. Unlike SK-containing lytic agents, its use does not result in the development of specific antibodies. It is available in vials of 20 mg and 50 mg and should be reconstituted using 20 ml and 50 ml water for injection BP, respect-ively. Further dilution, up to 1 : 5, if required, should be in 0.9% w/v sodium chloride; it should not be diluted in glucose-containing solutions. An initial portion of the dose can be given as a bolus, but thereafter the remainder should be administered as a continuous infusion. For details, see specific indications below. It is licensed only for the treatment of acute myocardial infarction and pulmonary embolism. It is being increasingly used for the treatment of peripheral arterial occlusion, for which it does not have a United Kingdom licence.

1.4 Urokinase

Following infusion, UK (Ukidan, Urokinase) binds preferentially to plasminogen and hence becomes concentrated in thrombus. It initiates fibrinolysis by promoting the conversion of plasminogen to plasmin. As it is of human origin, specific antibodies do not develop. It is available in vials of 5000, 25 000 and 100 000 iu as a freeze-dried powder. It should be reconstituted with sterile water; it should not be added to glucose infusions, as activation occurs. It is usually given as an initial bolus infusion over 10 min, followed by a continuous infusion. For details of infusion regimens, see Section 2. It is licensed for the treatment of DVT, pulmonary embolism and peripheral vascular occlusion; it can also be used to treat myocardial infarction, for which it does not have a United Kingdom licence.

Infusion of a plasminogen activator inhibits further thrombosis and hastens dissolution of thrombus by several different mechanisms. Firstly, activators diffuse into the thrombus to convert plasminogen, bound to fibrin, to plasmin. Secondly, alteplase and, to a lesser extent,

SK–plasminogen complex have affinity for fibrin, which further increases their local concentration in the thrombus. Thirdly, all the activators lead to enhanced proteolytic activity, which reduces the level of coagulant proteins, e.g. fibrinogen. Fourthly, the resultant fibrin degradation products have antithrombin and antiplatelet activity, which will help reduce the formation of further thrombus. In general, prolonged infusions, e.g. over 12 h, tend to result in a greater haemorrhagic tendency, due to the longer duration of enhanced fibrinolysis and also because there is greater depletion of circulating coagulation factors. Although alteplase might appear, on a theoretical basis, to be a safer drug than SK, clinical experience has demonstrated that, for an equivalent lytic dose, it is associated with a greater degree of intracranial haemorrhage, leading to stroke.

It is rational to aim to reduce systemic plasmin generation, with consequent hypofibrinogenaemia and its haemorrhagic risks. It is quite irrational to expect there to be no risk of haemorrhage. No currently available thrombolytic agent can distinguish between fibrin in an unwanted thrombus from fibrin in a haemostatic platelet plug. All patients will have such useful fibrin present. Some sealed wounds are clinically evident, e.g. line-insertion sites, surgical or biopsy wounds; others, e.g. intracranial aneurysms or peptic ulcers, may not be. Thrombolytic agents will seek these out, cause lysis and tend to produce bleeding, regardless of changes in the concentration of procoagulant plasma proteins.

2 Clinical indications for fibrinolytic therapy

2.1 Myocardial infarction
Following the definitive diagnosis of myocardial infarction, aspirin and a thrombolytic agent should be administered without delay, provided that there are no contraindications (Table 7.1). This form of therapy now constitutes the most important pharmacological intervention following acute infarction, and one which is associated with unequivocal benefit in terms of morbidity and mortality. Minimizing the delay to thrombolysis is of critical importance, and early treatment is associated with a more substantial improvement in ventricular function and clinical outcome. As a result of very large-scale studies, the methods of administration have been simplified for the respective thrombolytic agents and the guidelines for minimizing complications have been clarified.

The rationale for thrombolytic therapy in the treatment of myocardial infarction rests upon three established concepts: firstly, that acute myocardial infarction is associated with thrombotic coronary occlusion; secondly, that thrombolytic agents achieve a recanalization of coronary arteries and restoration of blood flow (reperfusion); and, thirdly, that thrombolytic therapy reduces the extent of myocardial injury, long-term heart failure and the risk of death (Serruys *et al.*, 1986; White *et al.*, 1989).

2.2 The impact of thrombolysis on vessel patency
Angiographic studies performed within the first 6 h of symptom onset demonstrate occlusion of the corresponding coronary artery in approximately 85% of patients in which infarction is associated with ST elevation. In some patients, a pattern of intermittent occlusion

Table 7.1 Major contraindications and risk factors for adverse events with thrombolytic therapy (modified from Lowe, 1991; Anderson & Willerson, 1993). The major contraindications are not absolute; the risks and benefits to each patient need to be considered on an individual basis

Risk category for bleeding	Peripheral or systemic bleeding	Intracranial bleeding
Major Thrombolytic therapy contraindicated	Major surgery or organ biopsy within 6 weeks Major trauma within 6 weeks Gastrointestinal or genitourinary bleeding within 6 months Pregnancy or recent delivery History of bleeding disorders, e.g. thrombocytopenia, haemophilia, hepatic or renal failure Known/suspected aortic dissection Known/suspected pericarditis	Stroke within 6 months Previous intracranial bleed Head trauma within 1 month Previous neurosurgery Known intracranial tumour Acute severe hypertension (systolic >200 mmHg or diastolic >120 mmHg) Recent transient ischaemic attack
Important	Puncture of non-compressible vessel (e.g. subclavian) Cardiopulmonary resuscitation for over 10 min Gastrointestinal or genitourinary active lesion, but no bleeding	

and spontaneous or partial recanalization occurs. Nevertheless, histopathological findings are of fissuring or rupture of an atheromatous plaque, with a variable extent of intraplaque haemorrhage and superimposed thrombus. Angiographic studies demonstrate that, following intravenous SK or alteplase, patency of the infarct-related arteries occurs in 61% and 80.8%, respectively, of patients at 90 min when the agent is administered with aspirin and intravenous heparin (TIMI grade 2 or 3 patency) (GUSTO Investigators, 1993). By 24 h, however, approximately 80% of patients have a patent infarct-related artery, irrespective of whether they have been treated with SK or alteplase with heparin. This compares with patency of approximately 25–35% in those treated with placebo.

2.3 Trials comparing thrombolytic therapy and control/placebo

Large-scale mortality trials have compared placebo and thrombolytic therapy with SK or alteplase (GISSI Study, 1986, 1987; AIMS, 1988; ISIS-2, 1988; Wilcox *et al.*, 1988; ISIS-3, 1992; Fibrinolytic Trialists, 1994). Furthermore, the Fibrinolytic Trials Collaboration has analysed all of the studies of more than 1000 patients in which thrombolytic therapy was compared with placebo controls. These amounted to 58 603 patients (Fibrinolytic Trialists, 1994). The mortality reduction was highly significant, with 25 lives saved per 1000 treated with thrombolysis alone (without aspirin). For those treated within 6 h, the mortality benefit was 30 lives saved and, from 7 to 12 h, the reduction corresponded to 17–20 lives saved per 1000 treated. There was no significant effect on mortality for those who presented more than 12 h after symptom onset who had received thrombolytic therapy. However, for those treated within the first 12 h of symptoms, the mortality reduction achieved by thrombolytic therapy is substantial, consistently established in large-scale studies and beyond reasonable doubt. The urgency for treatment is evident in the trials of early therapy and reinforced by the composite analysis. The greatest benefit occurs within the first 90 min of symptom onset and diminishes thereafter. For those treated within 6 h of initial symptoms with electrocardiogram (ECG) changes of ST segment elevation or bundle-branch block, the reduction in mortality is even greater and approaches 50 lives saved per 1000 patients treated (AIMS, 1988; ISIS-2, 1988). The Second International Study of Infarct Survival (ISIS-2) demonstrated that aspirin alone achieved a mortality reduction almost equivalent to that of SK and the benefit of the two combined was additive (35-day mortality for SK and aspirin 8%, SK alone 10.4%, aspirin alone 10.7% and double placebo 13.2%) (ISIS-2, 1988).

2.4 Risk categories

Provided the indications listed below are met, there is no evidence that the benefits are confined to specific risk groups and they are amplified in higher-risk patient populations; for example, similar proportional benefits, but larger absolute benefits, are seen in those with hypertension, diabetes, prior myocardial infarction and left bundle-branch block.

The mortality following acute myocardial infarction rises with age. In the absence of therapeutic thrombolysis, mortality within the first 35 days is 4.7% in those under 55 years, 9.3% for those aged 55–64, 16.5% for those aged 65–74 and 26.1% for those over 75 (who survive to reach hospital). These compare with 3.7%, 7.4%, 14.3% and 24.2% for those treated with therapeutic fibrinolysis in the respective groups. On account of the higher death rates in the elderly, more early deaths are saved by treating older patients in comparison with younger groups. Thus, there is no upper age limit for thrombolysis, provided that no other contraindications pertain.

2.5 Comparison of thrombolytic agents

Very large-scale comparisons of the three most widely used thrombolytic agents (SK, alteplase and anistreplase) revealed identical early and later mortality figures when the agents were administered with or without subcutaneous heparin (ISIS-3, 1992). These findings are supported by the pooled analysis of all of the published trials comparing one thrombolytic agent with another (Fibrinolytic Trialists, 1994). In this comparison, a total of 63 143 patients were investigated in trials that compared one fibrinolytic agent with another or fibrinolytic vs. control. The GUSTO trial was performed subsequently and employed an accelerated administration of tPA. It specifically compared intravenous or subcutaneous heparin in conjunction with SK against alteplase or the combination of SK and alteplase (GUSTO Investigators, 1993). The study indicated that there was no evidence of benefit for intravenous heparin in comparison with subcutaneous heparin when given with SK (30-day mortality rates 7.4% and 7.2%, respectively). The combination of alteplase and intravenous heparin revealed a mortality rate of 6.3%, compared with 7.3% in the SK pooled data. In those presenting after 4 h of symptom onset, there were identical mortality rates for the pooled SK data and for alteplase. Prior to 4 h, mortality rates were approximately 1% lower for the alteplase-treated group.

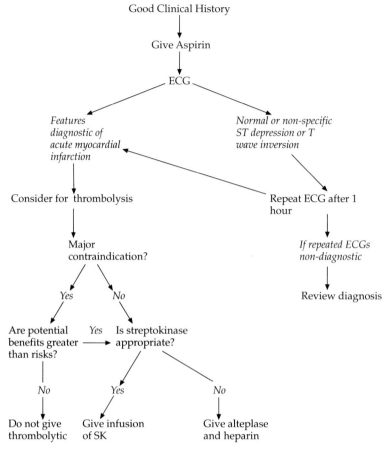

Fig. 7.2 Management of patient with clinical syndrome of myocardial infarction.

2.6 Indications in myocardial infarction

All patients developing symptoms suggestive of myocardial infarction should immediately be given aspirin 300 mg and transferred quickly to hospital, where they should be seen rapidly for diagnosis and consideration for fibrinolytic therapy. A management scheme is given in Fig. 7.2.

1 Unless clearly contraindicated, patients with infarction, as diagnosed by 1 mm or more ST elevation in two or more contiguous leads, or left bundle-branch block should receive aspirin and thrombolytic therapy with a minimum of delay. If the first ECG does not show diagnostic changes in the presence of a clinical syndrome of infarction, follow-up ECGs should be performed after an interval of approximately 1 h and the diagnosis reviewed. The latest British Heart Foundation guidelines aim for thrombolysis initiation within 90 min of the patient calling for medical treatment (call to needle time), but therapy may still be effective up to 12 h after the onset of symptoms (Weston *et al.*, 1994).

2 Those individuals with slowly evolving or stuttering myocardial infarction should have serial ECGs and, if the criteria for infarction (see above) are fulfilled, thrombolytic therapy should be given immediately.

Table 7.2 Fibrinolytic regimens for acute myocardial infarction

	Initial treatment	Further therapy	Specific contraindications
Streptokinase	1.5 million units over 1 h in 100 ml of 5% dextrose or 0.9% saline	None	Prior SK within 5 days to 2 years Known allergy to SK/anistreplase
Alteplase*	15 mg i.v. bolus	0.75 mg/kg over 30 min, then 0.5 mg/kg over 60 min i.v. Total dose not to exceed 100 mg	
Anistreplase	30 units in 3–5 min i.v.		Prior SK within 5 days to 2 years Known allergy to SK/anistreplase
Urokinase†	2 million units in 3–5 min i.v.		

* Patients weighing less than 67 kg should receive a total dose of 1.5 mg/kg.
† Not licensed for use in treatment of myocardial infarction in the United Kingdom.
i.v., intravenously.

Thrombolytic therapy should not be given to patients in whom: (i) the ECG remains normal or demonstrates only minor or non-specific T-wave inversion or ST segment depression, as there is no evidence of benefit and, furthermore, these patients experience all of the hazards of therapy (Blankenship & Almquist, 1989); and (ii) infarction has been established for more than 12 h.

2.7 Drugs and methods of administration (Table 7.2)

2.7.1 Aspirin
In patients not receiving regular aspirin, this should be administered as soon as possible after the diagnosis has been made. The first dose should be 300 mg (chewed), followed by 150 mg/day. In those already receiving aspirin therapy, it should be continued in a dose of 150 mg/day.

2.7.2 Streptokinase
An infusion of 1.5 million units (MU) SK should be given over 1 h in 100 ml of 5% dextrose or 0.9% saline. More rapid administration has been associated with marked hypotension. Severe allergic reactions are rare. Routine administration of hydrocortisone is not indicated, but it should be readily available in case of a severe reaction.

Hypotension is occasionally observed following thrombolytic therapy, and more frequently following SK-containing agents. It should be managed by temporarily halting the infusion, lying the patient flat or elevating the foot of the bed. Occasionally, atropine is required.

Heparin therapy may be indicated for some patients (Table 7.3). There is no evidence that routine intravenous or subcutaneous heparin improves mortality following SK, but subcutaneous heparin (5000–12 500 iu 12-hourly) should be considered for patients at risk of other thrombosis, e.g. those with atrial fibrillation, large anterior infarct, heart failure,

Table 7.3 Situations in which heparin is used in patients with myocardial infarction

	Heparin dose
In conjunction with alteplase	Bolus 5000 iu plus infusion 1000 iu/h (1200 iu/h if >70 kg) adjusted to give APTT ratio of 1.5–2.5
Prevention of venous thrombosis in those with heart failure, prolonged immobilization, obesity	5000 iu subcutaneously 8-hourly (or LMWH)
Previous DVT/pulmonary embolus or known thrombophilic condition	5000 iu subcutaneously 8-hourly (or LMWH)
Prevention of systemic embolism in those with large anterior infarct, atrial fibrillation, known left-ventricular thrombus	12 500 iu subcutaneously 12-hourly

previous venous thromboembolism, prolonged immobilization and obesity, the lower dose being appropriate to prevent venous thrombosis (Colvin & Barrowcliffe, 1993).

2.7.3 Alteplase

A bolus of 15 mg alteplase intravenously should be given, followed by 0.75 mg/kg intravenously (in 0.9% w/v sodium chloride) over 30 min (not to exceed 50 mg) and then 0.5 mg/kg over 60 min (not to exceed 35 mg). The total dose should not exceed 100 mg. This is the regimen used in GUSTO I, although the data sheet currently indicates that the infusion period should be 3 h.

Following the initial bolus of alteplase, 5000 iu of heparin should be given intravenously, as soon as possible, to reduce hypercoagulability and rethrombosis. This should be followed by an infusion of 1000 iu per hour (1200 iu per hour for patients over 80 kg). Full-dose heparin should be continued for 48 h to give an activated partial thromboplastin time (APTT) ratio of 1.5–2.5. Those at continued risk of venous thrombosis should thereafter receive heparin 7500 iu 12-hourly subcutaneously.

2.7.4 Anistreplase

This may have a place in the immediate out-of-hospital treatment of definitively diagnosed myocardial infarction, when a dose of 30 units infused over 3–5 min may be appropriate.

2.7.5 Urokinase

Although not licensed in the UK for use in myocardial infarction, there may be a place for its use in those in whom non-SK-mediated lysis is indicated. A dose of 1.5–2 MU in 3–5 min has been used to good effect, along with intravenous heparin (Neuhaus *et al.*, 1988; Gallagher *et al.*, 1992).

2.7.6 Oral anticoagulation

Although some studies have investigated oral anticoagulation, its role has not been defined and currently it is not recommended on a routine basis. It should be considered in patients at risk of arterial or venous thromboembolism (BCSH, 1990).

2.8 Readministration of a thrombolytic agent

Streptokinase-containing agents should not be readministered between approximately 3 days and a minimum of 2 years following initial treatment. Antibodies to SK persist for at least 2 years, at levels which impair SK activity. Alteplase and UK do not result in antibody formation and can be readministered at any time.

3 Peripheral arterial thromboembolism

3.1 Introduction

Local arterial thrombolytic therapy is an established and effective treatment for acute or subacute critical limb ischaemia due to arterial thrombosis or thromboembolism (Serkizowskyj, 1993).

The first British treatments by thrombolysis in peripheral arterial occlusion were performed in 1963 (McNicol *et al.*, 1963). Following the introduction of the Fogarty embolectomy catheter, interest in lysis waned until the early 1980s, when the value of fibrinolysis was again demonstrated (Katzen & van Breda, 1981; Hess *et al.*, 1987).

There are many different regimens for local arterial thrombolysis and results are not directly comparable. In the best studies, the maximum overall primary success rates range from 69 to 85% (McNamara & Fischer, 1985; Lammer *et al.*, 1986; Earnshaw *et al.*, 1987; McNamara *et al.*, 1991). Early recurrent thrombosis occurs in 9%, although half of these respond to further lysis. After successful lysis, a 2-year cumulative patency rate of 81% can be achieved (Lammer *et al.*, 1986). Around 8% of patients do not respond and require amputation. The overall incidence of significant complications, particularly bleeding from catheter sites and haematoma, is 12%, and there is a mortality of 1.6% (McNamara *et al.*, 1991), mostly due to haemorrhagic stroke.

Alteplase has been shown to be more effective than SK in achieving complete lysis (Lonsdale *et al.*, 1992). More importantly, alteplase achieved lysis in 22 h, compared with an average of 40 h for SK. As the risk of complication increases with the duration of therapy, alteplase would therefore appear to confer significant advantage.

3.2 Indications in peripheral arterial thromboembolism

The main indications are set out in Table 7.4 and include acute or subacute critical ischaemia of a limb due to thrombosis or, in certain cases, embolism. As 25% of acute arterial thrombosis is clinically misdiagnosed as 'embolus', preliminary angiography is worthwhile in cases of acute limb ischaemia. Thrombolytic therapy should only be considered when immediate backup is available from a vascular surgeon, because of the potential complications of arterial catheterization and intrathrombus injection of lytic agents. A most important contribution to a high success rate is therefore a close working relationship between vascular radiologist and vascular surgeon.

If there is irreversible ischaemic damage to the limb, as evidenced by total limb anaesthesia, paralysis, swollen or tense muscles or persistent skin discoloration, thrombolytic therapy is contraindicated.

Table 7.4 Indications for fibrinolytic therapy in peripheral arterial thromboembolism

- Arterial thrombosis
- Embolism from a known thrombotic source, e.g. atrial fibrillation
- Embolism older than 5 and less than 14 days (surgical embolectomy should be attempted within 5 days of the acute event)
- Failed embolectomy
- Occluded popliteal aneurysm
- Iatrogenic embolism (e.g. postangioplasty)
- Vascular graft occlusion (but not in the immediate postoperative period)

3.3 Angiographic appearance

The angiographic appearance of an occlusion correlates well with its clinical appearance and the outcome of lysis. The ideal lesion is a short, e.g. 10–20 cm, acutely occluded segment, with good reconstitution and run-off distally. Absence of distal arterial filling is a poor prognostic sign; if there is coexistent evidence of permanent ischaemic damage clinically, thrombolysis is unlikely to succeed.

Established occlusions, diagnosed as having a rounded or tapered proximal end and developed collaterals on the angiogram, are unlikely to respond to SK therapy. Alteplase may effect lysis, but, if such occlusions are less than 10 cm in length, simple recanalization by balloon angioplasty is indicated. The complication rates for thrombolysis are far greater than for angioplasty alone. Thrombolysis should not be performed if balloon angioplasty alone is likely to succeed.

Established occlusions over long segments of more than 10 cm should be considered for bypass graft surgery. Thrombolysis, angioplasty and surgery are most likely to succeed where there are good-quality distal vessels with run-off.

3.4 Use of arterial catheters

Access may be obtained from the ipsilateral or contralateral common femoral artery, depending on the site of occlusion. Using a standard Seldinger technique, an angiographic catheter is manipulated to the proximal end of the thrombus and its tip embedded. As lysis proceeds, frequent angiograms are performed and the catheter tip advanced distally into the remaining thrombus.

An increasing number of customized catheters, hollow guide-wires and mechanical devices are available for thrombolysis. These include multiple-channelled and side-holed catheters, side-holed and end-holed hollow guide-wires and mechanical devices to spray jets of thrombolytic agents into the thrombosed vessel (pulse-spray lysis). Open-ended hollow guide-wires (e.g. Sos wire) are of great benefit for distal lysis, as their small diameter and flexibility are ideally suited to arteries beyond the knee.

3.5 Drugs and methods of administration

The main agents are SK, UK and alteplase (which does not have a licence for use in arterial thromboembolism). There are many therapeutic regimens, and the following examples illustrate the use of each drug.

3.5.1 Standard infusion therapy

Streptokinase
A low-dose regimen is 5000 units/h SK, along with an initial 1000 iu heparin/h (which should subsequently be adjusted to give an APTT ratio of 1.5–2.5). Streptokinase should not be given for more than 3–5 days. Angiography should be repeated twice daily during treatment, unless there is clinical deterioration of the limb, when it should be repeated immediately.

Alternatively, a high-dose infusion of 3000 units SK/min can be given, up to a total of 20 000–30 000 units over 1–2 h (Lammer *et al.*, 1986; Earnshaw *et al.*, 1987; Hess *et al.*, 1987). During this period, frequent angiography is required to monitor progress; if lysis is not achieved, surgery should be considered.

Alteplase
An infusion of 0.5 mg/h alteplase should be started. Angiography should be repeated at 4 h and the catheter advanced. Further examinations should be twice daily and the infusion continued so long as there is continuing angiographic improvement. The average time to achieve reperfusion is 22 h (Lonsdale *et al.*, 1992). If higher doses of alteplase are used, the total dose should not exceed 100 mg and angiography should be repeated 4-hourly. Higher doses are associated with increased risk of haemorrhage (Earnshaw *et al.*, 1987).

Alteplase has also been used to treat intracardiac, aortic and venous thrombosis in neonates as a regional infusion at a dose of 0.01–0.05 mg/kg/h. Careful monitoring of both the efficacy of the treatment and the changes in haemostatic system is recommended. Lysis may be enhanced either by increasing the dose of alteplase or by giving fresh-frozen plasma as a source of plasminogen.

Urokinase
An infusion of 4000 iu/min UK can be given until antegrade flow is established; this requires 2-hourly angiography and catheter advancement. Thereafter, the dose can be reduced to 1000 iu/min until lysis is completed. The total dose should not usually exceed 500 000 iu. Heparin, initially at 1000 iu/h, should be given concurrently and the dose adjusted to give an APTT ratio of 1.5–2.0. The mean time to complete lysis is 18 h (McNamara & Fischer, 1985).

3.5.2 Pulse-spray thrombolysis
As an alternative to infusion therapy, many centres are switching to the more rapid pulse-spray technique, with either alteplase or UK. This involves embedding a catheter with a large number of side holes into the thrombus, until all the side holes in the shaft are covered by thrombus. Aliquots of lytic agent are then rapidly sprayed into the thrombus through these side holes, either by hand or via a specially adapted pump. The rapid spray has two advantages: it increases the surface area of thrombus exposed to lytic agent and simultaneously disrupts the thrombus (Bookstein *et al.*, 1989). Alteplase may be given as a 1–5 mg bolus, followed by an infusion of 0.5–1.0 mg/h.

The main advantages of this technique are its speed and high success rates. Successful lysis is reported in between 74 and 96% of arterial occlusions (Valji *et al.*, 1991; Yusuf *et al.*, 1994). Mean treatment time is from 65 to 120 min, compared with a median duration of 25.75 h with the slow continuous-infusion technique (Yusuf *et al.*, 1994). As a result of the faster time, there is a lower complication rate and major savings are made in in-patient and intensive-care costs.

As lysis is more rapid and predictable, a trial of lysis can be afforded in patients with possible reversible ischaemic damage. If there is no improvement after 1–2 h of treatment, surgical exploration can proceed with little fear of deterioration during the trial period. Such an option is not possible with the more conventional infusion method, where several hours may be needed before any improvement is noted. By this time, ischaemic damage may be irreversible.

3.6 Follow-on procedures

Often an underlying causal lesion will be revealed on successful completion of thrombolysis. Usually this will be a local stenosis, which can be treated by angioplasty. Following thrombolysis, distal stenosis or false aneurysm may be the underlying cause. Such lesions require immediate angioplasty or surgery; delay will simply risk reocclusion.

Unless specifically contraindicated, 300 mg aspirin should be given to all patients having angioplasty. In the majority of patients, it should be continued indefinitely. For patients undergoing angioplasty without a thrombolytic being administered, heparin 3000 iu, as a bolus, should be given. If arterial surgery is considered necessary, the patient should be maintained on intravenous or intra-arterial heparin to give an APTT ratio of 1.5–2.5.

All patients with indwelling catheters should receive heparin therapy; those with one in an upper limb or the aortic arch should receive intravenous heparin at a dose of 1000 iu/h to prevent catheter-related thrombus, which may subsequently embolize. For those with a catheter in the femoral artery, low-dose heparin at a rate of 250 iu/h intra-arterially should be given, usually via the side port of the introducing sheath.

4 Venous thromboembolic disease

While thrombolytic therapy with each of the currently available thrombolytic agents has been shown by repeated angiography to lyse both deep-vein thrombi and pulmonary thromboemboli, published randomized controlled trials have not been sufficiently large to show whether or not there is clinical benefit in the form of reductions in mortality, the chronic post-thrombotic leg syndrome or chronic pulmonary hypertension (Lowe, 1991; Carson *et al.*, 1992; Hyers *et al.*, 1992; ten Cate, 1993; Mosser *et al.*, 1994). In a multicentre study of clinically apparent pulmonary embolism in the USA, only 6% of patients received thrombolytic therapy (Carson *et al.*, 1992).

4.1 Indications in venous thromboembolic disease

Thrombolytic therapy is currently used on the anecdotal basis of perceived clinical benefit in the minority of patients with venous thromboembolism who have severe clinical symptoms due to massive pulmonary embolism, causing haemodynamic instability, or DVT, causing critical limb ischaemia (impending venous gangrene or phlegmasia dolens).

In these two groups of patients, when the physician perceives that life or limb is threatened despite achieving therapeutic target levels of heparin and despite other supportive measures, thrombolytic therapy is the only specific treatment, apart from pulmonary embolectomy (Gray *et al.*, 1989) or venous thrombectomy (Brady *et al.*, 1991). The evidence for clinical benefit from such surgical procedures is, likewise, only anecdotal. The choice between surgery and thrombolysis may often depend on the locally available investigative and therapeutic facilities.

Clinically suspected venous thromboembolism should be confirmed by an objective diagnostic method (venography, ultrasonography or plethysmography for suspected DVT; lung scanning and/or pulmonary angiogram for suspected pulmonary thromboembolism) prior to initiation of thrombolytic therapy, because, in the majority of patients, venous thromboembolism is not confirmed and these patients should not be exposed to the risks of thrombolytic agents.

Patients with clinically suspected and objectively confirmed venous thromboembolism, treated conventionally with heparin and oral anticoagulants, have mortality rates of 10–19% in the subsequent year, a prognosis similar to that of patients with acute myocardial infarction (ten Cate, 1993). Only part of this mortality is due to loss of life or limb from the haemodynamic effects of acute thromboembolism, which might be reduced by acute thrombolysis; much is due to recurrent thromboembolism or to the progression of underlying cancer or chronic heart or lung disease.

4.2 Drugs and methods of administration

1 Initiate standard intravenous heparin therapy with a loading dose of 5000 iu and an infusion of 1500 iu/h heparin to achieve a target APTT ratio of 1.5–2.5. Institute general supportive measures (oxygen, intensive-care and haemodynamic/respiratory support in massive pulmonary embolism; leg elevation and a vascular-surgical opinion in critical limb ischaemia due to DVT).

2 If general or limb circulatory deterioration progresses despite adequate heparinization and general supportive measures, consider the relative practicality, risks and benefits of thrombolytic therapy and surgical measures: pulmonary embolectomy (Gray *et al.*, 1989) or percutaneous catheter fragmentation (Brady *et al.*, 1991) for massive pulmonary embolism, or venous thrombectomy for massive venous thrombosis (Browse *et al.*, 1988). In DVT, the major determinant of successful thrombolysis is a short history of symptoms – less than 7 days and, optimally, less than 2 days (Rogers & Lutcher, 1990).

3 If the perceived benefits of thrombolytic therapy outweigh the apparent risks in the individual patient, the intravenous heparin infusion should be stopped prior to administration of the thrombolytic agent. The regimens in Table 7.5 should be considered (Hyers *et al.*, 1992; Goldhaber *et al.*, 1993; Association of the British Pharmaceutical Industry, 1994).

Table 7.5 Thrombolytic therapy for proved pulmonary embolus or deep venous thrombosis

	Initial treatment	Further therapy
Streptokinase	600 000 units over 30 min	100 000 units/h for 24 h for pulmonary embolus, 72 and 48 h for DVT
Urokinase	4400 iu/kg over 10 min	4400 iu/kg over 12 h for pulmonary embolus and for 12–24 h for DVT
Alteplase*	100 mg over 2 h (10 mg over 1–2 min, 90 mg over 2 h)	Heparin i.v. to give APTT ratio 1.5–2.5

* Licensed for treatment of pulmonary embolus but not DVT in the United Kingdom. Total dose of alteplase should not exceed 1.5 mg/kg in patients with body weight below 67 kg.
i.v., intravenously.

4.3 Treatment of venous thrombosis in other sites

There are anecdotal reports of successful thrombolytic therapy in venous thrombosis of the retinal, renal, portal, hepatic and mesenteric veins. The only randomized controlled trial in any of these situations is a trial of SK in central retinal-vein thrombosis. This showed an overall increase in visual acuity, but at the cost of blinding intraocular haemorrhage in two of 20 cases (Kohner *et al.*, 1976). In general, the guidelines for treatment of DVT and pulmonary embolism can be applied when there is thrombosis in these unusual sites.

4.4 Vena-caval filters for venous thromboembolism

As an alternative to anticoagulation, a metal filter may be inserted percutaneously into the inferior vena cava (IVC), either from the right internal jugular vein or the right femoral vein. This filter will then catch embolizing thrombus from the deep veins of the leg or pelvis and prevent it reaching the lungs. The indications for the insertion of an inferior vena-caval filter include patients with recurrent pulmonary embolism despite full anticoagulation, those with contraindication to or complications from anticoagulation or individuals with massive pulmonary embolism (as any further embolism may be fatal). Patients with large free-floating thrombus in iliac veins or IVC or those requiring preoperative prophylaxis, e.g. with pelvic malignancy, may also benefit from insertion of a filter.

In addition to a permanent filter, temporary devices are now available. These are usually inserted via the jugular vein and remain attached to a catheter, which can also be used to infuse lytic therapy. The main indications for such devices are to cover a period of high risk, e.g. obstetric delivery or orthopaedic surgery. A temporary filter can remain in position for up to 2 weeks.

The permanent caval filters do have complications. Incomplete opening, fracture of the filter and migration represent failure of the device. Perforation of the cava by the filter legs, thrombosis of the IVC and recurrent pulmonary embolism represent failure of technique. Fortunately, these complications are rare and there is a good long-term patency rate of up to 96% at 12 years (Greenfield, 1988).

4.5 Thrombosed arteriovenous haemodialysis shunts, Hickman lines and intravenous catheters

Urokinase (5000–25 000 iu in 2–3 ml of 0.9% w/v sodium chloride or sterile water for injection BP) is instilled into the thrombosed vessel, which is then clamped off for 2–4 h. The lysate is then aspirated and patency checked. The procedure may be repeated, if necessary. For treatment of thrombosed catheters in neonates, see use of alteplase in peripheral arterial disease (above).

5 Contraindications to thrombolytic therapy

Thrombolytic therapy is contraindicated in any patient who already has a haemorrhagic disorder or an anatomical lesion which may bleed. The major contraindications are set out in Table 7.1 and are not absolute; the risks and benefits to a patient need to be considered on an individual basis. More minor risk factors for bleeding include older age, female sex and lower body weight. There is a risk of systemic embolus in those with a left-heart thrombosis.

5.1 Measures to reduce bleeding during thrombolytic therapy

A balance has to be achieved between giving sufficient therapy to accomplish lysis and this being accomplished without an appreciable increase in serious haemorrhage. The following measures should be considered to reduce the risk of haemorrhage.

1 Avoid intramuscular injections; use the intravenous or subcutaneous routes.

2 Keep arterial and venous punctures to a minimum. Avoid sites that cannot be readily accessed or have pressure applied, e.g. subclavian vein.

3 Leaving an indwelling arterial cannula or sheath in place will help reduce bleeding, this being preferable to repeated punctures.

6 Control of prolonged thrombolytic therapy infusions

Sustained infusions of thrombolytic agents are normally employed in management of major vascular occlusions, usually venous, threatening viability of a limb or life. Monitoring of such infusions has two major aims: (i) monitoring of efficacy; and (ii) measurements designed to demonstrate fibrinolytic state.

6.1 Monitoring of efficacy

Except in the case of myocardial infarction, the efficacy of thrombolytic therapy should be monitored by repeat angiograms, as described above. When no improvement appears to be observed between consecutive angiograms, thrombolytic therapy should be stopped. It may be appropriate, however, to continue intravenous heparin.

Simple clinical observation of reduced swelling in a limb or reduced jugular venous pressure indicates that flow has been re-established. Clinical observation, however, does not establish degree of thrombus lysis, as considerable clinical improvement may occur via narrow channels or collaterals.

6.2 Measurements designed to demonstrate fibrinolytic state

The short-term administration of thrombolytic agents does not require monitoring blood tests, because there is usually only relatively little reduction in coagulant proteins and because there is no correlation between clinical bleeding and haemostatic abnormality as measured *in vitro*.

During a prolonged infusion (over more than 1 day) of a plasminogen activator, however, one of the following coagulation tests should be performed prior to starting therapy and serially thereafter. Blood should be anticoagulated with citrate in the presence of a fibrinolytic inhibitor (aprotinin 250 units/ml or ε-aminocaproic acid (EACA) 0.07 mol/l whole blood) to prevent continued lysis occurring *in vitro*.

6.2.1 Activated partial thromboplastin time

This becomes prolonged because of depletion of fibrinogen and factors V and VIII and the appearance of anticoagulant fibrin(ogen) degradation products. Development of an APTT ratio of 1.5 indicates significant systemic fibrinolytic activation.

6.2.2 Plasma fibrinogen

With systemic activation of fibrinolysis, the fibrinogen concentration falls, indicating the presence of free plasminogen activator within the circulation. It should be measured by a technique dependent on assessment of clottable fibrinogen, e.g. Clauss, and not on an indirect method from an automated coagulometer.

6.2.3 Full blood count

This will allow the platelets to be monitored, to give forewarning of developing thrombocytopenia, and the haemoglobin, to ensure the patient does not have significant, clinically inapparent, internal haemorrhage.

The systemic fibrinolytic state can also be assessed by the thrombin time, which becomes prolonged, due to the reduction in the plasma fibrinogen and the presence of its degradation products. Plasminogen activator activity can also be measured by the euglobulin lysis time or the fibrin-plate lysis test, but these are not necessary to monitor thrombolytic therapy routinely.

In about 10% of patients receiving standard doses of intravenous SK or UK, a fall in fibrinogen or prolongation of the APTT is not detected and there is a risk of venous thrombotic extension (Marder & Sherry, 1988). In this situation, the choices are: (i) increase the dose of the thrombolytic agent; (ii) change to another thrombolytic agent; or (iii) stop thrombolytic agents and substitute heparin; this will at least reduce the risk of thrombus extension.

Following cessation of the thrombolytic agent, intravenous heparin should be restarted when the APTT ratio is less than 2.0.

6.3 Bleeding and its management

Fibrinolytic therapy predisposes to bleeding, due to the depletion of the plasma concentration of procoagulants, as well as the generation of anticoagulant fibrin(ogen) degradation products. However, bleeding may occur when the coagulation screening tests are normal. This reflects the fact that plasminogen activators do not distinguish between fibrin in the thrombus and fibrin in a wound. Thus, high levels of free plasminogen activator may be absorbed on to any fibrin deposit, generate plasmin and lyse the deposit locally before systemic fibrinogen depletion occurs. The laudable aim of producing a perfect thrombolytic that has no haemorrhagic effect assumes absence of 'useful fibrin' sealing recent wounds. No blood test will predict this type of bleeding and, as a result, sustained thrombolytic therapy must be approached with very careful consideration of the risks of bleeding from recent wounds, surgery or other invasive procedures (Lowe & Rumley, 1991).

Haemorrhage is an inescapable complication in a proportion of patients. It is less common in those being treated for myocardial infarction than in those receiving prolonged infusions for venous thromboembolic disease. It is essential that patients are regularly monitored for clinical signs of bleeding, so that appropriate action can be taken. If internal bleeding is suspected, it is essential to consider whether the infusion of lytic therapy should be halted and definitive investigations undertaken. A computer-assisted tomography (CT) scan is necessary if intracranial bleeding is suspected; an abdominal ultrasound examination is invaluable for diagnosis of a retroperitoneal haematoma.

1   If bleeding is local and minor, e.g. persistent oozing from a venepuncture site, sustained local pressure should be applied.

2   For more serious bleeding the infusion of fibrinolytic activator (and heparin) should be stopped. Both these therapeutic agents are quickly cleared by the liver, which will restore the depleted fibrinogen and factors V and VIII over 12–24 h.

3   For severe, life-threatening bleeding, a fibrinolytic inhibitor should be given immediately. Aprotinin, which inhibits plasmin directly, should be given intravenously (500 000 kallikrein inactivator units over 10 min, followed by 200 000 units over 4 h) (Efstratiadis *et al.*, 1991). Alternatively, tranexamic acid, which inhibits the binding of plasminogen and plasmin to fibrin, can be given (1 g intravenously over 15 min, repeated every 8 h, as necessary). Depleted clotting factors should be replenished by use of fresh-frozen plasma and/or cryoprecipitate, depending upon the results of a coagulation screen.

4   Red cells should be transfused as clinically indicated.

5   If haematoma is life-threatening, e.g. intracranial, consider measures either to evacuate or relieve pressure effects.

References

AIMS Trial Study Group (1988) Effect of intravenous APSAC on mortality after acute myocardial infarction: preliminary report of a placebo-controlled clinical trial. *Lancet* **i**, 545–549.

Anderson H.V. & Willerson J.T. (1993) Thrombolysis in acute myocardial infarction. *New England Journal of Medicine* **329**, 703–709.

Association of the British Pharmaceutical Industry (ABPI) (1994) *Data Sheet Compendium (1994/95)*. Datapharm, London.

BCSH Haemostasis and Thrombosis Task Force of the British Society for Haematology (1990) Guidelines on oral anticoagulation: second edition. *Journal of Clinical Pathology* **43**, 177–183.

Blankenship J.C. & Almquist A.K. (1989) Cardiovascular complications of thrombolytic therapy in patients with a mistaken diagnosis of acute myocardial infarction. *Journal of the American College of Cardiologists* **14**, 1579–1582.

Bookstein J.J., Fellmeth B., Roberts A. *et al.* (1989) Pulse-spray pharmacomechanical thrombolysis: preliminary clinical results. *American Journal of Roentgenology* **152**, 1097–1100.

Brady A.J.B., Crake T. & Oakley C.M. (1991) Percutaneous catheter fragmentation and distal dispersion of proximal pulmonary embolus. *Lancet* **388**, 1186–1189.

Browse N.L., Burnand K.G. & Lea Thomas M. (1988) *Diseases of the Veins*. Edward Arnold, London.

Carson J.L., Kelley M.A., Duff A. *et al.* (1992) The clinical course of pulmonary embolism. *New England Journal of Medicine* **326**, 1240–1245.

Colvin B.T. & Barrowcliffe T.W., on behalf of BCSH Haemostasis and Thrombosis Task Force (1993) The British Society for Haematology Guidelines on the use and monitoring of heparin 1992: second revision. *Journal of Clinical Pathology* **46**, 97–103.

Earnshaw J.J., Gregorn R.H.S., Makin G.S. & Hopkinson B.R. (1987) Early results of low dose intra-arterial SK therapy in acute and subacute lower limb arterial ischaemia. *British Journal of Surgery* **74**, 504–507.

Efstratiadis T., Munsch C., Crossman D. & Taylor K. (1991) Aprotinin used in emergency coronary operation after streptokinase treatment. *Annals of Thoracic Surgery* **52**, 1320–1321.

Fibrinolytic Trialists (FTT) Cooperative Group (1994) Indications for fibrinolytic therapy in suspected acute myocardial infarction: collaborative overview of mortality and major morbidity results from all randomised trials of more than 1000 patients. *Lancet* **343**, 311–322.

Gallagher D., O'Rourke M., Healy J. *et al.* (1992) Paramedic-initiated, prehospital thrombolysis using urokinase in acute coronary occlusion (TICO 2). *Coronary Artery Disease* **3**, 605–609.

GISSI Study (1986) Effectiveness of intravenous thrombolytic treatment in acute myocardial infarction. *Lancet* **i**, 397–402.

GISSI Study (1987) Long term effects of intravenous thrombolysis in acute myocardial infarction. *Lancet* **ii**, 871–874.

Goldhaber S.Z., Haire W.D., Feldstein M.L. *et al.* (1993) Alteplase versus heparin in acute pulmonary embolism: randomised trial assessing right-ventricular function and pulmonary perfusion. *Lancet* **341**, 507–511.

Gray H.H., Miller G.A.H., Clarke D.B. & Oakley C.M. (1989) Is there a place for acute pulmonary embolectomy? *British Journal of Hospital Medicine* **41**, 467–469.

Greenfield L.K. (1988) 12 year clinical experience with the Greenfield vena caval filter. *Surgery* **104**, 706–712.

GUSTO Investigators (1993) An international randomized trial comparing four thrombolytic strategies for acute myocardial infarction. *New England Journal of Medicine* **329**, 673–682.

Hess H., Mietaschk A. & Bruckl R. (1987) Peripheral arterial occlusions: a 6 year experience with local low-dose thrombolytic therapy. *Radiology* **163**, 753–758.

Hyers T.M., Hull R.D. & Weg J.G. (1992) Antithrombotic therapy for venous thromboembolic disease. *Chest* **102** (Suppl.), 408S–425S.

ISIS-2 Collaborative Group (1988) Randomised trial of intravenous SK, oral aspirin, both, or neither among 17 187 cases of suspected acute myocardial infarction. *Lancet* **ii**, 349–360.

ISIS-3 (Third International Study of Infarct Survival) Collaborative Group (1992) ISIS-3: a randomised comparison of SK vs. tissue plasminogen activator vs. anistreplase and of aspirin plus heparin vs. aspirin alone among 41 299 cases of suspected acute myocardial infarction. *Lancet* **339**, 753–770.

Jalihal S. & Morris G.K. (1990) Antistreptokinase titres after intravenous streptokinase. *Lancet* **335**, 184–185.

Katzen B.T. & van Breda A. (1981) Low dose SK in the treatment of arterial occlusions. *American Journal of Roentgenology* **136**, 1171–1178.

Kohner E.M., Pettiot J.E., Hamilton A.M. *et al.* (1976) SK in central retinal vein occlusion: a controlled clinical trial. *British Medical Journal* **i**, 550.

Lammer J., Pilger E., Neumayer K. & Schreyner H. (1986) Intra-arterial fibrinolysis: long-term results. *Radiology* **161**, 159–163.

Lee H.S., Cross S., Davidson R. *et al.* (1993) Raised levels of antistreptokinase antibody and neutralization titres from 4 days to 54 months after administration of streptokinase or anistreplase. *European Heart Journal* **14**, 84–89.

Lonsdale R.J., Berridge D.C., Earnshaw J.J. *et al.* (1992) Recombinant tissue type plasminogen activator is superior to SK for local intra-arterial thrombolysis. *British Journal of Surgery* **79**, 272–275.

Lowe G.D.O. (1991) Clinical and laboratory aspects of thrombolytic therapy. In Poller L. (ed.) *Recent Advances in Blood Coagulation*, Vol. 5, pp. 265–291. Churchill Livingstone, Edinburgh.

Lowe G.D.O. & Rumley A. (1991) Laboratory aspects of thrombolytic therapy. In Thomson J.M. (ed.) *Blood Coagulation and Haemostasis: a Practical Guide*, pp. 171–208. Churchill Livingstone, Edinburgh.

McNamara T.O. & Fischer J.R. (1985) Thrombolysis of peripheral arterial and graft occlusions; improved results using high-dose urokinase. *American Journal of Roentgenology* **144**, 769–775.

McNamara T.O., Bomberger R.A. & Merchant R.F. (1991) Intra-arterial urokinase as the initial therapy for acutely ischaemic lower limbs. *Circulation* **83** (Suppl. I), I106–I119.

McNicol G.P., Reid W., Bain W.M. & Douglas A.S. (1963) Treatment of peripheral arterial occlusion by SK therapy. *British Medical Journal* **1**, 1508–1512.

Marder V.J. & Sherry S. (1988) Thrombolytic therapy: current status. *New England Journal of Medicine* **318**, 1512–1520, 1585–1595.

Mosser K.M., Fedullo P.F., Littejohn J.K. & Crawford R. (1994) Frequent asymptomatic pulmonary embolism in patients with deep venous thrombosis. *Journal of the American Medical Association* **271**, 223–225.

Neuhaus K.L., Tebbe U., Gottwik M. *et al.* (1988) Intravenous recombinant tissue plasminogen activator (rt-PA) and urokinase in acute myocardial infarction: results of the German activator urokinase study (GAUS). *Journal of the American College of Cardiologists* **12**, 581–587.

Rogers L.Q. & Lutcher C.L. (1990) SK therapy for deep vein thrombosis: a comprehensive review of the English literature. *American Journal of Medicine* **88**, 389–395.

Serkizowskyj I.M. (1993) The use of intra-arterial thrombolysis in acute limb ischaemia. *British Journal of Intensive Care* 400–405.

Serruys P.W., Simoons M.L., Suryapranata H. *et al.* (1986) Preservation of global and regional left ventricular function after early thrombolysis in acute myocardial infarction. *Journal of the American College of Cardiologists* **7**, 729–742.

ten Cate J.W. (1993) Thrombolytic treatment of pulmonary embolism. *Lancet* **341**, 1315–1316.

Valji K., Roberts A.C., Davis G.B. & Bookstein J.J. (1991) Pulse-spray thrombolysis of arterial and bypass graft occlusions. *American Journal of Roentgenology* **156**, 617–621.

Weston C.F.M., Penny W.J. & Julian D.G., on behalf of British Heart Foundation Working Group (1994) Guidelines for the early management of patients with myocardial infarction. *British Medical Journal* **308**, 767–771.

White H.D., Rivers J.T., Maslowski A.H. *et al.* (1989) Effect of intravenous streptokinase as compared with that of tissue plasminogen activator on left ventricular function after first myocardial infarction. *New England Journal of Medicine* **320**, 817–821.

Wilcox R.G., von der Lippe G., Olsson G.G. *et al.* for the ASSET Study Group (1988) Trial of tissue plasminogen activator for mortality reduction in acute myocardial infarction: Anglo-Scandinavian Study of Early Thrombolysis (ASSET). *Lancet* **ii**, 525–530.

Yusuf S.W., Whittaker S.C., Gregson R.H.S., Wenham P.W., Hopkinson B.R. & Makin G.S. (1994) Experience with pulse-spray technique in peripheral thrombolysis. *European Journal of Vascular Surgery* **8**, 270–275.

8 Guidelines on the Investigation and Management of Thrombocytopenia in Pregnancy and Neonatal Alloimmune Thrombocytopenia

Prepared by the Haemostasis and Thrombosis Task Force

1 Introduction

Maternal thrombocytopenia is a frequent finding in pregnancy. Appropriate assessment and investigation are crucial, as much to prevent unnecessary and potentially hazardous intervention as to identify a remediable cause and are the subject of these guidelines. Fetal/neonatal thrombocytopenia of immune origin is also considered.

2 Thrombocytopenia in pregnancy

The clinically important causes of maternal thrombocytopenia in pregnancy are: (i) spurious; (ii) gestational thrombocytopenia (incidental thrombocytopenia of pregnancy); (iii) autoimmune thrombocytopenia: idiopathic, drug-related, human immunodeficiency virus (HIV)-related; (iv) pre-eclampsia and HELLP syndrome; (v) disseminated intravascular coagulation (DIC); (vi) haemolytic uraemic syndrome (HUS), thrombotic thrombocytopenic purpura (TTP); (vii) folate deficiency; (viii) other: congenital, e.g. May–Hegglin anomaly, hereditary macrothrombocytopenia, coincidental marrow disease, hypersplenism.

3 Platelet count in normal pregnancy

Although in most instances remaining in the non-pregnant range of normal, the blood platelet count tends to fall during healthy pregnancy (Sill et al., 1985; Burrows & Kelton, 1988). Mild thrombocytopenia ($120–150 \times 10^9$/l) is a not uncommon finding, especially in the third trimester. It is, however, important that significant underlying disease be excluded as far as possible, particularly if a sudden fall in the count is detected. Greater degrees of thrombocytopenia require thorough clinical and laboratory assessment and consultation with a haematologist is indicated.

Reprinted with permission from *British Journal of Haematology*, 1996, **95**, 21–26.

4 Spurious thrombocytopenia

Apparent thrombocytopenia must be confirmed by repeating the blood count on a fresh sample and examination of the blood film to exclude laboratory error, sample clotting and ethylenediaminetetra-acetic acid (EDTA)-induced platelet agglutination. If the film appearances suggest the latter, performance of the automated platelet count on citrated blood will be informative.

5 'Benign' gestational thrombocytopenia (incidental thrombocytopenia of pregnancy)

In about 7% of pregnancies, mild to moderate thrombocytopenia is detected but appears to be clinically inconsequential for mother and fetus (Burrows & Kelton, 1990a, 1993). There is no prior history of autoimmune disease and the other causes of thrombocytopenia listed are not demonstrable. The platelet count may be as low as 80×10^9/l and, rarely, as low as 50×10^9/l. An initial normal platelet count with subsequent fall supports the diagnosis of benign gestational thrombocytopenia. Because the outcome is uniformly favourable (Aster, 1990), recognition of gestational thrombocytopenia is important in order to avoid unnecessary intervention. Diagnosis depends on the above features and exclusion, as far as possible, of other causes, as described below. It may be impossible to distinguish between gestational thrombocytopenia and immune thrombocytopenia (ITP), but clearly, where the platelet count is known to have been subnormal before pregnancy or during the first trimester, benign gestational thrombocytopenia is unlikely to be the cause.

6 Autoimmune thrombocytopenia

Autoimmune thrombocytopenia is less common than benign gestational thrombocytopenia. There is no reliable confirmatory laboratory test. Management decisions should be made in the light of the following observations.

1   Available treatments to raise the platelet count in the mother all carry some risk of significant side-effects.

2   Haemorrhage due to thrombocytopenia in the mother is unlikely if the platelet count is >50×10^9/l at the time of delivery.

3   The incidence of severe (platelets <50×10^9/l) fetal thrombocytopenia in presumed maternal ITP is low ($\leq$10%: Burrows & Kelton, 1993), although it may be higher in women known to have had ITP before the pregnancy (13–30%: Samuels *et al.*, 1990) and in those with symptomatic ITP during the index pregnancy.

4   The nadir of the platelet count in the affected fetus occurs 2–5 days after delivery, when the splenic circulation becomes established.

5   The risk of spontaneous fetal haemorrhage *in utero* and during normal vaginal delivery is low (Burrows & Kelton, 1990b; Samuels *et al.*, 1990).

6.1 Management

Close liaison should be maintained between obstetrician, haematologist and paediatrician. A thorough clinical assessment and examination of the blood film and measurements of KCCT, prothrombin time, fibrinogen concentration and that of fibrin/fibrinogen split products are mandatory. Particular attention should be paid to the exclusion of features that could favour an alternative diagnosis, including those listed in Section 2 – for example, the presence of splenomegaly, features of pre-eclampsia, poor nutrition, anaemia, schistocytes and/or white-cell abnormalities on the blood film and blood coagulation test results inappropriate for the gestational status. If there is no suspicious clinical feature and the blood count and film reveal thrombocytopenia only, bone-marrow examination is unnecessary. Laboratory testing for platelet autoantibodies remains unsatisfactory, despite the introduction of improved serology techniques (Kiefel *et al.*, 1992), and they are not of proved predictive value in pregnancy (Aster, 1990; Burrows & Kelton, 1990b; Bussel *et al.*, 1991). If a likely diagnosis of ITP is made, consideration should be given to the presence of associated autoimmune disease, especially systemic lupus erythematosus (SLE) and the antiphospholipid syndrome, because these diagnoses may carry prognostic and therapeutic implications.

If the maternal platelet count is $>50 \times 10^9/l$, fortnightly monitoring of clinical status and full blood count is the only requirement. Vaginal delivery should be allowed and decisions regarding operative delivery based on obstetric considerations only. Epidural/spinal anaesthesia is best avoided if the platelet count is $<80 \times 10^9/l$, because there is a theoretical risk of haematoma formation and neurological complications. There is no evidence that the skin bleeding time predicts haemorrhage in this situation and the test is not indicated.

If the maternal platelet count is $<50 \times 10^9/l$, there may be an increased risk of bleeding at delivery and it is therefore recommended that treatment is given to raise the platelet count to $>50 \times 10^9/l$ for delivery. If Caesarean section is contemplated, raising the platelet count to $>80 \times 10^9/l$ may allow all forms of anaesthesia to be considered. Treatment is also required earlier in pregnancy in a woman with symptomatic thrombocytopenia, usually present only when the count falls below $20 \times 10^9/l$. The primary treatment options are corticosteroids and high-dose intravenous human immunoglobulin G (IgG). If the duration of therapy is likely to be brief, corticosteroid treatment is an effective option (Carloss *et al.*, 1980). Fetal side-effects are unlikely, because approximately 90% of a dose of prednisolone is metabolized in the placenta (Smith & Torday, 1982), and concerns regarding suppression of the fetal adrenal glands are therefore unwarranted. Maternal side-effects are a potential problem, including hypertension, hyperglycaemia, osteoporosis, weight gain, acne and psychosis. Treatment should therefore be carefully monitored. A starting dose of oral prednisolone of 1 mg/kg/day, based on the pregestational weight, is appropriate, and the lowest maintenance dose at which the platelet count remains at $\geq 50 \times 10^9/l$ should be selected.

If the duration of therapy is likely to be prolonged or if an unacceptably high maintenance dose is required (perhaps >10 mg daily of prednisolone), intravenous immunoglobulin therapy is the preferred option. A dose of 0.4 g/kg/day for 5 days, by intravenous infusion, results in a clinically important effect in around 80% of subjects. In some cases, 3 days of treatment are sufficient. The duration of response is variable but is often 2–3 weeks or more, and the treatment can be safely and effectively repeated. An alternative regimen, which may be more convenient for the recipient and requires a smaller total dose, is the administration of 1 g/kg over 8 h, repeated 2 days later if there is no or an inadequate response (Burrows & Kelton, 1992). Side-effects are uncommon; an anaphylactic response in subjects congenitally deficient in IgA may preclude further treatment and, because of this risk, the initial dosage should be administered cautiously and under close supervision. It is noteworthy that hepatitis C has recently been transmitted through use of intravenous immunoglobulin preparations (Yap *et al.*, 1994). It is therefore recommended that preparations with a validated viral inactivation procedure should be used. The aim of treatment should be to alleviate haemorrhagic symptoms and ensure a platelet count of $>50 \times 10^9/l$ for delivery. Whether intravenous immunoglobulin can have a beneficial effect on the fetal platelet count remains open to doubt (Nicolini *et al.*, 1990).

The management of cases in which there is significant haemorrhage, due to ITP resistant to corticosteroid and intravenous immunoglobulin therapy, is problematic. One recommendation has been the use of 1 g of intravenous methylprednisolone, combined with intravenous immunoglobulin, 1 g/kg, possibly repeated after 3 weeks, if necessary. Other therapeutic options used in the non-pregnant subject, such as danazol and vinca alkaloids, cannot be recommended in pregnancy. Immunosuppresion with azathioprine has been safely achieved in transplant patients during pregnancy and is a therapeutic option in intractable ITP. Splenectomy should only be considered as a last resort in intractable and symptomatic ITP, although it is feasible (Martin *et al.*, 1984). It is best performed before the third trimester. Platelet concentrate should be available to control surgical haemorrhage but should be withheld until after the splenic vascular pedicle has been clamped and only administered if surgical bleeding is excessive. Clearly, close liaison between surgeon, obstetrician, paediatrician and haematologist is essential.

6.2 Management of the fetus and neonate

Historically, recommendations have included attempts to predict the fetal platelet count from clinical and haematological parameters, cordocentesis to determine the fetal platelet count *in utero* (Scioscia *et al.*, 1988), scalp-blood sampling to determine the fetal platelet count in early labour (Ayromlooi, 1978; Scott *et al.*, 1980) and delivery in every case by Caesarean section (Murray & Harris, 1976) to minimize the risk of fetal head trauma. Accurate prediction of the fetal platelet count, based on maternal count, antibody tests or maternal splenectomy status, is not possible; cordocentesis carries a risk of around 1% of fetal demise or the need for urgent delivery (Scioscia *et al.*, 1988) and fetal-scalp sampling is technically difficult, may result in haemorrhage in the thrombocytopenic infant and often yields false-positive results, due to clotting in the sample (Burrows & Kelton, 1992). Because of these considerations, as well as the low risk of important fetal thrombocytopenia and associated haemorrhage, Caesarean section is now recommended only when obstetric considerations dictate this mode of delivery (Bussel *et al.*, 1991).

A cord-blood sample should be obtained for measurement of the fetal platelet count in all instances. If thrombocytopenia is detected, close clinical and haematological observation is indicated, as the count is likely to fall further for 2–5 days. If the count falls to $<20 \times 10^9/l$ or if clinical haemorrhage is apparent, intravenous IgG (IVIgG), 1 g/kg, usually produces a rapid response in the platelet count. Intravenous hydrocortisone therapy is an alternative approach, but steroids are generally best avoided in the neonate, due to concerns regarding sepsis. Platelet transfusion (cytomegalovirus (CMV)-negative) should be reserved for life-threatening haemorrhage and combined with steroid and immunoglobulin therapy.

7 Thrombocytopenia in pre-eclampsia

The maternal platelet count is frequently reduced in pre-eclampsia, occasionally falling to $<50 \times 10^9/l$, although haemorrhagic manifestations are uncommon (Romero *et al.*, 1989). The fall in platelet count occurs early in the disorder (Redman *et al.*, 1978) and may precede any evidence of coagulation activation from clotting times, fibrinogen assay and tests for fibrin/fibrinogen split products. The thrombocytopenia may, occasionally, only develop in the early post-partum phase. It is important to recognize that severe thrombocytopenia may result from platelet consumption in pre-eclampsia without abnormal coagulation, because misdiagnosis, for example as ITP, could lead to deferment of the decision to deliver the fetus (Thiagarajah *et al.*, 1984). In some instances, evidence for DIC is clearly detectable, especially if, in interpretation of test results, it is acknowledged that the clotting times are normally short and fibrinogen concentration elevated in mid and late healthy pregnancy. The HELLP syndrome is part of this spectrum of platelet consumption and coagulation activation in pregnancy, in which Haemolysis, liver dysfunction with Elevated Liver enzymes in serum and Low Platelet count predominate.

The thrombocytopenia is unlikely to resolve before delivery and should be regarded as a marker of ongoing platelet consumption. Rapid progression of the coagulation activation, which may be life-threatening, is possible, and the situation must be closely monitored by the haematologist, in close liaison with the obstetrician and paediatrician. Careful monitoring of full blood count and coagulation tests is indicated. These should be interpreted alongside a careful clinical assessment, in order to make rational decisions regarding early delivery.

8 Thrombocytopenia due to disseminated intravascular coagulation

The pregnancy-related triggers for development of DIC are well recognized and include pre-eclamptic toxaemia, placental abruption, amniotic-fluid embolism and retention of dead fetus. The DIC may be chronic and subclinical in the last instance. The management is along the lines used in DIC from other causes and depends on the particular trigger and manifestation. Delivery of the fetus is indicated. It may be safe to delay this in pre-eclampsia, for reasons of fetal immaturity, but only if the pre-eclampsia can be vigorously managed, the coagulopathy is mild and the situation is monitored carefully, including performance of daily full blood count and clotting times and fibrinogen assay. Again, it must be acknowledged that any prolongation of clotting times or reduction of fibrinogen concentration below 2 g/l due to DIC in the third trimester of pregnancy represents a highly significant degree of coagulation activation.

Blood components should be administered on clinical grounds. In the face of haemorrhage and a fibrinogen concentration of <1 g/l, use of cryoprecipitate may be considered. Fresh-frozen plasma is indicated for treatment of bleeding if the clotting times are prolonged (BCSH Guidelines, 1992a). Platelet transfusions can be considered in the bleeding patient with platelets $<80 \times 10^9/l$ (BCSH Guidelines, 1992b). In many instances, blood-transfusion support is not required. The coagulation disturbance usually resolves within 24–48 h after delivery, although thrombocytopenia may persist for up to 7 days.

Use of heparin and other anticoagulants is generally contraindicated in DIC. Exceptions may be DIC due to amniotic-fluid embolism and where the major manifestations are secondary to tissue ischaemia, including digital ischaemia and major-organ (cerebral, renal) dysfunction without haemorrhage, when carefully monitored heparin therapy may be considered.

9 Thrombocytopenia in thrombotic thrombocytopenic purpura and haemolytic uraemic syndrome

The life-threatening disorders TTP and HUS very occasionally complicate pregnancy and the post-partum period (Weiner, 1987). The central feature is microangiopathic haemolysis, with platelet consumption and thrombocytopenia. Schistocytes are prominent in the blood film. In HUS, the kidney is the organ that is predominantly affected and renal impairment may be severe. In TTP, a more widespread systemic involvement is typical, particularly including neurological dysfunction, with manifestations ranging from headache through fluctuating disturbance of consciousness and sensorimotor dysfunction to fits and coma. The pentad of fever, microangiopathic haemolysis, renal impairment, thrombocytopenia and neurological features is highly suggestive of TTP. In HUS and TTP, evidence of DIC is absent; clotting times are normal and the fibrinogen concentration is in the normal pregnancy range. A modest increase in the concentration of fibrin/fibrinogen split products may be detected, especially in pregnancy. It is probable that HUS and TTP represent part of a clinical spectrum of disease for which the pathogenesis is unclear, but the thrombocytopenia and red-cell fragmentation must relate to a diffuse vascular endothelial insult; unusual large forms of von Willebrand factor multimers have been detected and a calcium-dependent cysteine protease in plasma has been implicated in the pathogenesis (Moake *et al.*, 1982; Moore *et al.*, 1990).

It is essential to differentiate HUS and TTP in pregnancy from DIC or thrombocytopenia due to pre-eclampsia, because the latter are likely to be strong indications for prompt delivery. There is no evidence that delivery affects the course of TTP and HUS, although, when present in late pregnancy, the option of early delivery may allow vigorous treatment of the mother without harm to the fetus.

Treatment by plasma exchange is largely empirical, although the concept of increased plasma levels of a pathogenic enzyme and abnormal von Willebrand factor multimers, with increased platelet reactivity, gives some support to this approach. Clinical studies in non-pregnant subjects with TTP suggest high-intensity plasma exchange, with replacement of 3 l or more daily, is more effective than plasma infusion (Rock *et al.*, 1991). This treatment should be combined with supportive therapy for the renal, cerebral and other manifestations. Corticosteroids are usually given, although there is no evidence for efficacy.

10 Neonatal alloimmune thrombocytopenia

Alloimmune thrombocytopenia, due to fetomaternal incompatibility for platelet antigens, is a serious fetal disorder with no maternal consequences, in contrast to ITP, which is a maternal disorder with rare fetal consequences. Most cases are diagnosed after birth, affecting around 1 in 2000 live births and responsible for about 10% of all instances of neonatal thrombocytopenia with platelets $<100 \times 10^9/l$ (Blanchette *et al.*, 1990). However, the condition develops *in utero* and the fetus may be severely affected.

In Caucasian women, the most frequently implicated antibody is anti-human platelet antigen (HPA)-1a (Pl^{A1}), accounting for 80–90% of cases. Anti-HPA-5b(Br^a) is responsible for a further 5–15%, other antibodies rarely being important. Less than 10% of HPA-1a-negative women who are exposed to HPA-1a become immunized, because the maternal immune response is, in part, determined by genes located in the major histocompatibility complex. Women with human leucocyte antigen (HLA)-B8, HLA-DR3 and HLA-DR52a antigens who are HPA-1a-negative are at increased risk of alloimmunization.

In contrast to haemolytic disease of the newborn, the first-born is affected in 40–60% of cases. This is usually unexpected, because as yet there is no routine antenatal screening for the condition. Importantly, subsequent pregnancies are affected in 75–90% of cases, with similar or increasing severity. There is a broad spectrum of clinical presentation (Kaplan *et al.*, 1992). The unexpected first case may be symptomless, with thrombocytopenia discovered incidentally. More commonly, a purpuric rash may alert the paediatrician to the presence of thrombocytopenia and investigations reveal intracranial haemorrhage (ICH), porencephaly or evidence of old haemorrhage (DeVries *et al.*, 1988). In the most severe cases, there may be marked neurological impairment, including motor dysfunction, blindness and mental retardation. Developmental abnormalities have been reported in up to 25% of cases (Pillai, 1993). Intrauterine death due to massive ICH has been described during labour, but spontaneous ICH *in utero* may occur in about 10% of cases, most commonly between 30 and 35 weeks, but occasionally before 20 weeks (Waters, 1991). Where anti-HPA-5b is responsible, the clinical picture is similar but less severe, although ICH may occur (Mueller-Eckhardt *et al.*, 1989).

Diagnosis requires laboratory confirmation. This depends on the demonstration of a maternal platelet alloantibody against the father's platelets, which are a convenient source of the relevant antigen. It is important to differentiate reactions due to HLA antibodies and to exclude a maternal platelet autoantibody. The allospecificity of the platelet antibody and the platelet antigen phenotype of both parents should be determined, and the help of a reference laboratory should be sought.

A maternal platelet alloantibody may not be detectable in up to 20% of cases (Kaplan *et al.*, 1991). Nevertheless, it will often be possible to demonstrate incompatibility between mother and father for the HPA-1a antigen. Failure to demonstrate the causative antibody may be due to an inappropriate assay procedure. It is therefore essential to combine a sensitive binding assay, such as the platelet immunofluorescence test, with an antigen capture method, e.g. monoclonal antibody immobilization of platelet antigens (MAIPA), to detect weak antibodies or antibodies that react with relatively few antigen sites, such as anti-HPA-5b. This is especially important if multispecific HLA antibodies are also present.

Any difficulties in confirming the diagnosis should not delay therapy, especially when there is a risk of life-threatening haemorrhage and there are sufficient grounds for a provisional diagnosis.

10.1 Neonatal management

As there is no routine antenatal screening, the first affected baby is usually diagnosed after birth. The platelet count may continue to fall during the first 48 h after birth and should be monitored daily. Significant thrombocytopenia warrants an ultrasound scan for possible ICH.

If there is a risk of bleeding, a compatible platelet transfusion should be given. Compatible donor platelets or washed (irradiated) maternal platelets can be used. More than one transfusion of compatible platelets may be needed before the platelet count reaches a satisfactory level. If platelets are not available, high-dose IVIgG (1 g/kg/day for 1–3 days) may be used; in one study, it was effective in 75% of cases, although the effect on the platelet count was delayed for 24–48 h (Mueller-Eckhardt *et al.*, 1989).

10.2 Antenatal management

For subsequent pregnancies, antenatal management can be planned in advance. The family at risk should be referred, ideally before embarking on a further pregnancy, to a specialist centre, where informed counselling can be given about the risk of haemorrhage in subsequent pregnancies and the benefits and risks of various diagnostic and management strategies. Part of the assessment of risk involves determining whether the father is homozygous or heterozygous for the relevant platelet antigen.

The introduction of ultrasound-guided cordocentesis for fetal blood sampling (FBS) has made it possible to diagnose alloimmune thrombocytopenia *in utero* and to assess its severity by directly measuring the fetal platelet count. In addition, cordocentesis can be used to transfuse compatible platelets to the fetus to reduce the risk of thrombocytopenic bleeding, but the short survival of transfused platelets (about 1 week) presents a special problem in maintenance of the platelet count for a prolonged period. The first FBS in an at-risk pregnancy is planned for between 20 and 24 weeks, depending on the history and time of presentation of the previously affected infant. The procedure is covered by transfusion of compatible platelets (see above), as the degree of thrombocytopenia, if present, cannot be predicted.

Management of the pregnancy at risk has concentrated on attempts to protect the fetus from thrombocytopenic bleeding, in particular serious ICH. Maternal administration of IVIgG and/or steroids may be effective in some mildly affected cases, but serial fetal platelet transfusions are the preferred therapy for severely affected cases (Kaplan *et al.*, 1991; Lynch *et al.*, 1992; Murphy *et al.*, 1994).

There is no generally agreed approach to antenatal management and at present a successful outcome cannot be guaranteed.

Antenatal screening for the most common form of alloimmune neonatal thrombocytopenia, due to anti-HPA-1a, is under consideration, but there is no established method at present (Reesink & Engelfriet, 1993; Flug *et al.*, 1994).

11 Acknowledgements

Dr M.F. Murphy and Professor A.H. Waters have made an invaluable contribution to the section on alloimmune neonatal thrombocytopenia.

References

Aster R.H. (1990) 'Gestational' thrombocytopenia: a plea for conservative management. *New England Journal of Medicine* **323**, 264–266.

Ayromlooi J. (1978) A new approach to the management of immunologic thrombocytopenic purpura in pregnancy. *American Journal of Obstetrics and Gynecology* **130**, 235–236.

BCSH Guidelines (1992a) The use of fresh-frozen plasma. *Transfusion Medicine* **2**, 57–63.

BCSH Guidelines (1992b) Platelet transfusions. *Transfusion Medicine* **2**, 311–318.

Blanchette V.S., Chen L., Salomon de Friedberg Z., Hogan V.A., Trudel E. & Decary F. (1990) Alloimmunization to the Pl^A1^ platelet antigen: results of a prospective study. *British Journal of Haematology* **74**, 209–215.

Burrows R.F. & Kelton J.G. (1988) Incidentally detected thrombocytopenia in healthy mothers and their infants. *New England Journal of Medicine* **319**, 142–145.

Burrows R.F. & Kelton J.G. (1990a) Thrombocytopenia at delivery: a prospective survey of 6715 deliveries. *American Journal of Obstetrics and Gynecology* **162**, 731–734.

Burrows R.F. & Kelton J.G. (1990b) Low fetal risks in pregnancies associated with idiopathic thrombocytopenic purpura. *American Journal of Obstetrics and Gynecology* **163**, 1147–1150.

Burrows R.F. & Kelton J.G. (1992) Thrombocytopenia in pregnancy. In Greer I.A., Turpie A.G.G. & Forbes C.D. (eds) *Haemostasis and Thrombosis in Obstetrics and Gynaecology*, pp. 407–429. Chapman and Hall, London.

Burrows R.F. & Kelton J.G. (1993) Fetal thrombocytopenia and its relation to maternal thrombocytopenia. *New England Journal of Medicine* **329**, 1463–1466.

Bussel J., Kaplan C., McFarland J. and the Working Party on Neonatal Immune Thrombocytopenia of the Neonatal Hemostasis Subcommittee of the Scientific and Standardization Committee of the ISTH (1991) Recommendations for the evaluation and treatment of neonatal autoimmune and alloimmune thrombocytopenia. *Thrombosis and Haemostasis* **65**, 631–634.

Carloss H.W., McMillan R. & Crosby W.H. (1980) Management of pregnancy in women with immune thrombocytopenic purpura. *Journal of the American Medical Association* **244**, 2756–2758.

DeVries L.S., Connell J., Bydder G.M. *et al.* (1988) Recurrent intracranial haemorrhages *in utero* in an infant with alloimmune thrombocytopenia: case report. *British Journal of Obstetrics and Gynaecology* **95**, 299–302.

Flug F., Karpatkin M. & Karpatkin S. (1994) Should all pregnant women be tested for their platelet PLA (Zw, HPA-1) phenotype? *British Journal of Haematology* **86**, 1–5.

Kaplan C., Daffos F., Forrestier F., Morel M.-C., Chesnel N. & Tchernia G. (1991) In Kaplan-Gouet C., Schlegel N., Salmon C. & McGregor J. (eds) *Platelet Immunology: Fundamental and Clinical Aspects*, pp. 267–268. John Libbey, Paris.

Kaplan C., Morelkopp M.C., Clemenceau S., Daffos F., Forestier F. & Tchernia G. (1992) Fetal and neonatal alloimmune thrombocytopenia: current trends in diagnosis and therapy. *Transfusion Medicine* **2**, 265–271.

Kiefel V., Santoro S. & Mueller-Eckhardt C. (1992) Serological, biochemical and molecular aspects of platelet autoantigens. *Seminars in Hematology* **29**, 26–33.

Lynch L., Bussel J.B., McFarland J.G., Chitkara U. & Berkowitz R.L. (1992) Antenatal treatment of alloimmune thrombocytopenia. *Obstetrics and Gynecology* **80**, 67–71.

Martin J.N., Morrison J.C. & Files J.C. (1984) Autoimmune thrombocytopenic purpura: current concepts and recommended practices. *American Journal of Obstetrics and Gynecology* **150**, 86–96.

Moake J.L., Rudy L.K., Troll J.H. *et al.* (1982) Unusually large plasma factor VIII : vWF multimers in chronic relapsing TTP. *New England Journal of Medicine* **307**, 1432–1435.

Moore J.C., Murphy W.G. & Kelton J.G. (1990) Calpain proteolysis of vWF enhances its binding to platelet membrane glycoprotein IIb/IIIa: an explanation for platelet aggregation in TTP. *British Journal of Haematology* **74**, 457–464.

Mueller-Eckhardt C., Kiefel V., Grubert A. *et al.* (1989) 348 cases of suspected neonatal alloimmune thrombocytopenia. *Lancet* **i**, 363–366.

Murphy M.F., Waters A.H., Doughty H.A. *et al.* (1994) Antenatal management of fetomaternal alloimmune thrombocytopenia: report of 15 affected pregnancies. *Transfusion Medicine* **4**, 281–292.

Murray J.M. & Harris R.E. (1976) The management of the pregnant patient with idiopathic thrombocytopenic purpura. *American Journal of Obstetrics and Gynecology* **12**, 449–451.

Nicolini U., Tannirandorn Y., Gonzalez P. *et al.* (1990) Continuing controversy in alloimmune thrombocytopenia: fetal hyperimmunoglobulinemia fails to prevent thrombocytopenia. *American Journal of Obstetrics and Gynecology* **163**, 1144–1146.

Pillai M. (1993) Platelets and pregnancy. *British Medical Journal* **100**, 201–204.

Redman C.W.G., Bonnar J. & Bellin C. (1978) Early platelet consumption in pre-eclampsia. *British Medical Journal* **i**, 467–469.

Reesink W. & Engelfriet C.P. (1993) Prenatal management of fetal alloimmune thrombocytopenia. *Vox Sanguinis* **65**, 180–197.

Rock G.A., Shumack K.H., Buskard N.A. *et al.* (1991) Canadian Apheresis Study Group. Comparison of plasma exchange with plasma infusion in the treatment of thrombotic thrombocytopenic purpura. *New England Journal of Medicine* **325**, 393–397.

Romero R., Mazor M. & Lockwood C.J. (1989) Clinical significance, prevalence and natural history of thrombocytopenia in pregnancy-induced hypertension. *American Journal of Perinatology* **6**, 32–38.

Samuels P., Bussel J.B., Braitman L.E. *et al.* (1990) Estimation of the risk of thrombocytopenia in the offspring of pregnant women with presumed immune thrombocytopenic purpura. *New England Journal of Medicine* **323**, 229–235.

Scioscia A.L., Grannum P.A.T., Copel J.A. & Hobbins J.C. (1988) The use of percutaneous umbilical blood sampling in immune thrombocytopenic purpura. *American Journal of Obstetrics and Gynecology* **159**, 1066–1068.

Scott J.R., Cruikshank D.P. & Kochenour N.K. (1980) Fetal platelet counts in the obstetric management of immunologic thrombocytopenic purpura. *American Journal of Obstetrics and Gynecology* **136**, 495–499.

Sill P.R., Lind T. & Walker W. (1985) Platelet values during normal pregnancy. *British Journal of Obstetrics and Gynaecology* **92**, 480–483.

Smith B.T. & Torday J.S. (1982) Steroid administration in pregnant women with autoimmune thrombocytopenia. *New England Journal of Medicine* **306**, 744–745.

Thiagarajah S., Bourgeois F.J., Harbert G.M. & Caudle M.R. (1984) Thrombocytopenia in pre-eclampsia: associated abnormalities and management principles. *American Journal of Obstetrics and Gynecology* **150**, 1–6.

Waters A. (1991) In Nance S.J. (ed.) *Clinical and Basic Science Aspects of Immunohaematology*, pp. 155–177. American Association of Blood Banks.

Weiner C.P. (1987) Thrombotic microangiopathy in pregnancy and the postpartum period. *Seminars in Hematology* **2**, 119–129.

Yap P.L., McOmish F., Webster O.D.B. *et al.* (1994) Hepatitis C virus transmission by intravenous immunoglobulin. *Journal of Hepatology* **21**, 455–460.

9 Guidelines on Oral Anticoagulation
Prepared by the Haemostasis and Thrombosis Task Force

1 Introduction

The revision of the 1990 oral anticoagulant guidelines by the British Committee for Standards in Haematology (BCSH) (British Committee for Standards in Haematology, 1990) has been undertaken to reflect changes in the current medical literature and to incorporate the outcomes of medical audit. Guidelines on heparin were published by the BCSH in 1993 (British Committee for Standards in Haematology, 1993a). These present guidelines include indications for oral anticoagulation and suggested arrangements for the management of an anticoagulant service.

These new guidelines aim to take account of the current practical difficulties involved in the safe monitoring of the rapidly expanding numbers of patients on long-term anticoagulant therapy. With patient numbers more than doubling in most anticoagulant clinics in the past 5 years and the trend set to continue, the organizational problems are immense (Baglin, 1994; Rose, 1996). However, it remains the haematologist's responsibility to ensure that local arrangements for laboratory testing and dosage of oral anticoagulant therapy are satisfactory. This involves regular participation in national/regional quality assessment schemes and audit of clinical practice.

The third edition of these guidelines has been prepared by the Haemostasis and Thrombosis Task Force of the British Society for Haematology. The document has been circulated to members of the BCSH. Relevant scientific papers from systematic literature review were identified from Medline for 1965 to July 1996, using the index terms oral anticoagulation or warfarin and venous thromboembolism, deep vein thrombosis, pulmonary embolus, stroke, heart valve(s), prosthesis, atrial fibrillation, peripheral vascular disease, grafts, coronary artery, myocardial infarction, coronary artery graft, angioplasty and stents, central venous catheters and chemotherapy. Further publications were obtained from the references cited and reviews known to members of the task force. Evidence and graded recommendations are according to the US Agency for Health Care Policy and Research (US Department of Health and Human Services, 1992; see Appendix 9.1).

Reprinted with permission from *British Journal of Haematology*, 1998, **101**, 374–387.

2 Target international normalized ratio

The international normalized ratio (INR) is a recommended method for reporting prothrombin time (PT) results for control of oral anticoagulation (British Committee for Standards in Haematology, 1990). Since adoption of the INR system, it has been usual practice to adjust the dose of warfarin, or other oral vitamin K antagonist, to maintain the INR within a therapeutic range. The range was often one INR unit, e.g. INR between 2.0 and 3.0. However, in practice many clinicians and computer support systems regulate dosage according to deviation of INR from a single target, taken as the mid-point of the designated range, e.g. target INR of 2.5 for a range of 2.0–3.0. Furthermore, extensive audit indicates that only 50% of INRs in a population of patients taking warfarin are usually within the range at any one time, i.e. 0.5 INR units of the target (Rose, 1996), whereas 80% of patients are within 0.75 INR units of the target. With this experience, it now seems more practical to designate a target INR and encourage dose adjustment dependent on deviation of INR from the target and also individual patient characteristics, such as reason for anticoagulation, stability of INRs over time, previous bleeding and thrombotic events.

In view of this, we have elected to recommend target INRs throughout these guidelines. We recommend that appropriate dose adjustment is made dependent on deviation of INR from the target. An INR within 0.5 INR units of the target is generally satisfactory and deviations of 0.5 and 0.75 INR units can be used as standards for audit (see also Section 11).

3 Indications for anticoagulation

The indications for oral anticoagulation and recommended target INRs are summarized in Table 9.1 for ease of access. The evidence basis for these recommendations is summarized within the chapter.

3.1 Venous thromboembolism in non-pregnant patients

First event of pulmonary embolus or proximal-vein thrombosis: INR 2.5 for 6 months (grade A, level Ib). Calf-vein thrombosis in non-surgical patients with no persistent risk factors: INR 2.5 for 3 months (grade A, level Ib). Postoperative calf-vein thrombosis without persistent risk factors: INR 2.5 for 6 weeks (grade A, level Ib). Continued treatment should be considered if risk factors are persistent (grade B, level IIb). A recurrence after stopping warfarin requires a further episode of treatment, INR 2.5. A recurrence on treatment requires intensification of treatment, INR 3.5 (grade C, level IV), or alternative anticoagulant treatment.

Initial anticoagulation with heparin and a period of at least 6 weeks' oral anticoagulant therapy is necessary dependent on the extent of thrombus, on whether the thrombotic event was triggered by a precipitating event, such as surgery, and on the existence of risk factors for recurrence (Hull *et al.*, 1979; Francis, 1994; Weinmann & Salzman, 1994).

Table 9.1 Indications for oral anticoagulation, target INR and grade of recommendation

Indication	Target INR	Grade of recommendation
Pulmonary embolus	2.5	A
Proximal deep-vein thrombosis	2.5	A
Calf-vein thrombus	2.5	A
Recurrence of venous thromboembolism when no longer on warfarin therapy	2.5	A
Recurrence of venous thromboembolism while on warfarin therapy	3.5	C
Symptomatic inherited thrombophilia	2.5	C
Antiphospholipid syndrome	3.5	B
Non-rheumatic atrial fibrillation	2.5	A
Atrial fibrillation due to rheumatic heart disease, congenital heart disease, thyrotoxicosis	2.5	C
Cardioversion	2.5	B
Mural thrombus	2.5	B
Cardiomyopathy	2.5	C
Mechanical prosthetic heart valve	3.5	B
Bioprosthetic valve	Not indicated	A (see text)
Ischaemic stroke without atrial fibrillation	Not indicated	A (see text)
Retinal-vessel occlusion	Not indicated	C (see text)
Peripheral arterial thrombosis and grafts	Not indicated	A (see text)
Coronary-artery thrombosis	Not indicated	A (see text)
Coronary-artery graft thrombosis	Not indicated	A (see text)
Coronary angioplasty and stents	Not indicated	A (see text)

Pulmonary embolus is strongly associated with proximal deep-vein thrombosis (DVT) of the lower limb (Sandler & Martin, 1989), but occurs infrequently when thrombosis remains confined to the calf (Hirsh, 1990; Ginsberg, 1996). There has been no randomized study to determine the optimum intensity or duration of oral anticoagulant therapy after an episode of pulmonary embolism. Recommendations are therefore derived from the results of treatment of proximal-vein thrombosis in the lower limb, where pulmonary embolism is typically regarded as an end-point in interventional studies. Fatal recurrence of pulmonary embolism is extremely rare when DVT is treated with heparin initially, followed by a prolonged period of treatment with warfarin (Coon *et al.*, 1969; Hull *et al.*, 1979; Carson *et al.*, 1992; Schulman *et al.*, 1995). An INR of 2.0–3.0 gives the lowest recurrence and bleeding rates (Hull *et al.*, 1982) and is the recommended range for venous thromboembolism.

Retrospective studies gave conflicting results as to the optimal duration of oral anticoagulant therapy, ranging from 6 weeks (Petiti *et al.*, 1986) to 6 months (Coon *et al.*, 1969). A series of small studies showed no difference in recurrence rates for patients treated for 4 weeks (Holmgren *et al.*, 1985) or 6 weeks (O'Sullivan, 1972), compared with 6 months' therapy, but not all patients had an objectively confirmed diagnosis. In addition, these studies either combined or did not distinguish between patients with proximal thrombosis and those with thrombus confined to the calf. A review of duration of therapy in 1988 recommended at least 6 weeks' therapy and indicated the need for prospective randomized studies. This review did not indicate the methods used for evaluating studies, but stated that the confidence intervals (CIs) for recurrence rates after only 6 weeks' therapy were wide (Fennerty *et al.*, 1988). Since then, two prospective studies have randomized patients with proximal-vein thrombosis to different durations of anticoagulation, one comparing 4 weeks with 3 months (Levine *et al.*, 1995) and the other comparing 6 weeks with 6 months (Schulman *et al.*, 1995). In the 4-week/3-month study, recurrence rates were 8.6% in the 4-week group compared with 0.9% in the 3-month group (OR = 10.1, 95% CI 1.3–81.4) (Levine *et al.*, 1995). In the 6-week/6-month study, recurrence rates after 2 years were 18.1% after 6 weeks' treatment and 9.5% after 6 months' treatment (OR = 2.1, 95% CI 1.4–3.1). In the 6-week group, there was a sharp increase in the recurrence rate immediately after cessation of oral anticoagulant therapy (Schulman *et al.*, 1995). Further clarification of the optimal duration of therapy will be obtained from the Durée optimale du traitement antivitamine K (DOTAVK) study, in which patients with proximal DVT are randomized to 3 or 6 months' therapy. Therefore, the present recommendation for duration of treatment of proximal DVT or symptomatic pulmonary embolism is 6 months (grade A recommendation, level Ib evidence). There is an opinion, based on subgroup analysis, that a period of 6 weeks' therapy is adequate for proximal-vein thrombosis in patients without permanent risk factors (grade C, level IV) (Hirsh, 1995; Ginsberg, 1996).

Thrombi below the level of the popliteal vein are not usually detected by compression ultrasound examination. Although these calf-vein thrombi do not typically cause symptomatic pulmonary emboli, they may extend into the popliteal and femoral veins and then cause significant emboli (Hirsh, 1990). Calf-vein thrombi detected by contrast venography should be either treated with anticoagulant therapy or monitored with serial non-invasive tests, such as compression ultrasound examination (Cogo *et al.*, 1998), and treated as for a proximal thrombus if extension occurs. Untreated symptomatic calf-vein thrombosis in non-surgical patients is associated with a recurrence rate of >25% and the risk of proximal extension and pulmonary embolization (Lagerstedt *et al.*, 1985; Lohr *et al.*, 1991; Raskob, 1996). Treatment with warfarin to maintain an INR of 2.0–3.0 for 3 months reduces these risks to 7.6% or less (Lagerstedt *et al.*, 1985; Research Committee of the British Thoracic Society, 1992). This rate is lower than that achieved with 4 weeks' (12.4%) (Research Committee of the British Thoracic Society, 1992) or 6 weeks' anticoagulation (11.8%) (Schulman *et al.*, 1995) and comparable to that achieved with 6 months' treatment (5.8%) (Schulman *et al.*, 1995). Therefore, the best general recommendation at the present time is that symptomatic calf-vein thrombosis in non-surgical patients without predisposing factors, such as cancer or thrombophilia, should be treated for 3 months (grade A, level Ib).

Postoperative calf-vein thrombosis is also associated with proximal extension and pulmonary embolus (Kakkar *et al.*, 1969; Pellegrini *et al.*, 1993). However, a shorter period of anticoagulation appears to be sufficient to prevent recurrence after the initial precipitating event. In the British Thoracic Society Research Committee (BTSRC) study, recurrence rates in surgical patients were low in patients assigned to 4 weeks' (1.7%) as well as 3 months' treatment (1.8%) (Research Committee of the British Thoracic Society, 1992).

However, 26% of patients randomized to 4 weeks' treatment actually received 6 weeks' therapy, so it is prudent to recommend 6 weeks' therapy until the results of further randomized studies are available (grade A, level Ib).

Continued treatment should be considered for patients with persistent risk factors for recurrence, e.g. cancer, thrombophilia (grade B, level IIb) (Research Committee of the British Thoracic Society, 1992; Hirsh, 1995; Levine *et al.*, 1995; Schulman *et al.*, 1995).

Patients with recurrent venous thromboembolism after stopping warfarin require further treatment with warfarin to maintain an INR of 2.5. The risk of further recurrence is high and the optimum duration of therapy is currently unknown (Schulman *et al.*, 1997). Patients who have a recurrence while anticoagulated with warfarin should be considered for higher-intensity therapy with warfarin, INR 3.5 (British Committee for Standards in Haematology, 1990) (grade C, level IV), or alternative anticoagulant therapy and evaluation for carcinoma or the antiphospholipid syndrome (Ginsberg, 1996).

3.2 Inherited thrombophilia

No episode of thromboembolism–antithrombotic prophylaxis for high-risk periods (grade C, level IV). After an episode of venous thromboembolism, evidence of thrombophilia lowers the threshold for long-term anticoagulant therapy: INR 2.5 (grade C, level IV).

For these guidelines, the term thrombophilia is used to refer to inherited disorders of the haemostatic system that result in an increased risk of venous thromboembolism (Cavenagh & Colvin, 1996; De Stefano *et al.*, 1996; Lane *et al.*, 1996), namely deficiencies of anti-thrombin, protein C and protein S and the factor V Leiden mutation (FV : R506Q). Acute thrombotic events should be treated with initial heparinization and oral anticoagulation to achieve an INR of 2.5 (Cavenagh & Colvin, 1996; De Stefano *et al.*, 1996; Lane *et al.*, 1996). It is not yet known if, after the initial treatment episode, this level of anticoagulation is required long-term or whether lower-intensity warfarin regimens or aspirin will give equivalent protection. Until this information is available, a target INR of 2.5 is recommended for those patients receiving anticoagulant therapy (grade C, level IV). Recommendations on the duration of therapy cannot be given, as this will vary with the genetic defect and according to whether more than one defect is present, whether previous events were precipitated and whether other family members with the defect are thrombosis-prone. Guidelines on the investigation and management of thrombophilia are currently being prepared by the Haemostasis and Thrombosis Task Force.

3.3 Antiphospholipid syndrome

Guidelines on the investigation and management of the antiphospholipid syndrome are currently being prepared by the Haemostasis and Thrombosis Task Force. It should be noted, however, that patients with arterial thrombosis associated with this syndrome should be treated immediately with heparin initially and then warfarin (grade C, level V) (Greaves & Preston, 1991). The target INR has not been clarified. A target of 2.5 has often been used, but a non-randomized comparative study supported a target of 3.5 (Khamashta *et al.*, 1995) (grade B, level III).

3.4 Atrial fibrillation

3.4.1 Non-rheumatic atrial fibrillation

INR 2.5 (grade A, level Ia).

In five randomized primary-prevention trials comparing oral anticoagulation with placebo or no treatment, anticoagulation prevented two-thirds of fatal or disabling strokes due to major thromboembolism (Peterson *et al.*, 1989; Boston Area Anticoagulation Trial for Atrial Fibrillation Investigators, 1990; Connolly *et al.*, 1991; Stroke Prevention in Atrial Fibrillation Investigators, 1991; Ezekowitz *et al.*, 1992; Atrial Fibrillation Investigators, 1994). In these studies, the target INR ranged from 1.5 to 4.5. Thromboembolic event rates were relatively higher with INRs <2.0 (European Atrial Fibrillation Trial Study Group, 1995). These studies indicate a beneficial effect of warfarin in carefully selected patients in whom anticoagulation is expertly controlled.

The atrial fibrillation investigators established a common database to identify subgroups of patients whose risk of stroke was so low that warfarin is not justified. They identified patients under 65 years of age without diabetes, a history of hypertension or a previous stroke or transient ischaemic attack (TIA) as low-risk. These patients had an annual event rate of 1.0%, which was not reduced by warfarin (European Atrial Fibrillation Trial Study Group, 1993; Hylek *et al.*, 1996). The Second Study of Stroke Prevention in Atrial Fibrillation (SPAF II) was the first primary-prevention study in which patients were randomized to either anticoagulation (target INR 2.0–4.5) or aspirin 325 mg/day, and, overall, aspirin was as effective as warfarin (Stroke Prevention in Atrial Fibrillation Investigators, 1994). However, the rate of intracranial haemorrhage in patients >75 on warfarin was higher than in previous studies and it is not clear if the results of SPAF II were due to patient characteristics or chance.

In SPAF III, patients at high risk of thromboembolism (congestive heart failure, left-ventricular dysfunction on echocardiography, previous thromboembolism, systolic hypertension at enrolment or being a woman over 75 years) had a lower primary-event rate with adjusted-dose warfarin (INR 2.0–3.0), compared with combined low-dose warfarin and aspirin (Stroke Prevention in Atrial Fibrillation Investigators, 1996).

Warfarin should be considered as first-line therapy in patients with atrial fibrillation and at least one risk factor (previous thromboembolism, hypertension, heart failure, abnormal left-ventricular function on echocardiography) for thromboembolism. However, patients should be reviewed, as the benefit/risk ratio may alter with increasing age or the development of additional illness. Low-risk patients may be treated with aspirin alone (grade A, level Ia). The Dutch PATAF (Primary Prevention of Arterial Thrombo-embolism in Non-rheumatic Atrial Fibrillation) study and AFASAK II (Atrial Fibrillation, Aspirin,

Anticoagulation Study) will further evaluate the effectiveness of aspirin and different intensities of anticoagulant therapy (Laupacis & Albers, 1995).

3.4.2 Rheumatic heart disease

INR 2.5 (grade C, level IV).

The risk of stroke is three times greater in patients with atrial fibrillation with mitral stenosis than in those without valve disease (Wolf *et al.*, 1978). Based on its apparent effectiveness in non-randomized studies and its effect in non-rheumatic atrial fibrillation, warfarin is usually given to maintain an INR of 2.5.

3.4.3 Congenital heart disease and thyrotoxicosis

INR 2.5 (grade C, level IV).

The risk of embolic stroke in patients with atrial fibrillation due to congenital heart disease and thyrotoxicosis is unknown. Given the benefit in other patients with atrial fibrillation, warfarin is usually given to prevent stroke.

3.4.4 Cardioversion

INR 2.5 for 3 weeks before and 4 weeks after cardioversion (grade B, level III).

No randomized study has determined if anticoagulation reduces the risk of systemic embolization when atrial fibrillation is terminated, although non-randomized reports indicate a reduced risk with anticoagulant therapy (grade B, level III) (Bjerkelund & Orning, 1969; Weinberg & Mancini, 1989; Arnold *et al.*, 1992). Embolic risk is associated with both electrical and pharmacological termination of atrial fibrillation. Therefore, warfarin is typically given for 3 weeks prior to and 4 weeks after termination of fibrillation (Laupacis, 1996).

3.5 Heart-valve disease without atrial fibrillation

Mitral-valve prolapse, mitral annular calcification and aortic-valve disease in the absence of atrial fibrillation or previous embolic events are associated with a low risk of stroke and are not routine indications for anticoagulant therapy. Rheumatic mitral-valve disease is associated with a high risk of stroke, even in the absence of atrial fibrillation, and is an indication for anticoagulation, INR 2.5 (Levine *et al.*, 1992) (grade C, level IV).

3.6 Mural thrombus

INR 2.5 for 3 months (grade B, level III).

Patients with mural thrombus after myocardial infarction are at greatest risk of embolization in the first 3 months, especially in the presence of a left-ventricular aneurysm. Following initial heparin therapy, warfarin is recommended for 3 months to achieve an INR of 2.5 (Schecter *et al.*, 1996) (grade B, level III).

3.7 Cardiomyopathy

INR 2.5 (grade C, level IV).

Dilated cardiomyopathy is associated with a 30–50% risk of thrombus formation and a high risk of systemic embolization (Fuster *et al.*, 1981). Prolonged anticoagulant therapy is recommended (Schecter *et al.*, 1996) (grade C, level IV).

3.8 Heart-valve prostheses

3.8.1 Mechanical prosthetic valves

INR 3.5 (grade B, level IIa).

The recommended intensity of anticoagulation varies with different consensus statements (British Committee for Standards in Haematology, 1990; Ad Hoc Committee of the Working Group on Valvular Heart Disease, European Society of Cardiology, 1993; Stein *et al.*, 1995). Recent recommendations for INR ranges of 2.0–3.0 (Ad Hoc Committee of the Working Group on Valvular Heart Disease, European Society of Cardiology, 1993) and 2.5–3.5 (Stein *et al.*, 1995) are based on prospective randomized studies, but these studies have limitations (Turpie, 1996) and none had a group of patients randomized to a range of 2.0–3.0 without additional antiplatelet therapy. An effective, relatively low-intensity regimen (INR 3.0–4.0) is supported by the latest analysis of a large Dutch study equating actual INRs to events (Cannegieter *et al.*, 1995) (grade B, level IIa). This study also indicated the need to allow for the significant number of patients who are inadequately anticoagulated when the target INR is low. There was a clear relationship between event rates and actual INRs, with a sharp rise in embolism rates with an INR <2.5 and haemorrhagic rates with an INR >5.0. Actual INRs were lower than the target range 31% of the time, so the target should be above 2.5. A target of 3.5 would maintain the majority of patients >2.5 and <5.0 and therefore maximize efficacy. The position and age of the prosthesis are also factors that determine thrombotic risk.

3.8.2 Bioprosthetic valves

Long-term warfarin not required in absence of atrial fibrillation (grade A, level Ib).

Oral anticoagulants are not required for valves in the aortic position in patients in sinus rhythm, although many centres anticoagulate patients for 3–6 months after any tissue-valve implant (Turpie, 1996). Patients with bioprostheses in the mitral position should receive oral anticoagulants to achieve an INR of 2.5 for the first 3 months (Turpie *et al.*, 1988) (grade A, level Ib). After 3 months, patients with atrial fibrillation should receive lifelong therapy to achieve an INR of 2.5. Patients with bioprosthetic valves with a history of systemic embolism and those with intracardiac thrombus should also be anticoagulated to achieve an INR of 2.5. Patients who do not require oral anticoagulants after the first 3 months may be considered for antiplatelet therapy, e.g. aspirin (Nunez *et al.*, 1984; Stein *et al.*, 1992).

3.9 Ischaemic stroke (see also Section 8.2 on stroke as a contraindication to warfarin)

Aspirin should be considered as secondary prophylaxis (grade A, level Ia).

Anticoagulant therapy reduces the risk of stroke in patients with atrial fibrillation (see Section 3.4), but it has also been considered for patients without atrial fibrillation who suffer TIAs, stroke in evolution and completed stroke.

There have been no randomized double-blind studies to evaluate the effect of oral anticoagulants in patients with TIAs. Several small studies have given insignificant and contrasting results. Given the clear risk reduction with aspirin therapy, warfarin should not be given as first-line therapy (del Zoppo, 1994; Hart *et al.*, 1996), unless there is a potential cardiac source of embolism. There is no evidence for a beneficial effect of warfarin in patients with carotid-artery stenosis.

No recommendation can be given for warfarin for stroke in evolution, as appropriately sized, randomized trials have not been performed (del Zoppo, 1994; Hart *et al.*, 1996).

There is no evidence to support the use of warfarin in completed stroke. In a small randomized study, the outcome of patients receiving anticoagulants was worse than those receiving placebo, with more episodes of further stroke and death due to intracerebral haemorrhage (Baker *et al.*, 1962). The results of other small studies support the observation that warfarin does more harm than good in patients with stroke (Genton *et al.*, 1977; Sherman *et al.*, 1992).

If warfarin is given, the recommended INR is unknown. Given the effectiveness of low-intensity anticoagulation, INR 2.0–3.0, in patients with atrial fibrillation and other cardiac sources of emboli and the effectiveness of an INR >3.0 in patients with coronary thrombosis, it is reasonable to adopt an INR between 2.0 and 4.0 if patients are to receive warfarin (grade C, level IV). Evidence-based guidelines may be facilitated by results from ongoing trials, such as the Stroke Prevention in Reversible Ischaemia Trial (SPIRIT), warfarin to INR of 3.0–4.5 versus aspirin 30 mg daily) and the Warfarin–Aspirin Reinfarction Study (WARS), warfarin to INR of 1.4–2.8 versus aspirin 325 mg.

3.10 Retinal-vein thrombosis

The value of anticoagulant therapy in retinal-vein thrombosis has not been evaluated. When retinal-vein thrombosis complicates the antiphospholipid syndrome, anticoagulation is recommended (grade C, level V; see Section 3.3).

3.11 Peripheral-arterial thrombosis and grafts

Aspirin should be considered as secondary prophylaxis (grade A, level Ia).

Uncontrolled surveys suggest that oral anticoagulants may reduce the risk of acute thrombotic arterial occlusion without any effect on the progress of atherosclerosis (Tillgren, 1965; Gallus, 1988). Likewise, the effect of anticoagulation following peripheral-arterial reconstructive surgery is not established, but it may be beneficial (Kretschmer *et al.*, 1988). Based on the intensity of anticoagulation required to prevent coronary-artery thrombosis, an INR of 3.5 is usually recommended if warfarin is given (grade C, level IV). However, these patients have widespread atherosclerosis and treatment with aspirin should be considered, as the risk of acute peripheral-arterial occlusion, coronary thrombosis and ischaemic stroke is reduced by one-third (Antiplatelet Trialists Collaboration, 1994). Large-scale studies comparing anticoagulation with aspirin after bypass surgery are now being conducted (Clagett, 1992).

3.12 Coronary-artery thrombosis (see also Section 3.6)

Aspirin should be considered as secondary prophylaxis (grade A, level Ia).

Oral anticoagulant therapy to achieve an INR >2.8 reduces the risk of reinfarction following a first event (Report of the Sixty-Plus Reinfarction Study Research Group, 1980; Smith *et al.*, 1990; Anticoagulants in the Secondary Prevention of Events in Coronary Thrombosis (ASPECT) Research Group, 1994) (level Ib). Earlier meta-analysis had revealed a 20% reduction in mortality with anticoagulant therapy during the immediate postinfarction period (Chalmers *et al.*, 1977), but the management of myocardial infarction has changed dramatically with the widespread adoption of thrombolysis and aspirin therapy and, at the moment, oral anticoagulation cannot be generally recommended in preference to aspirin, except in patients with mural thrombus (Vaitkus & Barnathan, 1993). The effect of warfarin to achieve an INR >3.0 is not apparently superior to the beneficial effect of aspirin, and bleeding rates in anticoagulated patients are higher (EPSIM Research Group, 1982). At present, all patients should receive aspirin at 150 mg daily following coronary thrombosis or the development of angina. Low-dose warfarin (INR 1.5) to reduce factor VII coagulant activity as primary prevention of infarction is being evaluated, but no recommendation can yet be given (Meade *et al.*, 1988). A large number of randomized studies combining anti-coagulant and antiplatelet therapy are now being conducted (Becker & Ansell, 1996), and further meta-analysis by the Antithrombotic Trialists Collaboration will become available. At the present time, if warfarin is given, an INR of 3.5 is recommended (grade A, level Ib).

3.13 Coronary-artery graft thrombosis

Aspirin should be considered as secondary prophylaxis (grade A, level Ib).

Vein-graft occlusion occurring in the first month is due to thrombosis. The frequency of thrombosis is 10–20% and this is reduced by aspirin, but warfarin has not been shown to be effective (Van der Meer, J. *et al.*, 1993). Late occlusion is due to atherosclerosis with super-imposed thrombosis. Although aspirin plus oral anticoagulation may reduce the risk of late occlusion, the value of warfarin alone is not known and anticoagulation is not routinely recommended (Pfisterer *et al.*, 1989). If warfarin is given, an INR of 3.5 is recommended, based on the results of reinfarction studies. A lower intensity of anticoagulation has not been evaluated.

3.14 Coronary angioplasty and coronary stents

Aspirin should be considered as first-line therapy (grade A, level Ib).

Both aspirin and heparin reduce the risk of acute occlusion following angioplasty. Oral anti-coagulation has not been shown to reduce the incidence of late stenosis (Thorton *et al.*, 1984). Coronary stents do not require oral anticoagulation, but aspirin is recommended after angioplasty and stent insertion to prevent coronary and other thrombotic events in this high-risk population.

3.15 Vena-caval filters

Filters are used to prevent pulmonary emboli in patients in whom anticoagulation is con-traindicated or in whom it has failed. The use of anticoagulation in patients with filters must be determined by individual risk–benefit analysis. There are no prospective randomized studies. Vena-caval thrombosis can occur in up to 20% of patients and therefore, in the absence of either bleeding or high bleeding risk, anticoagulation is justified (Elliott & Eklof, 1996). Contraindications to anticoagulation may resolve after insertion of a filter, allowing introduction of warfarin with a target INR of 2.5 at that stage (grade C, level IV).

3.16 Low-dose warfarin

Minidose warfarin has been evaluated in gynaecological and orthopaedic surgery. It did reduce the risk of DVT in a small study of patients having gynaecological surgery (Poller *et al.*, 1987), but it did not reduce the risk of venous thrombosis in hip-replacement sur-gery (Fordyce *et al.*, 1991). A two-step warfarin regimen has been shown to be effective in hip surgery, but it was not monitored with INR (Francis *et al.*, 1983). The effectiveness of fixed minidose warfarin at 1 mg/day to reduce the risk of central venous catheter-associated thrombosis is unproved. In a randomized study of 121 patients, final analysis was only available for 80 patients. These patients were not representative of the complete group and no recommendation can be given until further studies are completed (Bern *et al.*, 1990). A very-low-dose warfarin regimen to keep the INR at 1.3–1.9 has been used to reduce the risk of venous thromboembolism in patients with advanced breast cancer (Levine *et al.*, 1994).

Absolute recommendations on the indications, duration and intensity of low-dose warfarin regimens cannot be given at present.

4 Commencement of oral anticoagulant therapy

It is important to confirm objectively the diagnosis for which anticoagulant treatment is to be given. However, this should not delay the start of therapy. Where possible, routine blood samples for PT and activated partial thromboplastin time (APTT), platelet count and liver function tests should be taken before starting treatment, but the results are rarely needed immediately (McLinley & Wrenn, 1993). Oral anticoagulation can be commenced on day 1 in conjunction with heparin in most patients with DVT. Five days of heparin treatment is as effective as a longer period of heparin in patients with venous thromboembolism (grade A, level Ib) (Gallus *et al.*, 1986; Rosiello *et al.*, 1987; Hull *et al.*, 1990; Mohiuddin *et al.*, 1992). As the initial period of treatment with warfarin may be associated with a procoagulant state, due to a rapid reduction in protein-C levels, it is recommended that patients receive heparin therapy for at least 4 days and it should not be discontinued until the INR has been in the therapeutic range for 2 consecutive days (Ginsberg, 1996) (grade C, level IV). In patients with large thromboses, a longer period of heparin, up to 10 days, may be administered (Hull *et al.*, 1990; Mohiuddin *et al.*, 1992). A standard protocol for the commencement of anticoagulant treatment is recommended (grade B, level IIb) (Fennerty *et al.*, 1984; see Appendix 9.2).

For in-patient anticoagulation, a specific anticoagulant treatment chart is recommended, containing the treatment protocol, the results of coagulation tests (INR and APTT ratios) and the prescribed doses based on these results. This chart can then form the basis of the anticoagulant referral form for out-patient follow-up. A standard chart is being prepared by the task force.

Modifications to the oral anticoagulant loading dose may be necessary if baseline coagulation results are abnormal. Some patients may be particularly sensitive to warfarin. These include the elderly and those with high-risk factors, such as congestive cardiac failure and liver disease or those on drug therapy known to potentiate oral anticoagulants. A loading dose of < 10 mg daily is recommended under these circumstances.

For rapid anticoagulation with warfarin, daily INR measurement for a minimum of 4 days is recommended (see Appendix 9.2). Having achieved an INR in the desired therapeutic range, the INR should continue to be monitored weekly until control is stable. Thereafter, the frequency of recall can be extended. Extension of recall up to 12 weeks is acceptable. In the out-patient setting or the community, when rapid anticoagulation is not required, loading doses of <10 mg daily are recommended. A slow induction of anticoagulation with warfarin can be achieved by starting at a dose of 2 mg daily and increasing this slowly until the target INR is achieved (grade C, level IV).

It is important that discharge arrangements for anticoagulant follow-up are detailed in the hospital notes and that patients receive the yellow Department of Health anticoagulant booklets (obtained from: England, The Stationary Office, Broadway, Chadderton, Oldham, Lancashire OL9 6QH; Scotland, The Stationary Office, 21 South Gyle Crescent, Edinburgh EH12 9EB; Northern Ireland, Northern Ireland Office, Central Sources Agency, 27 Adelaide Street, Belfast BT2 8FH). At discharge, an appointment should be made for further INR measurement (this should not normally exceed 7 days). Responsibility for the discharge arrangements lies with the clinician referring the patient.

4.1 Thrombophilia

Patients with protein-C deficiency are at risk of developing skin necrosis during commencement of oral anticoagulation. Introduction of warfarin therapy should proceed without a loading dose of warfarin, even when heparin is given. Patients with protein-S deficiency may also be at risk. Skin necrosis has not yet been reported in patients with resistance to activated protein C. It would be prudent to introduce anticoagulation with warfarin slowly in all patients and to withdraw warfarin slowly at the end of treatment (grade C, level IV).

5 Managing anticoagulation in the perioperative period

Stop anticoagulation or perform surgery with the INR <2.5. If there is a risk of dangerous bleeding, e.g. internal, then stop anticoagulation at least 3 days before surgery or reverse anticoagulation with low-dose vitamin K (see Section 6) (grade B, level III).

The short-term risk of thromboembolism in patients with mechanical heart valves when not anticoagulated is very small. Therefore these patients should be managed in the same way (grade B, level IIb).

In rare circumstances where it is necessary to continue anticoagulation, e.g. life-threatening thromboembolism in patients with adenocarcinoma, then reduce INR to <2.5 and start heparin (British Committee for Standards in Haematology, 1993a) (grade C, level IV).

For minor surgical procedures, the oral anticoagulant dose should be stopped or adjusted to achieve a target INR of approximately 2.0 on the day of surgery (Taberner *et al.*, 1978; Francis *et al.*, 1983) (grade B, level III). The INR should be checked preoperatively and, if <2.5, the patient can proceed to surgery. If the INR is >2.5, the surgeon and haematologist must decide if the level of anticoagulation is safe for surgery to take place.

Prevention of bleeding with oral tranexamic acid mouthwash (4.8%) can be achieved after dental extraction without dose modification of oral anticoagulants (Ramstrom *et al.*, 1993) (grade A, level Ib).

For major surgery, oral anticoagulants should be stopped at least 3 days prior to surgery and, depending on the thrombotic risk of the condition for which the patient is receiving anticoagulant therapy, the INR can be monitored and, if necessary, heparin instituted once the INR is below the lower limit of the therapeutic range (e.g. <2.0 for a target of 2.5) (grade C). After warfarin is stopped, it typically takes about 4 days for the INR to reach 1.5 (White *et al.*, 1995). The threshold for institution of heparin and the dose required will depend on the underlying condition, e.g. secondary prevention of venous thrombosis is low-risk after the first month of anticoagulation and warfarin could be replaced with low-dose subcutaneous heparin preoperatively. A caged-ball metal mitral valve prosthesis is relatively high-risk and warfarin might be replaced with a continuous infusion of heparin once the INR is <3.0. There is, of course, a risk of bleeding associated with heparin during surgery, and some experts consider that the risk of heparin is greater than the risk of stopping anticoagulation for 4 days before surgery and restarting as soon as possible after surgery in patients with mechanical heart valves (Kearon & Hirsh, 1997) (see below).

The timing for reinstitution of oral anticoagulants will depend on the risk of post-operative haemorrhage. The 48–72 h delay for achievement of anticoagulation with oral vitamin K antagonists will also influence this decision. In many instances, oral anticoagulants can be started again as soon as the patient has an oral intake.

Certain types of surgery, such as neurosurgery, are particularly high-risk for bleeding complications and a period without any anticoagulant is preferable (Cannegieter *et al.*, 1994) (grade B). Anticoagulant therapy in patients with metal heart-valve prostheses can be temporarily discontinued. A meta-analysis of studies covering a period of 53 647 patient-years indicated that the risk of all thromboembolic events when not on oral anticoagulant therapy was only 8 per 100 patient-years. This equates to a risk of <0.2% over a 7-day period (Cannegieter *et al.*, 1994). However, this study did not specifically address the perioperative period, when the risk may be higher, due to the prothrombotic state associated with surgery. In a retrospective analysis of 180 non-cardiac operations in 159 patients with valve prostheses (170 Starr–Edwards, 59 mitral and 108 aortic), 153 operations were performed >12 months after valve replacement. In 62% of patients anticoagulation was discontinued 1–3 days before surgery and in 23% more than 3 days before. Anticoagulation was resumed 1–3 days later in 60% and after 4 days in 24%. Total perioperative cessation averaged 6.6 days. No postoperative thromboembolic events occurred in relation to the surgical procedure (level III) (Tinker & Tarhan, 1978). In another study, in which patients with metal prostheses underwent non-cardiac surgery with cessation of oral anticoagulation, two of 10 procedures in patients with mitral prostheses were complicated by perioperative thromboembolism, compared with 0 of 25 procedures in patients with aortic prostheses (level III) (Kathol *et al.*, 1976).

6 Managing bleeding and excessive anticoagulation

Bleeding while on oral anticoagulants increases significantly with INR results >5.0 (Eckman *et al.*, 1993; Cannegieter *et al.*, 1995). Therapeutic decisions are dependent on the INR and whether there is minor or major bleeding. The dose of vitamin K used to reverse overanticoagulation depends on the INR (Shetty *et al.*, 1992). Recommendations for management are given in Table 9.2.

INR >8.0, no bleeding or minor bleeding.

Stop oral anticoagulants. If no other risk factors for haemorrhage, stop treatment until INR <5.0. If risk factors for haemorrhage or minor bleeding (e.g. age >70 years, previous bleeding complications, epistaxis), give vitamin K. Due to near-complete absorption, oral vitamin K is as effective as intravenous, with the delay in action hardly influenced by the absorption time. However, only 0.5 mg is required to reduce the INR from >5.0 to a target

Table 9.2 Recommendations for management of bleeding and excessive anticoagulation

3.0 < INR <6.0 (target INR 2.5)	**1** Reduce warfarin dose or stop	
4.0 < INR <6.0 (target INR 3.5)	**2** Restart warfarin when INR <5.0	
6.0 < INR <8.0, no bleeding or minor bleeding	**1** Stop warfarin **2** Restart when INR <5.0	
INR >8.0, no bleeding or minor bleeding	**1** Stop warfarin **2** Restart warfarin when INR <5.0 **3** If other risk factors for bleeding, give 0.5–2.5 mg of vitamin K (oral)	Level III, grade B
Major bleeding	**1** Stop warfarin **2** Give prothrombin complex concentrate 50 units/kg or FFP 15 ml/kg **3** Give 5 mg of vitamin (oral or i.v.)	Level III, grade B

FFP, fresh-frozen plasma; i.v., intravenous.

level of 2.0–3.0 (Shetty *et al*., 1992). Vitamin K tablets usually contain >5 mg, which will completely reverse anticoagulation. Therefore, when partial correction is required, it may be necessary to give intravenous vitamin K or, alternatively, give the intravenous preparation orally. Allergic reactions following intravenous administration are rare with new preparations of vitamin K. If the INR is still too high at 24 h, the dose of vitamin K can be repeated.

Major bleeding.

Resuscitate and transfer to hospital for reversal of anticoagulation with vitamin K and pro-thrombin complex concentrates (PCC) or fresh-frozen plasma (FFP). Anticoagulation can be effectively reversed with 50 units/kg prothrombin complex concentrate, PCC (factors II, VII, IX and X or factor II, IX and X concentrate and factor VII concentrate) (Makris *et al*., 1996) and vitamin K 5 mg by slow intravenous injection (grade B, level III). However, patients receiving warfarin may have an underlying hypercoagulable state and infusion of prothrombin complex concentrate may exacerbate this. Further studies are required to determine the minimum dose of concentrate required to restore thrombin generation to normal and the safety of concentrates used for this purpose. In the absence of available concentrate licensed for this emergency use, treatment with 15 ml/kg of FFP and intravenous vitamin K 5 mg will partially reverse anticoagulation, although the levels of individual factors will typically remain <20% (Makris *et al*., 1996) and larger doses should be given if possible.

For patients with prosthetic heart valves, full reversal of oral anticoagulants with vitamin K may result in prolonged oral anticoagulant resistance and the possibility of valve thrombosis and thromboemboli. The degree of reversal must therefore be decided on an individual basis. All patients with bleeding should be evaluated to identify if there is a local anatomical reason for bleeding.

Bleeding may occur when patients are not overanticoagulated. In these circumstances, it may still be necessary to reverse anticoagulation and identify the cause of bleeding.

7 Drug interactions

If the drug change lasts <5 days, either no change, minor dose reduction or omit one complete dose of warfarin if known potentiating drug given (grade C, level IV). If the drug change lasts >5 days, check INR after start of new drug and adjust warfarin dose on basis of result (grade C, level IV).

Almost any drug can interact with oral anticoagulants, the majority potentiating the anticoagulant effect (notable exceptions which reduce the effect are antiepileptics, barbiturates, sucralfate, Rowachol, rifampicin). For further details, see relevant appendix in the current *British National Formulary*. When prescribing, a non-interacting drug should be chosen, when possible.

For short courses of new drug therapy, oral anticoagulant dose adjustment is not essential, but a slight dose reduction or omission of one dose could be recommended if a known potentiator is prescribed (grade C). If medication is for >5 days, the INR should be checked 1 week after commencement and the oral anticoagulant dose adjusted accordingly, returning to the normal maintenance dose after stopping the new drug.

8 Contraindications to anticoagulation

These are seldom absolute. The risk of haemorrhage is multifactorial, although increasing age is often found to be associated with an increased risk of major bleeding (Landefeld *et al.*, 1989; Fihn *et al.*, 1993; Van der Meer, F. *et al.*, 1993; Hylek & Singer, 1994; Stroke Prevention in Atrial Fibrillation Investigators, 1994; Palareti *et al.*, 1996). The following situations deserve specific mention.

8.1 Pregnancy

Organogenesis occurs during the sixth to twelfth weeks of gestation and exposure to warfarin at this time may be associated with embryopathy (Hall *et al.*, 1980; Iturbe-Alessio *et al.*, 1986; Wong *et al.*, 1993). However, due to immaturity of the fetal liver, there is a continuing risk of fetal bleeding throughout pregnancy. Avoiding oral anticoagulants reduces the risk of embryopathy, but heparin can cause maternal osteoporosis and thrombocytopenia. Furthermore, heparin may not be as effective during pregnancy in preventing thromboembolic events in patients with mechanical valves (Sbarouni & Oakley, 1994). Patients receiving warfarin should be told of the risk before conception and advised to have early pregnancy tests to detect pregnancy before 6 weeks' gestation. The possible need for alternative treatment with heparin in the first trimester and for 2–3 weeks before delivery (British Committee for Standards in Haematology, 1993b; Ginsberg & Barron, 1994) should be explained in advance (British Committee for Standards in Haematology, 1993b) Guidelines on management of anticoagulant therapy in pregnancy have been published (British Committee for Standards in Haematology, 1993b).

8.2 Stroke

Haemorrhagic stroke is a contraindication to oral anticoagulant therapy (Lowe, 1996). In patients with ischaemic strokes, anticoagulation increases the risk of secondary haemorrhage into the infarcted brain. In patients with atrial fibrillation, long-term warfarin therapy is beneficial, but the risk of early recurrent embolism is low and initial heparin is not required. Start warfarin 48 h to 14 days after ischaemic stroke, without initial heparin therapy, dependent on size of infarct and blood pressure. In patients with large embolic strokes or uncontrolled hypertension, anticoagulation should be postponed for 14 days. Patients with small- to moderate-sized ischaemic strokes without evidence of haemorrhage on computer-assisted tomography (CT) scanning 48 h after the onset of the event can be anticoagulated without delay.

9 Organization

Responsibility for ensuring a safe anticoagulant service and organizational procedures should be documented. The level of personnel involved in an anticoagulant service will be determined by local circumstances. Increasingly, pharmacists, nurses, clinical scientists and technologists are involved in providing anticoagulant care. With the development of local guidelines and computer decision-support systems, some duties may be devolved at the discretion of the local hospital or trust. The following organizational issues are recommended.

A lead clinician should be nominated who should be in charge of the anticoagulant service. Responsibilities are outlined in Table 9.3.

Where non-medical personnel are involved in anticoagulant care, they should have a strong clinical background with appropriate clinical qualifications, e.g. nurse practitioner, senior pharmacist. Recommendations regarding non-medical personnel are listed in Table 9.4.

The devolvement of anticoagulant services away from a hospital setting, using a postal service for collection of samples and return of dosage recommendations, has been practised for many years in some areas. Particular care is needed, however, to ensure that patients can

Table 9.3 Responsibilities of lead clinician for anticoagulant service

1	Receive referrals and approve need for anticoagulation
2	Give advice on duration and intensity of anticoagulation
3	Ensure system is in place for patients to receive urgent medical advice relating to anticoagulation
4	Ensure participation in national laboratory quality assurance scheme and monitor performance
5	Ensure regular clinical audit
6	Ensure anticoagulant guidelines are available, including the management of overanticoagulation
7	Provide general practitioners involved in anticoagulant care with advice and guidelines
8	Approve computer-assisted management programmes prior to implementation
9	Ensure adequate training is available for all personnel
10	Provide written approval for personnel, detailing levels of responsibility

Table 9.4 Recommendations for non-medical personnel involved in anticoagulant service

1 Personnel should be responsible to the lead clinician organizing the anticoagulant service
2 Personnel should have received adequate training and should be approved prior to commencement of duties
3 Dose recommendations and recall should be made according to written protocols or computer-assisted guidelines
4 Recommendations should be available for review by the clinician
5 The clinician should be alerted to patients with an INR >8 and those with bleeding problems
6 Personnel should provide patient education regarding anticoagulant therapy

Table 9.5 Recommendations for implementation of computer-assisted anticoagulation

1 Rapid retrieval of data to screen or printer
2 Data storage in chronological order
3 Dosage recommendations according to algorithm or guidelines approved by consultant in charge of the service; this should include evaluation of results over the full range of INR results
4 An alerting system for patient results which fall outside defined criteria
5 A facility to override computer recommendations
6 Patient recall for testing according to agreed criteria based on previous stability with invalid-date alerts
7 An alerting system for non-attendees
8 An alerting system for discontinuation of treatment
9 A prompt system to check for bleeding problems when high INR values are obtained
10 A system to record bleeding/thrombotic events or other rare side-effects
11 A facility to audit results

be quickly contacted regarding any change of dose. It is essential that patients managed in this way know how to report any complications of treatment and how to get urgent clinical advice. A system using trained staff to provide a peripatetic service to the home or general practice maintains a direct route for good communication with the patient. All previous patient results should be readily accessible, with full documentation of the clinical condition and duration of treatment, before further instructions are given. Records should be regularly audited.

10 Computer support systems

The computerization of anticoagulant management offers practical benefits for the laboratory and clinical staff, with standardization and continuity of recommendations. The standardization of anticoagulant control according to previous BCSH guidelines has been achieved using computer programs (Ryan *et al.*, 1989; Hunt, 1993). Table 9.5 indicates facilities for inclusion when considering implementing a computer system.

Organizational advantages may include automatic generation of clinic lists, transport lists and letters to GPs/colleagues regarding commencement and discontinuation of treatment. A database of drug interactions with warfarin is a helpful additional facility.

Table 9.6 Standards for audit

1	Provision of adequate data for safe transfer of anticoagulant follow-up
2	Provision of anticoagulant cards for patients on hospital discharge
3	Patient information: awareness of need for anticoagulation and possible side-effects of treatment
4	Hospital notes contain information that the patient is currently on warfarin
5	The use of heparin/warfarin dosage schedules in hospital setting (see Appendix 9.2)
6	Follow-up arrangements for patients failing to attend appointments
7	Achievement of target INR: 50% of INRs within 0.5 INR units and 80% within 0.75 INR units of target

11 Clinical audit

Routine audit of clinic management, with review of overanticoagulated patients, should be an integral part of the anticoagulant service. Review of patient outcome of INR values >8 (Philips *et al.*, 1993) or of patients requiring therapeutic interventions to reverse anticoagulant effect is a useful criterion for audit. Potential outcomes of audit may include better use of consultant time, reduction of in-patient stay to achieve stable anticoagulation, reduction in surgery-related thromboembolic problems and reduction in near-miss events and potential litigation problems. Table 9.6 indicates some standards for audit.

12 Laboratory control

The INR system is used to standardize variability of response of different thromboplastin reagents to warfarin (WHO Expert Committee on Biological Standardization, 1983). The INR is calculated from the PT ratio of test plasma to the geometric mean normal PT (GMNPT), to the power of the international sensitivity index (ISI) of the thromboplastin.

$$INR = (patient\ PT/GMNPT)^{ISI}$$

Two important sources of variability remain in the INR calculation: the measurement of the GMNPT and the ISI determination of the thromboplastin reagent (Taberner *et al.*, 1989; Peters *et al.*, 1991). The GMNPT should be derived from the geometric mean of 20 healthy adult plasma samples or the use of validated lyophilized normal control plasma. Low-ISI thromboplastins are recommended for monitoring oral anticoagulant therapy (Moriarty *et al.*, 1988). Local estimation of ISI values is not recommended, and ISI values of each thromboplastin batch should be assigned by manufacturers by comparison with an international standard. Unfortunately, there remains a problem that is partly due to the source of reference material (human or non-human) used in the calibration. Furthermore, problems with coagulometers producing shorter PT times than manual methods are well recognized (Poller *et al.*, 1989). Local calibration of coagulometers can be achieved by using plasma calibrants with manually certified PT values (Poller *et al.*, 1995). Participation in a Clinical Pathology Accreditation (CPA)-accredited external quality assurance scheme (EQAS) for anticoagulation is essential for monitoring laboratory performance

(Preston, 1995). Participants are encouraged to discuss technical problems with the EQAS coordinators.

There is no clinically significant change in INR when analysis is delayed for up to 3 days. Off-site blood sampling can accommodate a large increase in patient workload without a major revenue increase in primary care and with continued total quality management and central expert advice (Baglin & Luddington, 1997).

13 Near-patient testing

There are now several near-patient testing systems available for monitoring oral anticoagulant control (Machin *et al.*, 1996). These have generally shown a good correlation with manual and automated methods. The advantages include a rapid result without centrifugation of samples, using portable equipment that is easy to use by non-scientific staff. The monitoring of quality control may be more difficult, due to lack of appropriate quality-control material. Furthermore, the ISI values of some reagents incorporated in the disposable cards are higher than recommended. When near-patient testing is to be used, it is recommended that this is established in conjunction with local pathology services, in order to overview quality control (British Committee for Standards in Haematology, 1995) (see Chapter 1).

14 Acknowledgement

The task force are grateful to Professor Gordon Lowe for helpful advice.

Appendix 9.1: Graded recommendations

Grade of recommendation

A (Evidence levels Ia, Ib)	Requires at least one randomized controlled trial as part of the body of literature of overall good quality and consistency addressing the specific recommendation
B (Evidence levels IIa, IIb, III)	Requires availability of well-conducted clinical studies but no randomized clinical trials on the topic of recommendation
C (Evidence level IV)	Requires evidence from expert committee reports or opinions and/or clinical experience of respected authorities; indicates absence of directly applicable studies of good quality

Levels of evidence

Ia. Meta-analysis of randomized controlled trials

Ib. At least one randomized controlled trial

IIa. At least one well-designed controlled study without randomization

IIb. At least one other type of well-designed quasi-experimental study

III. Well-designed non-experimental descriptive studies, such as comparative studies, correlation studies and case–control studies

IV. Expert committee reports or opinions and/or clinical experience of respected authorities

Appendix 9.2: Warfarin loading schedule

Day	INR	Warfarin dose (mg)
First	<1.4	10
Second	<1.8	10
	1.8	1
	>1.8	0.5
Third	<2.0	10
	2.0–2.1	5
	2.2–2.3	4.5
	2.4–2.5	4
	2.6–2.7	3.5
	2.8–2.9	3
	3.0–3.1	2.5
	3.2–3.3	2
	3.4	1.5
	3.5	1
	3.6–4.0	0.5
	>4.0	0
		(Predicted maintenance dose)
Fourth	<1.4	>8
	1.4	8
	1.5	7.5
	1.6–1.7	7
	1.8	6.5
	1.9	6
	2.0–2.1	5.5
	2.2–2.3	5
	2.4–2.6	4.5
	2.7–3.0	4
	3.1–3.5	3.5
	3.6–4.0	3
	4.1–4.5	Miss out next day's dose, then give 2 mg
	>4.5	Miss out 2 days' doses, then give 1 mg

References

Ad Hoc Committee of the Working Group on Valvular Heart Disease, European Society of Cardiology (1993) Guidelines for prevention of thromboembolic events in valvular heart disease. *Journal of Heart Valve Disease* **2**, 398–410.

Anticoagulants in the Secondary Prevention of Events in Coronary Thrombosis (ASPECT) Research Group (1994) Effect of long-term oral anticoagulant treatment on mortality and cardiovascular morbidity after myocardial infarction. *Lancet* **343**, 499–503.

Antiplatelet Trialists Collaboration (1994) Collaborative overview of randomised trials of antiplatelet therapy. II. Maintenance of vascular graft or arterial patency by antiplatelet therapy. *British Medical Journal* **308**, 159–168.

Arnold A., Mick M., Mazurek R., Loop F. & Trohman R. (1992) Role of prophylactic anticoagulation for direct current cardioversion in patients with atrial fibrillation or atrial flutter. *Journal of the American College of Cardioligists* **19**, 851–855.

Atrial Fibrillation Investigators (1994) Risk factors for stroke and efficacy of antithrombotic therapy in atrial fibrillation: analysis of pooled data from five randomised controlled trials. *Archives of Internal Medicine* **154**, 1449–1457.

Baglin T. (1994) Decentralised anticoagulant care. *Clinical and Laboratory Haematology* **16**, 327–329.

Baglin T. & Luddington R. (1997) Reliability of delayed INR determination: implications for decentralized anticoagulant care with off-site blood sampling. *British Journal of Haematology* **96**, 431–434.

Baker R., Broward J., Fang H. *et al.* (1962) Anticoagulant therapy in cerebral infarction. *Neurology* **12**, 823–835.

Becker R. & Ansell J. (1996) Oral anticoagulants (antithrombotic agents) for cardiovascular disorders. In *Disorders of Thrombosis*, (Hull R. & Pineo G.F. eds), pp. 75–89. Saunders, Philadelphia.

Bern M., Lokich J., Wallach S. *et al.* (1990) Very low doses of warfarin can prevent thrombosis in central venous catheters. *Annals of Internal Medicine* **112**, 423–428.

Bjerkelund C. & Orning O. (1969) The efficacy of anticoagulant therapy in preventing embolism related to DC electrical conversion of atrial fibrillation. *American Journal of Cardiology* **23**, 208–216.

Boston Area Anticoagulation Trial for Atrial Fibrillation Investigators (1990) The effect of low-dose warfarin on the risk of stroke in patients with nonrheumatic atrial fibrillation. *New England Journal of Medicine* **323**, 1505–1511.

British Committee for Standards in Haematology (1990) Guidelines on oral anticoagulation: second edition. *Journal of Clinical Pathology* **43**, 177–183.

British Committee for Standards in Haematology (1993a) Guidelines on the use and monitoring of heparin 1992: second edition. *Journal of Clinical Pathology* **46**, 97–103.

British Committee for Standards in Haematology (1993b) Guidelines on the prevention, investigation, and management of thrombosis associated with pregnancy. *Journal of Clinical Pathology* **46**, 489–496.

British Committee for Standards in Haematology (1995) Guidelines for near patient testing. *Clinical and Laboratory Haematology* **17**, 301–310.

Cannegieter S., Rosendaal F. & Briet E. (1994) Thromboembolic and bleeding complications in patients with mechanical heart valve prostheses. *Circulation* **89**, 635–641.

Cannegieter S., Rosendaal F., Wintzen A., Van Der Meer F., Vandenbroucke J. & Briet E. (1995) Optimal oral anticoagulant therapy in patients with mechanical heart valves. *New England Journal of Medicine* **333**, 11–17.

Carson J., Kelley M., Duff A. *et al.* (1992) The clinical course of pulmonary embolism. *New England Journal of Medicine* **326**, 1240–1245.

Cavenagh J. & Colvin B. (1996) Guidelines for the management of thrombophilia. *Postgraduate Medical Journal* **72**, 87–94.

Chalmers T., Matta R., Smith H. & Kunzler A. (1977) Evidence favoring the use of anticoagulants in the hospital phase of acute myocardial infarction. *New England Journal of Medicine* **297**, 1091–1096.

Clagett G. (1992) Antithrombotic therapy for lower extremity bypass. *Journal of Vascular Surgery* **15**, 867–875.

Cogo A., Lensing A., Koopman M. *et al.* (1998) Compression ultrasonography for diagnostic management of patients with clinically suspected deep vein thrombosis: prospective cohort study. *British Medical Journal* **316**, 17–20.

Connolly S., Laupacis A., Gent M. *et al.* (1991) Canadian Atrial Fibrillation Anticoagulation (CAFA) Study. *Journal of the American College of Cardiologists* **18**, 349–355.

Coon W., Willis P. & Symons M. (1969) Assessment of anticoagulant treatment of venous thromboembolism. *Annals of Surgery* **170**, 559–568.

del Zoppo G. (1994) Antithrombotic therapy in cerebrovascular disease. In *Thrombosis and Haemorrhage*, pp. 1225–1252. Blackwell Scientific Publications, Boston.

De Stefano V., Finazzi G. & Mannucci P. (1996) Inherited thrombophilia. *Blood* **87**, 3531–3544.

Eckman M., Levine H. & Pauker S. (1993) Effect of laboratory variation in the prothrombin-time ratio on the results of oral anticoagulant therapy. *New England Journal of Medicine* **329**, 696–702.

Elliott G. & Eklof B. (1996) Vena caval filters. In *Disorders of Thrombosis*, pp. 329–335. Saunders, Philadelphia.

EPSIM Research Group (1982) A controlled comparison of aspirin and oral anticoagulants in prevention of death after myocardial infarction. *New England Journal of Medicine* **307**, 701–708.

European Atrial Fibrillation Trial Study Group (1993) Secondary prevention in non-rheumatic atrial fibrillation after transient ischaemic attack or minor stroke. *Lancet* **ii**, 1255–1262.

European Atrial Fibrillation Trial Study Group (1995) Optimal oral anticoagulant therapy in patients with non-rheumatic atrial fibrillation and recent cerebral ischemia. *New England Journal of Medicine* **333**, 5–10.

Ezekowitz M., Bridgers S., James K. *et al.* (1992) Warfarin in the prevention of stroke associated with non-rheumatic atrial fibrillation. *New England Journal of Medicine* **327**, 1406–1412.

Fennerty A., Dolben J., Thomas P. *et al.* (1984) Flexible induction dose regimen for warfarin and prediction of maintenance dose. *British Medical Journal* **288**, 1268–1270.

Fennerty A., Campbell I. & Routledge P. (1988) Anticoagulants in venous thromboembolism. *British Medical Journal* **297**, 1285–1288.

Fihn S., McDonell M., Martin D. *et al.* (1993) Risk factors for complications of chronic anticoagulation: a multicenter study: warfarin optimised outpatient follow-up study group. *Annals of Internal Medicine* **118**, 511–520.

Fordyce M., Baker A. & Staddon G. (1991) Efficacy of fixed minidose warfarin prophylaxis in total hip replacement. *British Medical Journal* **303**, 219–220.

Francis C. (1994) Prevention and treatment of venous thromboembolic disease. In *Thrombosis and Haemorrhage*, pp. 1287–1311. Blackwell Scientific Publications, Boston.

Francis C., Marder V., Evarts C. & Yaukoolbodi S. (1983) Two-step warfarin therapy: prevention of postoperative venous thrombosis without excessive bleeding. *Journal of the American Medical Association* **249**, 374–378.

Fuster V., Gersh B., Giulani E., Tajik A., Brandenburg R. & Frye R. (1981) The natural history of dilated cardiomyopathy. *American Journal of Cardiology* **47**, 525–531.

Gallus A. (1988) Long term warfarin in artery disease. *Blood Reviews* **2**, 95–101.

Gallus A., Jackaman J., Tillett J., Mills W. & Wycherley A. (1986) Safety and efficacy of warfarin started early after submassive venous thrombosis or pulmonary embolism. *Lancet* **ii**, 1293–1296.

Genton E., Barnett H., Fields W., Gent M. & Hoak J. (1977) Cerebral ischaemia: the role of thrombosis and of antithrombotic therapy. *Stroke* **8**, 150–175.

Ginsberg J. (1996) Drug therapy: management of venous thromboembolism. *New England Journal of Medicine* **335**, 1816–1828.

Ginsberg J. & Barron W. (1994) Pregnancy and prosthetic heart valves. *Lancet* **344**, 1170–1172.

Greaves M. & Preston F. (1991) Clinical and laboratory aspects of thrombophilia. In *Recent Advances in Blood Coagulation*, (Poller L. ed.), pp. 119–140. Churchill Livingstone, Edinburgh.

Hall J., Paul R. & Wilson K. (1980) Maternal and fetal sequelae of anticoagulation during pregnancy. *American Heart Journal* **68**, 122–140.

Hart R., Solomon D. & Anderson D. (1996) Oral anticoagulation for prevention of stroke and cerebral embolism. *Oral Anticoagulants*, pp. 150–166. Arnold, London.

Hirsh J. (1990) Anticoagulant therapy in venous thromboembolism. In *Antithrombotic Therapy*, (Poller L. & Hirsh J. eds), pp. 685–692. Baillière Tindall, London.

Hirsh J. (1995) The optimal duration of anticoagulant therapy for venous thrombosis. *New England Journal of Medicine* **332**, 1710–1711.

Holmgren K., Andersson G., Fagrell B. *et al.* (1985) One-month versus six-month therapy with oral anticoagulants after symptomatic deep vein thrombosis. *Acta Medica Scandinavica* **218**, 279–284.

Hull R., Delmore T., Genton E. *et al.* (1979) Warfarin sodium versus low-dose heparin in the long-term treatment of venous thrombosis. *New England Journal of Medicine* **301**, 855–858.

Hull R., Hirsh J., Jay R. *et al.* (1982) Different intensities of oral anticoagulant therapy in the treatment of proximal-vein thrombosis. *New England Journal of Medicine* **307**, 1676–1681.

Hull R., Raskob G., Rosenbloom D. *et al.* (1990) Heparin for 5 days as compared to 10 days in the initial treatment of proximal vein thrombosis. *New England Journal of Medicine* **322**, 1260–1264.

Hunt B. (1993) Development of a MUMPS-based anticoagulant management system. *British Journal of Biomedical Science* **50**, 117–124.

Hylek E. & Singer D. (1994) Risk factors for intracranial haemorrhage in outpatients taking warfarin. *Annals of Internal Medicine* **120**, 897–902.

Hylek E., Skates S., Sheehan M. & Singer D. (1996) An analysis of the lowest effective intensity of prophylactic anticoagulation for patients with nonrheumatic atrial fibrillation. *New England Journal of Medicine* **335**, 540–546.

Iturbe-Alessio I., del Carmen Fonseca M., Mutchinik O., Santos M., Zajarias A. & Salazaar E. (1986) Risks of anti-coagulant therapy in pregnant women with artificial heart valves. *New England Journal of Medicine* **315**, 1390–1393.

Kakkar V., Flanc C., Howe C. & Clarke M. (1969) Natural history of postoperative deep vein thrombosis. *Lancet* **ii**, 230–233.

Kathol R., Nolan S. & McGuire L. (1976) Living with prosthetic valves: subsequent non-cardiac operations and the risk of thromboembolism or hemorrhage. *American Heart Journal* **92**, 162–167.

Kearon C. & Hirsh J. (1997) Management of anticoagulation before and after elective surgery. *New England Journal of Medicine* **336**, 1506–1511.

Khamashta M., Cuadrado M., Mujic F., Taub N., Hunt B. & Hughes G. (1995) The management of thrombosis in the antiphospholipid syndrome. *New England Journal of Medicine* **332**, 993–997.

Kretschmer G., Wenzl E., Schemper M. *et al.* (1988) Influence of postoperative anticoagulant treatment on patient survival after femeropopliteal vein bypass surgery. *Lancet* **i**, 797–799.

Lagerstedt C., Olsson C., Fagher B., Oqvist B. & Albrechtsson U. (1985) Need for long-term anticoagulant treatment in symptomatic calf-vein thrombosis. *Lancet* **ii**, 515–518.

Landefeld C., Rosenblatt M. & Goldman L. (1989) Bleeding in outpatients treated with warfarin: relation to the prothrombin time and important remedial lesions. *American Journal of Medicine* **87**, 153–159.

Lane D., Mannucci P., Bauer K. *et al.* (1996) Inherited thrombophilia. *Thrombosis and Haemostasis* **76**, 824–834.

Laupacis A. (1996) Atrial fibrillation and oral anticoagulants. In *Oral Anticoagulants*, (Poller L. & Hirsh J. eds), pp. 123–129. Arnold, London.

Laupacis A. & Albers G. (1995) Atrial fibrillation. In *Disorders of Thrombosis*, pp. 106–115. Saunders, Philadelphia.

Levine H., Pauker S. & Eckman M. (1992) Antithrombotic therapy in valvular heart disease. *Chest* **102**, 434S–444S.

Levine M., Hirsh J., Gent M. *et al.* (1994) Double-blind randomised trial of a very-low-dose warfarin for prevention of thromboembolism in stage IV breast cancer. *Lancet* **343**, 886–889.

Levine M., Hirsh J., Gent M. *et al.* (1995) Optimal duration of oral anticoagulant therapy: a randomised trial comparing four weeks with three months of warfarin in patients with proximal deep vein thrombosis. *Thrombosis and Haemostasis* **74**, 606–611.

Lohr J., Kerr T., Lutter K., Cranley R., Spirtoff K. & Cranley J. (1991) Lower extremity calf thrombosis: to treat or not to treat? *Journal of Vascular Surgery* **14**, 618–623.

Lowe G. (1996) Acute stroke. In *Disorders of Thrombosis*, pp. 116–125. Saunders, Philadelphia.

Machin S., Mackie I., Chitolie A. & Lawrie A. (1996) Near patient testing (NPT) in haemostasis: a synoptic review. *Clinical and Laboratory Haematology* **18**, 69–74.

McLinley L. & Wrenn K. (1993) Are baseline prothrombin time/partial thromboplastin time values necessary before instituting anticoagulation? *Annals of Emergency Medicine* **22**, 697–702.

Makris M., Greaves M., Philips W., Kitchen S., Rosendaal F. & Preston F. (1996) Emergency oral anticoagulant reversal: the relative efficacy of infusions of fresh frozen plasma and clotting factor concentrate on correction of the coagulopathy. *Thrombosis and Haemostasis* **77**, 477–480.

Meade T., Wilkes H., Stirling Y., Brennan P., Kelleher C. & Browne W. (1988) Randomised controlled trial of low dose warfarin in the primary prevention of ischemic heart disease. *European Heart Journal* **9**, 836–843.

Mohiuddin S., Hilleman D., Destache C., Stoysich A., Gannon J. & Sketch M. (1992) Efficacy and safety of early versus late initiation of warfarin during heparin therapy in acute thromboembolism. *American Heart Journal* **123**, 729–732.

Moriarty H., Lam-Po-Tang P. & Anastas N. (1988) Comparison of thromboplastins using the ISI and INR system. *Pathology* **10**, 67–71.

Nunez L., Aguado G., Larrea J., Celemin D. & Oliver J. (1984) Prevention of thromboembolism using aspirin after mitral valve replacement with porcine bioprosthesis. *Annals of Thoracic Surgery* **37**, 84–87.

O'Sullivan E. (1972) Duration of anticoagulant therapy in venous thromboembolism. *Medical Journal of Australia* **ii**, 1104–1107.

Palareti G., Leali N., Coccheri S. *et al.* (1996) Bleeding complications of oral anticoagulant treatment: an inception-cohort, prospective collaborative study (ISCOAT). *Lancet* **348**, 423–428.

Pellegrini V., Langhans M., Totterman S., Marder V. & Francis C. (1993) Embolic complications of calf thrombosis following total hip arthroplasty. *Journal of Arthroplasty* **8**, 449–457.

Peters R., Van den Besselaar A. & Olthius F. (1991) Determination of mean normal prothrombin time for the assessment of INR. *Thrombosis and Haemostasis* **66**, 442–445.

Peterson P., Boysen G., Godtfredsen J., Andersen E. & Andersen B. (1989) Placebo-controlled, randomised trial of warfarin and aspirin for prevention of thromboembolic complications in chronic atrial fibrillation: the Copenhagen AFASAK study. *Lancet* **i**, 175–179.

Petiti O., Strom B. & Melmon K. (1986) Duration of warfarin anticoagulant therapy and the probabilities of recurrent thromboembolism and hemorrhage. *American Journal of Medicine* **81**, 255–259.

Pfisterer M., Burkart F., Jockers G. *et al.* (1989) Trial of low-dose aspirin plus anticoagulants for prevention of aortocoronary vein graft occlusion. *Lancet* **ii**, 1–7.

Philips W., Makris M. & Preston F. (1993) Audit of frequency and clinical response to excessive oral anticoagulation. *British Journal of Haematology* **84** (Suppl. 1), 57 (A129).

Poller L., McKernan A., Thomson J., Elstein M., Hirsch P. & Jones J. (1987) Fixed minidose warfarin: a new approach to prophylaxis against venous thrombosis after major surgery. *British Medical Journal* **295**, 1309–1312.

Poller L., Thomson J. & Taberner D. (1989) Effect of automation on the prothrombin time test in NEQAS surveys. *Journal of Clinical Pathology* **42**, 97–100.

Poller L., Triplett D., Hirsh J., Carroll J. & Clark K. (1995) The value of plasma calibrants in correcting coagulometer effects on international normalised ratios. *American Journal of Chemical Pathology* **103**, 358–365.

Preston F. (1995) Quality control and oral anticoagulation. *Thrombosis and Haemostasis* **74**, 515–520.

Ramstrom G., Sindet-Pederson S., Hall G., Blomback M. & Alander U. (1993) Prevention of postsurgical bleeding in oral surgery using tranexamic acid without dose modification of oral anticoagulants. *Journal of Oral and Maxillofacial Surgery* **51**, 1211–1216.

Raskob G. (1996) Calf-vein thrombosis. In *Disorders of Thrombosis*, (Hull R. & Pineo G.F. eds), pp. 398–405. Saunders, Philadelphia.

Report of the Sixty-Plus Reinfarction Study Research Group (1980) A double blind trial to assess long term anticoagulant therapy in elderly patients after myocardial infarction. *Lancet* **ii**, 989–993.

Research Committee of the British Thoracic Society (1992) Optimum duration of anticoagulation for deep-vein thrombosis and pulmonary embolism. *Lancet* **340**, 873–876.

Rose P. (1996) Audit of anticoagulant therapy. *Journal of Clinical Pathology* **49**, 5–9.

Rosiello R., Chan C., Tencza F. & Matthay R. (1987) Timing of oral anticoagulation therapy in the treatment of angiographically proven acute pulmonary embolism. *Archives of Internal Medicine* **147**, 1469–1473.

Ryan P., Gilbert M. & Rose P. (1989) Computer control of anticoagulant dose for therapeutic management. *British Medical Journal* **299**, 1207–1209.

Sandler D. & Martin J. (1989) Autopsy proven pulmonary embolism in hospital patients: are we detecting enough deep vein thrombosis? *Journal of the Royal Society of Medicine* **82**, 203–205.

Sbarouni E. & Oakley C. (1994) Outcome of pregnancy in women with valve prostheses. *British Heart Journal* **71**, 196–201.

Schecter A., Fuster V. & Chesebro J. (1996) Anticoagulants in cardiomyopathy. In *Oral Anticoagulants*, (Poller L. & Hirsh J. eds), pp. 258–263. Arnold, London.

Schulman S., Rhedin A., Lindmarker P. *et al.* (1995) A comparison of six weeks with six months of oral anticoagulant therapy after a first episode of venous thromboembolism. *New England Journal of Medicine* **332**, 1661–1665.

Schulman S., Granqvist S., Holmstrom M. *et al.* (1997) The duration of oral anticoagulant therapy after a second episode of venous thromboembolism. *New England Journal of Medicine* **336**, 393–398.

Sherman D., Dyken M., Fisher M., Gent M., Harrison M. & Hart R. (1992) Antithrombotic therapy for cerebrovascular disorders. *Chest* **102** (Suppl.), 529S–537S.

Shetty H., Backhouse G., Bentley D. & Routledge P. (1992) Effective reversal of warfarin-induced excessive anticoagulation with low dose vitamin K1. *Thrombosis and Haemostasis* **67**, 13–15.

Smith P., Arnesen H. & Holme I. (1990) The effect of warfarin on mortality and reinfarction after myocardial infarction. *New England Journal of Medicine* **323**, 147–152.

Stein P., Alpert J., Copeland C., Dalen J., Goldman S. & Turpie A. (1992) Antithrombotic therapy in patients with mechanical and biological prosthetic heart valves. *Chest* **102** (Suppl.), 445S–455S.

Stein P., Alpert J., Copeland J., Dalen J. & Turpie A. (1995) Antithrombotic therapy in patients with mechanical and bioprosthetic heart valves. *Chest* **108**, 371S–379S.

Stroke Prevention in Atrial Fibrillation Investigators (1991) Stroke prevention in atrial fibrillation study: final results. *Circulation* **84**, 527–539.

Stroke Prevention in Atrial Fibrillation Investigators (1994) Warfarin versus aspirin for prevention of thromboembolism in atrial fibrillation: Stroke Prevention in Atrial Fibrillation II Study. *Lancet* **343**, 687–691.

Stroke Prevention in Atrial Fibrillation Investigators (1996) Adjusted-dose warfarin versus low-intensity, fixed-dose warfarin plus aspirin for high-risk patients with atrial fibrillation: stroke prevention in atrial fibrillation III randomised clinical trial. *Lancet* **348**, 633–638.

Taberner D., Poller L., Burslem R. & Jones J. (1978) Oral anticoagulants controlled by the British Comparative Thromboplastin versus low-dose heparin prophylaxis of deep vein thrombosis. *British Medical Journal* **ii**, 272–274.

Taberner D., Poller L. & Thompson J. (1989) Effect of international sensitivity index (ISI) of thromboplastins on precision of international normalised ratios (INR). *Journal of Clinical Pathology* **42**, 1–3.

Thorton M., Gruentzig A., Hollman J., King S. & Douglas J. (1984) Coumadin and aspirin in the prevention of recurrence after transluminal coronary angioplasty: a randomised study. *Circulation* **69**, 721–727.

Tillgren C. (1965) Obliterative arterial disease of the lower limbs. IV. Evaluation of long-term anticoagulant therapy. *Acta Medica Scandinavica* **178**, 203–219.

Tinker J. & Tarhan S. (1978) Discontinuing anticoagulant therapy in surgical patients with cardiac valve prostheses. *Journal of the American Medical Association* **239**, 738–739.

Turpie A. (1996) Valvular heart disease and heart valve prostheses. In *Oral Anticoagulants*, pp. 143–149. Arnold, London.

Turpie A., Gunstensen J., Hirsh J., Nelson H. & Gent M. (1988) Randomised comparison of two intensities of oral anticoagulant therapy after tissue heart valve replacement. *Lancet* **i**, 1242–1245.

US Department of Health and Human Services, Public Health Service and Agency Care Policy and Research (1992) *Acute Pain Management: Operative or Medical Procedures and Trauma.* Report AHCPR Pub. 92-0038, Agency for Health Care Policy and Research Publications.

Vaitkus P. & Barnathan E. (1993) Embolic potential, prevention and management of mural thrombus complicating anterior myocardial infarction: a meta-analysis. *Journal of the American College of Cardiologists* **22**, 1004–1009.

Van der Meer F., Rosendaal F., Vandenbroucke J. & Briet E. (1993) Bleeding complications in oral anticoagulant therapy. *Archives of Internal Medicine* **153**, 1557–1562.

Van der Meer J., Hillege H., Ascoop C., Pfisterer M., Van Gilst W. & Lie K. (1993) Prevention of one-year vein-graft occlusion after aortocoronary bypass surgery: a comparison of low dose aspirin, low dose aspirin plus dipyridamole, and oral anticoagulants. *Lancet* **342**, 257–264.

Weinberg D. & Mancini J. (1989) Anticoagulation for cardioversion of atrial fibrillation. *American Journal of Cardiology* **63**, 745–746.

Weinmann E. & Salzman E. (1994) Deep-vein thrombosis. *New England Journal of Medicine* **331**, 1630–1641.

White R., McKittrick T., Hutchinson R. & Twitchell J. (1995) Temporary discontinuation of warfarin therapy: changes in the international normalised ratio. *Annals of Internal Medicine* **122**, 40–42.

WHO Expert Committee on Biological Standardization (1983) *Report 33*, pp. 81–105. World Health Organisation Technical Report Series no. 687. London.

Wolf P., Daeber T., Emerson T. & Krannel W. (1978) Epidemiological assessment of chronic atrial fibrillation and the risk of stroke: the Framingham Study. *Neurology* **28**, 973–977.

Wong V., Cheng C. & Chan K. (1993) Fetal and neonatal outcome of exposure to anticoagulants during pregnancy. *American Journal of Medical Genetics* **45**, 17–21.

10 Guidelines for Pretransfusion Compatibility Procedures in Blood Transfusion Laboratories
Prepared by the Blood Transfusion Task Force

1 Introduction

1.1 Purpose of pretransfusion guidelines

Technical errors and/or inappropriate test systems or administrative errors may result in immediate and delayed haemolytic transfusion reactions. The purpose of these guidelines, which replace those previously published (BCSH, 1991b), is to define organizational, documentation and technical procedures undertaken in hospital or regional transfusion-centre laboratories prior to blood transfusion.

1.2 Elements in pretransfusion testing

1   ABO and Rh D grouping of the recipient.
2   Antibody screen of the recipient, or mother in the case of neonatal transfusion, which, in the event of a positive screen, should be followed by antibody identification.
3   A computer or manual check of records.
(These three elements constitute a group and screen.)
4   Donor red-cell selection and cross-matching.
In certain emergencies, the recipient's need for immediate red-cell support may dictate that pretransfusion testing is abbreviated.

1.3 Clinical significance of red-cell antibodies (Table 10.1)

1   Clinically significant antibodies are those which are capable of giving rise to accelerated destruction of red cells bearing the relevant antigen.
2   Anti-A, anti-B and anti-A,B must always be regarded to be of clinical significance.
3   With few exceptions, irregular antibodies which are potentially clinically significant are only those which are reactive in the indirect antiglobulin test (IAT), performed strictly at 37°C.
4   In certain clinical emergencies, e.g. massive blood loss, the recipient's need for red-cell transfusion may necessitate the use of incompatible units.

Reprinted with permission from *Transfusion Medicine*, 1996, **6**, 273–283.

Table 10.1 The clinical significance of antibodies of given specificities and selection/testing of red-cell units prior to their issue

Specificity	Clinical significance	Selection of units
Rh antibodies (reactive in IAT)	Yes	Antigen-negative
Kell antibodies	Yes	Antigen-negative
Duffy antibodies	Yes	Antigen-negative
Kidd antibodies	Yes	Antigen-negative
Anti-S,-s	Yes	Antigen-negative
Anti-A_1, -P_1, -N	Rarely	IAT cross-match-compatible 37°C
Anti-M	Rarely	IAT cross-match-compatible 37°C
Anti-M reactive at 37°C	Sometimes	Antigen-negative
Anti-Le^a, Anti-Le^{a+b}	Rarely	IAT cross-match-compatible 37°C
Anti-Le^b	No	Not clinically significant and can be ignored
High-titre low-avidity antibodies (HTLA)	Unlikely	Seek advice from transfusion centre
Antibodies against low/high-frequency antigens	Depends on specificity	Seek advice from transfusion centre

2 Quality assurance in pretransfusion procedures

2.1 Role of the hospital transfusion committee

This chapter is primarily concerned with the laboratory aspect of pretransfusion testing. However, the provision of safe and effective red-cell transfusion support requires multidisciplinary collaboration. The hospital transfusion committee can help with the areas covered by this chapter, as follows: (i) training medical staff and designated phlebotomists in accordance with local written procedures for the generation of request forms and labelling of patient samples; (ii) supporting the consultant haematologist and transfusion laboratory in enforcing policies relating to the non-laboratory aspects of blood transfusion, e.g. documentation, identification of patients and labelling of blood samples for transfusion, required intervals between samples, verbal requests, the collection of blood from the blood-issue refrigerator and conditions of storage outside the transfusion laboratory; (iii) in the formulation and periodic review of maximum surgical blood-order schedules (MSBOS), the schedules being essential if donor blood and laboratory staff are to be utilized effectively; and (iv) audit of practice.

2.2 Laboratory aspects of quality assurance

The laboratory should document its quality system and include the following points.
1   The laboratory should participate in appropriate external quality assurance.
2   Transfusion laboratories should make use of systems validated against the documented requirements of the laboratory. They should also have written standards for the manual procedures that need to be followed when the computer system is unavailable.

3   Whether using a manual or semi-automated system, the laboratory must develop procedures to build in checks for all critical points in transfusion testing, e.g. preserving the identity of samples during separation and processing.

2.2.1 Reagents

1   The head of the laboratory should refer to the specifications for reagents given in the *Guidelines for the Blood Transfusion Services in the United Kingdom* (Department of Health, 1996).

2   All reagents or systems should be used in accordance with the manufacturer's instructions. If this is not appropriate, then the procedure should be validated in accordance with the guidelines of the British Committee for Standards in Haematology (BCSH, 1995).

3   There should be a record of all batch numbers and expiry dates of all reagents used in the laboratory.

2.2.2 Techniques

1   All procedures used should be in accordance with recommended practice, as outlined in Section 8.

2   It is imperative that the antiglobulin technique chosen has been validated against the documented requirements of the laboratory and has been subjected to a thorough field trial before being introduced into the laboratory (Voak, 1992).

3   All changes in techniques must also be thoroughly validated in accordance with BCSH (1995) before being introduced into routine use.

4   Written authorized standard operating procedures (SOPs), which cover all aspects of the laboratory work, must be available and reviewed regularly.

5   The regular checking and maintenance of all laboratory equipment must be documented. In particular, there should be a documented quality-assurance procedure for cell washers, e.g. using the National Institute for Biological Standards and Control (NIBSC) anti-D standard (Phillips *et al.*, 1993).

2.2.3 Staff training and proficiency

1   There must be a documented programme for training laboratory staff, which covers all SOPs in use and which fulfils the documented requirements of the laboratory.

2   Laboratory tasks should only be undertaken by appropriately trained staff.

3   There must be a documented programme for assessing staff proficiency, e.g. replicate testing for the IAT, which should include details of the action limits for retraining (Voak *et al.*, 1988).

2.2.4 Auditing and reviewing practice

1   There should be a system in place for documenting and reviewing all incidents of non-compliance with procedures. All serious incidents of non-compliance, near misses and adverse transfusion reactions should be reviewed by the hospital transfusion committee.

There should be a mechanism for reporting the adverse effects of transfusion to the consultant haematologist.

2   The systems should enable a full audit trail of laboratory steps, including the original results, interpretations, authorizations and all staff responsible for conducting each step.

3   A programme of independent audits should be conducted to assess compliance with documented 'in-house' laboratory procedures.

3 Samples/documentation

3.1 Introduction

The majority of ABO-incompatible transfusions are due to clerical/documentation/identification errors (Sazama, 1990).

3.2 Written/electronic requests

Transfusions must be prescribed by a medical officer. It is essential that the request form and sample contain the following minimum patient identification (PIN), as described in BCSH (1991a): (i) surname (correctly spelt); (ii) first name(s); (iii) date of birth (not age or year of birth); and (iv) hospital number/accident and emergency number. The sample should be labelled and signed by the person taking it. A local SOP should be in place for the procedure for dealing with inadequately labelled samples.

Information concerning the sex of the patient and obstetric and recent transfusion history should be obtained, wherever possible, and is essential when there are anomalous pretransfusion testing results. Requests should also include the date and time required, the number or volume and type of components required, the reason for the request and any other specific requirements relating to the patient or request.

Addressograph labels are more likely to result in inadequate checking of PIN at the bedside and it is therefore recommended that these are not accepted for grouping or pretransfusion testing samples. Electronic ward requesting should comply with all the same minimum standards mentioned above in this section.

Samples received from trauma or unconscious accident-and-emergency patients are unlikely to contain the full PIN. There must, however, be at least one unique identifier, usually an accident-and-emergency or trauma number and the sex of the patient. The sample should be taken and labelled and the form and sample signed by the prescribing medical officer as one continuous procedure.

In the event of there not being at least one unique identifier on the sample in a life-threatening situation, group O blood only must be issued until a suitably labelled sample is available. If the patient is a premenopausal female, group O RhD-negative blood should be given.

3.3 Telephone requests

There should be a policy for documenting telephone requests. The use of a telephone request pad is recommended. Requests must be made by a medical officer or delegated

Table 10.2 Timing of sample collection in relation to previous transfusions

Patient transfused within	Sample to be taken
3 to 14 days	24 h before transfusion
14 to 28 days	72 h before transfusion
28 days to 3 months	1 week before transfusion

individual. The identity of the person or people initiating and making the request should be documented. The following minimum information must be given and confirmed: (i) surname; (ii) forename; (iii) hospital/accident-and-emergency number/trauma number; (iv) location; (v) number/volume and type of product; (vi) reason for request; and (vii) date and time required.

3.4 Duplicate records

Duplicate patient records must be avoided; otherwise, essential transfusion or antibody history may be overlooked. It is therefore necessary, at the time of the request, to identify and link separate records that exist for each patient.

If a computer system is in use, the user must be alerted at the entry of a request that there are existing records for patients with the same name and date of birth. If a computer system is not in use, manual records need to be checked by name and date of birth for previous encounters.

3.5 Sample requirements

Clotted or ethylenediaminetetra-acetic acid (EDTA) samples may be used for pretransfusion testing. If a change in protocol is made from the use of serum to that of plasma, appropriate validation, using weak examples of antibodies, must be performed to ensure that the detection of clinically significant antibodies is not compromised.

3.6 Timing of sample collection in relation to previous transfusions

Transfusion or pregnancy may cause either a primary or secondary immune response, and samples selected for cross-matching or antibody screening must take account of this, so that any newly developed antibodies are detected. It is also important to note that any component containing residual red cells can elicit an immune response.

In situations in which patients are being repeatedly transfused, it is not necessary to require a daily sample. These patients should be screened for the development of irregular antibodies at least every 72 h.

If a transfusion has been given more than 72 h previously, a new sample is required in accordance with Table 10.2. It is recognized that for some individuals, e.g. thalassaemic patients who are repeatedly transfused and who have not had an antibody response, a more tolerant approach may be taken.

Table 10.3 Suggested storage limits for pretransfusion testing

	18–25°C	4°C	–30°C
EDTA whole blood	Up to 48 h	Up to 7 days	n/a
Separated plasma/serum	n/a	Up to 7 days	6 months

n/a, not applicable.

If there is no history of pregnancy or transfusion during the previous 6 months, stored plasma or serum may be used for cross-matching. Storage conditions will determine the length of storage (see Section 3.7).

It is recognized that there may be a problem obtaining samples from pregnant women – for example, when they are booked for elective Caesarean section, but may not arrive in the hospital until shortly before surgery. As immunization is more likely to occur during the last trimester of pregnancy, samples used for pretransfusion testing should never be more than 7 days old. Where possible, it is advisable that a sample taken immediately before transfusion is also available for retrospective testing in the event of a transfusion reaction occurring.

3.7 Storage of samples

Whole-blood samples will deteriorate over a period of time. Problems associated with storage include red-cell lysis, loss of complement in serum and decrease in potency of red-cell antibodies, particularly immunoglobulin M (IgM) antibodies and bacterial contamination.

There is a paucity of evidence concerning the use of stored samples for pretransfusion testing. Laboratories may wish to evaluate the stability of weak antibodies before making their local recommendations for storage conditions. However, Table 10.3 gives suggested working limits.

4 ABO and rhesus-D grouping

4.1 Introduction

Samples must be grouped for ABO and Rh D using a validated technique (see also Section 3.6). Testing of patient's red cells against blood grouping reagents and of patient's plasma/serum against known reagent red cells (reverse group) should be performed, wherever possible, to determine the ABO group of all patients over 6 months of age.

4.2 ABO grouping

Patient's red cells should be tested against monoclonal anti-A and anti-B blood-grouping reagents (see Section 4.8).

Patient's plasma or serum should be tested against A_1 and B reagent red cells. The reverse group should include a negative control, e.g. patient's own cells or group O cells, to exclude reactions with A and B cells due to cold antibodies in the patient's sample other than anti-A or anti-B. To prevent misinterpretation of results due to haemolysis where

Table 10.4 Positive and negative controls

Reagent	Positive control cells	Negative control cells
Anti-A	A	B
Anti-B	B	A
Anti-D	Rh D-positive	Rh D-negative

serum is used, it is recommended that the diluent used for resuspension of reverse-grouping cells contains EDTA (see Section 8.3.1).

4.3 Rh D grouping

Each sample must be tested in duplicate with IgM monoclonal anti-D blood-grouping reagents, which should not detect D^{VI}. The antiglobulin test should not be used for Rh D grouping.

4.4 Controls

Positive and negative controls must be included with each batch of tests, as shown in Table 10.4. A reagent control should be used where recommended by the manufacturer.

4.5 Interpretation of results

4.5.1 Manual reading

Documentation errors may occur during the manual reading and interpretation of ABO and Rh D groups. The risk of error can be minimized by separating the procedure into distinct tasks and, wherever possible, using different members of staff to perform each task. Suggested options for achieving this are: (i) separating the documentation of reaction patterns from the final interpretation; and (ii) separating the interpretation and documentation of the cell and reverse groups.

4.5.2 Automated reading

Automated readers are frequently used to interpret individual reactions and reaction patterns, when using microplate or microcolumn techniques. The system must be validated against manual systems prior to routine use.

In the absence of a fully automated system (e.g. where there is no integrated bar-code reader), procedures, including double-checking of samples and plates or cards, should be in place to prevent misidentification.

A visual inspection of results is still necessary when using automated readers that are unable to interpret mixed-field reactions.

4.6 Verification of results

The ABO and Rh D group must, wherever possible, be verified against previous results for the patient. Any discrepancies must be resolved prior to transfusion of red cells or red-cell contaminated components.

4.7 Grouping anomalies

The following are all examples of blood-group anomalies.

4.7.1 Cold autoantibodies

See Section 4.2.

4.7.2 Acquired B

Some anti-B reagents may react strongly with the acquired B antigen. This usually leads to a discrepancy between cell and reverse groups. If, however, the patient's own anti-B is only weakly detectable, an incorrect interpretation may result. Particular care must be taken if an antiglobulin test is not performed as part of the cross-match.

4.7.3 Unexpected mixed-field reactions

Any samples showing mixed-field reactions must be repeated and/or investigated prior to group authorization or issue of red cells.

4.7.4 Partial or weak D

See Section 4.9.

4.7.5 Intrauterine transfusions

For a period of several months post delivery, neonates who have received intrauterine transfusion may appear to be the same ABO and RhD group as that of the transfused red cells, due to bone-marrow suppression.

4.8 Repeating ABO and Rh D grouping

ABO and Rh D groups must be repeated when a discrepancy is found. Repeats should be performed using washed cells. To prevent the perpetuation of mistakes, the cells used should be taken from the original sample, rather than from a suspension made previously. An autocontrol should be included.

Repeatably anomalous results should be referred to a senior person in the laboratory. It may also be necessary to obtain a fresh sample and refer to a reference laboratory.

If it is not possible to obtain a reliable reverse-grouping result, due to the age of the patient or to insufficient sample, and there is no historical group against which to validate, the cell group must be repeated. Where verification checks against historical results reveal a discrepancy, a further sample must be obtained and tested immediately.

4.9 Partial and weak D

It is important to note that monoclonal anti-D reagents vary widely in their ability to detect both partial and weak D. It may be helpful to use reagents that give similar reactions. Where there is a discrepancy in typing, the patient should be treated as Rh D-negative until the D status is resolved. The sample may need to be sent to a reference laboratory for investigation.

Patients with a known partial D status should be regarded as Rh D-negative. Patients with a weak D status may be regarded as Rh D-positive.

Patients of category D^{VI} status are those most likely to make anti-D; reagents used for Rh D grouping of patients must not detect category D^{VI}.

4.10 Infants
It is important to distinguish cord samples from maternal samples to prevent mistyping.

4.11 ABO/Rh D grouping in urgent situations
When blood or blood products are required urgently, there may be insufficient time for routine ABO/Rh D grouping prior to selection of blood products. Emergency groups performed in these circumstances must include a test against anti-A, anti-B and anti-D, with appropriate controls or a reverse group. The result must be documented, and it must be confirmed as soon as possible by routine methods, if these differ from emergency procedures.

5 Antibody screening

5.1 Introduction
Antibody screening undertaken in advance of the requirement to provide blood for transfusion alerts the clinician to possible delay in the supply of compatible blood if the antibody screen is positive. It also provides the laboratory with time to identify irregular antibodies and select suitable units.

Antibody screening may be more reliable and sensitive than cross-matching against donor red cells and it is therefore recommended that antibody screening should be performed in all pretransfusion testing (see also Section 5.3).

5.2 Choice of techniques

5.2.1 Indirect antiglobulin test
The IAT, using red cells suspended in low-ionic-strength saline (LISS), is considered to be the most suitable for the detection of clinically significant antibodies, because of its speed, sensitivity and specificity. Liquid-phase tube and microplate, and solid-phase microplate and microcolumn ('column agglutination') antiglobulin methods have all been shown to be reliable. The use of normal-ionic-strength techniques (NISS) requires a minimum incubation time of 45 min and is therefore not recommended, but may be useful when particular problems with LISS are encountered – for example, when LISS-dependent autoantibodies are present or there are other non-specific reactions (see Section 6.3.3).

5.2.2 Antibody screening using the indirect antiglobulin test alone
Since IAT methods can detect almost all clinically significant antibodies, it is acceptable to use an IAT for pretransfusion antibody screening without any additional screening technique. The use of an unsupported IAT should only be implemented if: (i) the laboratory has implemented a documented programme for the assessment of worker proficiency in the IAT method; (ii) the laboratory has implemented a documented programme of replicate

testing to assure the efficacy of cell washers; (iii) the IAT method has been properly valid-ated against the documented requirements of the laboratory; and (iv) the laboratory has performed consistently well in the National External Quality Assessment Scheme (NEQAS) exercises using different workers and the IAT method in use.

A fully automated screening IAT method, including positive sample identification at the sampling and reading stages, provides a valuable additional security check if a single antibody-screening method is used. It should be recognized that non-automated methods are more liable to human error.

5.2.3 Additional techniques

Additional techniques, such as two-stage enzyme and Polybrene methods, may be used. However, it must be realized that these methods are unable to detect with an adequate level of sensitivity as wide a range of specificities as the IAT is capable of, and proficiency in the performance in the IAT is therefore of overriding importance.

References for these methods will be found in Mollison *et al.* (1993) and Scott *et al.* (1994).

5.3 Reagent red cells for use in antibody screening

Antibody screening provides the laboratory with the most reliable and sensitive method of detecting an irregular red-cell antibody. Cross-match methods using red cells from donor units are often less reliable, because the expression of blood-group antigens varies accord-ing to genotype; for example, the homozygous genotype Jk^aJk^a often results in a higher expression of the Jk^a antigen than the heterozygous genotype Jk^aJk^b. In addition, red cells for antibody screening should be preserved in a medium shown to minimize loss of blood-group antigens during the recommended storage period. For these reasons, an antiglobulin cross-match using donor cells is not the most effective way of detecting a serological incompatibility between patient and donor.

The specification for red cells suitable for use in antibody screening are summarized below.

1   The following antigens should be expressed: C, c, D, E, e, K, k, Fy^a, Fy^b, Jk^a, Jk^b, S, s, M, N, P_1, Le^a, Le^b. Reagent red cells should not be pooled.

2   At least one of the reagent red-cell samples should express the probable haplotype R_2.

3   Apparent homozygous expression of the following, in the stated order of priority, is desirable: D, c, Fy^a, Jk^a, Jk^b, S, s, Fy^b.

It is essential that, if an antiglobulin cross-match against donor red cells has been omitted, the sensitivity of the antibody screening system in use is at least equivalent to that obtained with a LISS-spin IAT test using reagent red cells having homozygous expression of all the antigens listed in **3**.

5.4 Autologous controls

An autologous control or direct antiglobulin test (DAT) need not form a part of antibody screening.

6 Antibody identification

When an irregular antibody is detected in the screening procedure, its specificity should be determined and its clinical significance assessed. If the patient is known to have a red-cell antibody, the serum/plasma should be checked on each occasion of testing to exclude the development of further alloantibodies.

A blood sample should be referred to a red-cell reference laboratory if there is any doubt concerning the identity of the antibody/ies present or lack of exclusion of clinically significant antibodies. Laboratories that are not registered for antibody identification in NEQAS should refer all sera that have given positive results in the antibody screen to a laboratory which is registered for antibody identification.

It is important to recognize the limitations of the panel in use. A single panel may be unable to identify some common combinations of antibodies, and the use of a second panel is strongly recommended for laboratories which do not refer samples to a reference laboratory, so that additional antibodies of clinical significance can be excluded.

6.1 Principles of antibody identification

The patient's serum should be tested by an appropriate technique against an identification panel of reagent red cells. As a starting-point, the technique by which the antibody was detected during screening should be used. Inclusion of the patient's own red cells may be helpful – for example, in the recognition of an antibody directed against a high-frequency antigen.

The specificity of the antibody should only be assigned when it is reactive with at least two examples of reagent red cells carrying the antigen and non-reactive with at least two examples of reagent red cells lacking the antigen. When one antibody specificity has been identified, it is essential that the presence of additional clinically significant antibodies has not been missed. Multiple antibodies can only be confirmed by choosing cells that are antigen-negative for the recognized specificity but positive for other antigens to which clinically significant antibodies may arise.

The use of additional techniques – for example, enzyme and low-temperature saline techniques – may be helpful in antibody identification, particularly when an antibody weakly reactive by the antiglobulin technique or a mixture of antibodies is present. The use of mono-specific antiglobulin reagents in place of a polyspecific reagent is beneficial when determining the presence of IgG antibodies in serum samples containing complement-binding antibodies.

Although most antibodies detectable only by an enzyme technique are unlikely to be of clinical significance, specific antibodies should not be ignored unless procedural errors in the antiglobulin test have been ruled out. This can be best achieved by retesting the serum/plasma against homozygous cells by an antiglobulin technique. The patient's red cells should be phenotyped using antiserum of appropriate specificity. The incorporation of a reagent control or AB serum control used by the same technique as the phenotyping serum is particularly important. A positive DAT will invalidate test results.

6.2 Reagent red cells for use in antibody identification

Specifications for suitable red cells for use in antibody identification are summarized below.

1 The panel should permit confident identification of those clinically significant alloantibodies which are most frequently encountered – for example, anti-D, anti-E, anti-c, anti-K and anti-Fy^a.

2 A distinct pattern of reactivity should be apparent for each of the commonly encountered alloantibodies.

3 The antigenic profile of the reagent red cells should, as far as possible, permit assignment of specificity in test sera containing more than one commonly encountered alloantibody – for example, anti-D + K.

Minimum characteristics are as follows.

1 One individual should be R_1R_1 and one $R_1{}^wR_1$. Between them, these two individuals should express the antigens: K, k, Fy^a, Fy^b, Jk^a, Jk^b, S, s.

2 One individual should be R_2R_2 and one r′r.

3 A minimum of four individuals should lack the Rh antigens C and D. One of these individuals should be K^+ and one should be E^+. Between them, these individuals should exhibit apparent homozygous expression of: c, k, Fy^a, Fy^b, Jk^a, Jk^b, S, s.

6.3 Autoantibodies

Many autoantibodies cause no clinical problems. In patients with autoimmune haemolytic anaemia (AIHA), autoantibodies directed against red-cell antigens are responsible for shortening red-cell survival, which may lead to severe anaemia. Serological investigations in AIHA should focus on the determination of the correct ABO and RhD group of the patient and determination of the presence of alloantibody. Autoantibody may 'mask' the presence of underlying alloantibody. It may be necessary to refer cases of AIHA to a red-cell reference laboratory, in view of the complexity of the investigations required.

Selection of blood for transfusion may be influenced by the presence of an autoantibody of 'simple' specificity, but extensive investigations to determine complex specificities of autoantibodies are rarely of value.

6.3.1 Cold-type autoimmune haemolytic anaemia or cold haemagglutinin disease

The red cells from the patient should be washed at 37°C for performing the DAT. The red cells from the patient will usually have a strongly positive DAT, due to coating with complement (C3d) components.

Reagent controls are particularly important when phenotyping the patient's red cells or performing the DAT, because of the possibility of autoagglutination.

It is important to exclude the presence of alloantibodies, using cells and serum separately prewarmed to 37°C; the use of anti-IgG in place of polyspecific antiglobulin reagent may also be helpful when serum, not plasma, is used. It should be noted that some antibodies of apparently clear-cut specificity – for example, anti-M – may be auto in nature.

6.3.2 *Warm-type autoimmune haemolytic anaemia*
The red cells from the patient will usually have a positive DAT, due to coating with IgG and sometimes complement components.

Phenotyping of the patient's red cells can only be performed using IgM or chemically modified IgG (complete) saline-reactive antisera. Reagent controls are essential. Immunoglobulin G antibody may be removed from the red cells by, for example, treatment with chloroquine diphosphate; however, results should be interpreted with caution, as antigens can be removed or destroyed (Edwards *et al.*, 1982).

Autoabsorption
Autoabsorption, using the patient's red cells, may be necessary to permit the recognition of underlying alloantibody. Removal of autoantibody from the patient's red cells and enzyme treatment of the cells improves the efficiency of autoabsorption and may be performed in a single stage, using the ZZAP method (Branch & Petz, 1982).

In some circumstances, autoabsorption may be difficult or undesirable (e.g. following a recent transfusion). Absorption with red cells which are Rh-identical, K– and, if possible, Fy^{a-} and Jk^{a-} should allow the exclusion of most antibodies of clinical significance. If a more complete phenotype of the patient's red cells is known, as close a match as possible for the absorbing red cells should be used.

6.3.3 '*LISS-dependent antibodies*'
Some sera/plasma will be found to contain an antibody, usually of no particular specificity, which reacts with red cells suspended in LISS but not in NISS. These antibodies may be directly agglutinating and are usually complement-binding. If plasma is used, subsequent serological work may be performed using NISS; if serum is used, anti-IgG should replace the polyspecific antiglobulin reagent.

7 Cross-matching

7.1 Introduction
The cross-match is defined in this chapter as a procedure to exclude incompatibility between donor and recipient. This may include serological tests or electronic cross-matching (see Section 7.4.3).

7.2 Selection of blood
Red-cell components of the same ABO and RhD group as the patient must be selected, whenever possible. If ABO-identical blood is not available, group O blood may be used, provided it is plasma-depleted or does not contain high-titre haemagglutinins. Group AB blood should be used for AB patients, but, if it is not available, group A or B red cells may be used.

When supplies of Rh D-negative blood are limited, Rh D-positive blood may be selected for Rh D-negative recipients. It is important that Rh D-positive cellular components should not be issued to Rh D-negative premenopausal females.

7.2.1 Patients with clinically significant red-cell antibodies

Blood should be selected which has been tested and found negative for the relevant antigen. If the antibodies are not clinically significant, it is not necessary to select antigen-negative blood (see Section 1.3).

7.2.2 Patients with autoimmune haemolytic anaemia

Except in emergency situations, patients should be investigated for the presence of alloantibodies, as in Section 6.3. It is unacceptable simply to cross-match and issue blood as compatible as the patient's own cells and serum.

7.2.3 Massive blood transfusion

Where the volume of blood transfused in any 24-h period is equivalent to the patient's own blood volume, ABO-group-identical blood can be issued without further serological testing. The laboratory staff must assure themselves of the validity of the ABO and RhD group of the donor blood. If ABO non-identical blood has to be transfused, blood of the same group as the patient should be used as soon as possible. There is no need to persist with the ABO group originally transfused.

7.2.4 Fetal/neonatal transfusions (BCSH, 1994)

Fetal transfusion

Blood should be cross-matched against the maternal serum/plasma; this should include an indirect antiglobulin test if the maternal serum/plasma contains clinically significant red-cell antibodies. The blood should be less than 5 days old, group O, of high haematocrit (0.55–0.75), cytomegalovirus (CMV)-negative and irradiated.

Neonatal exchange transfusion

If group O blood is selected irrespective of the baby's ABO group, the laboratory should seek assurance that high-titre anti-AB in the donation has been excluded. The blood should be used within 5 days of collection.

Neonatal top-up transfusion

In the absence of atypical maternal antibodies, blood may be given without prior cross-matching.

7.2.5 Sickle-cell disease

The incidence of alloimmunization in multiply transfused sickle-cell anaemia patients varies from about 10% in children to 50% is some adult populations, with a general range of

20–30% (Ness, 1994). It is desirable to phenotype sickle-cell patients as fully as possible prior to transfusion and to match for K, C and E antigens before the onset of alloimmunization. Other extended antigen matching may be required.

7.2.6 Chronically transfused patients

In contrast to patients with sickle-cell disease, other groups requiring chronic transfusion are not at excessive risk of alloimmunization, and phenotyping and antigen matching are not necessary.

7.2.7 Recipients of allogeneic haemopoietic stem-cell grafts

Recipients of allogeneic transplants present unusual grouping and cross-matching problems. The transplant may introduce a new ABO antigen (major mismatch) or a new ABO antibody (minor mismatch) or both. All cellular products should be irradiated to prevent graft-versus-host disease (BCSH, 1996).

Major ABO mismatch

Red cells should be of the patient's own ABO group until recipient ABO group is no longer detectable and the DAT is negative.

Minor ABO mismatch

Red cells should be of donor ABO group and plasma depleted until the original recipient red cells are no longer detectable.

Combined ABO mismatch

Red cells should be group O until recipient ABO group is no longer detectable.

Rh D-positive recipient with Rh D-negative donation or graft

Rh D-negative components should be transfused.

7.3 Procedure

It is preferable for one person to carry out the cross-matching procedure from beginning to end. Where this is not possible, there should be written auditable procedures to establish staff accountability.

7.3.1 Immediate-spin cross-match

The immediate-spin cross-match must not be used alone: (i) if the patient's serum/plasma contains or has been known to contain clinically significant antibodies; (ii) if the antibody-screening test does not conform to the recommendations in Section 5; (iii) if ABO grouping reveals macroscopically undetectable anti-A or anti-B, except in group AB patients; and (iv) except in emergency situations (see Section 7.3.4).

A short incubation time of 2–5 min before centrifugation is recommended to enhance the detection of weak ABO antibodies. The use of EDTA saline is recommended to overcome the potential problem of prozone if serum is used (Judd *et al.*, 1988).

7.3.2 Indirect antiglobulin test cross-match

A cross-match which includes an IAT must be used if: (i) the patient's plasma/serum contains or has been known to contain clinically significant red-cell alloantibodies; (ii) the antibody screen does not conform to the recommendations in Section 5; (iii) ABO grouping reveals macroscopically undetectable anti-A or anti-B, except in group AB patients; (iv) the patient has had an ABO-incompatible solid-organ transplant and is being transfused within 3 months of the transplant; this is necessary to detect IgG anti-A or anti-B produced by passenger lymphocytes in the transplanted organ.

7.3.3 Computer issue without a serological cross-match

A cautionary approach must be taken before considering the implementation of this innovation. See Appendix 10.2 for minimum recommendations.

7.3.4 Emergency situations

A correctly labelled blood sample must be obtained from the patient. If a correctly labelled sample is not immediately available and blood is required because of a life-threatening situation, group O blood must be issued. If the patient is a premenopausal female, group O Rh D-negative blood must be given.

The sample should be ABO- and Rh D-grouped by rapid techniques. Blood of appropriate ABO and Rh D group may be issued after completion of a reverse group, repeat cell group or immediate-spin cross-match. The laboratory must assure themselves of the validity of the ABO and Rh D group of the donor blood. This will require written verification from the supplying blood-transfusion centre or confirmatory testing within the hospital's laboratory.

An antibody screen should be performed as soon as possible. If this is negative, it is not necessary to carry out a retrospective IAT cross-match.

7.4 The compatibility report

A compatibility report must be issued before or with the first unit of blood. Information should include the location of the laboratory, the patient's surname, first name, hospital number, date of birth, ward and blood group of the patient and the donation number and blood group.

If standard pretransfusion testing has not been carried out, this should be stated in the report. The report may be used as a record in the patient's notes that pretransfusion testing has not been carried out in full.

7.4.1 The compatibility label

There must be a compatibility label, which should be securely attached to the blood bag. Information should include the patient's surname, first name, hospital number, donation number and group, and the date the blood is required/cross-matched.

7.5 Visual inspection of the red cell unit

Before the unit is placed in the blood-issue refrigerator, it should be inspected for: (i) integrity of the pack, by checking for leaks at the ports and seams; (ii) evidence of haemolysis in the plasma or at the interface between the plasma and red cells; (iii) evidence of discoloration of the red cells; and (iv) presence of large clots in the pack.

If there is any evidence of the above, the unit should not be used and should be returned to the issuing blood-transfusion centre.

Removal of blood from the issue refrigerator should be in accordance with a written procedure.

8 Techniques

8.1 Introduction

As new techniques are continually evolving, it is not possible to provide a comprehensive list of recommended methods. Users of new technologies should follow the manufacturer's instructions and should refer to the current BCSH guidelines (BCSH, 1995). Guidance for microplate methods may be found in the BCSH (1991c).

Particular emphasis must be placed on the interpretation of weak reactions when establishing or reviewing a procedure and during training, so that inconsistency is minimized. This must then be consolidated by ongoing quality assurance for staff, equipment and reagents (see Section 2).

8.2 Antiglobulin techniques

For the method, see Appendix 10.1.

Monospecific anti-IgG may be used in place of polyspecific anti-human globulin (AHG) for the LISS IAT, because of the higher sensitivity of the LISS IAT methods and because of the increased, undesirable susceptibility of these methods to interference from low-thermal-optimum and LISS-dependent antibodies, which are complement-binding. Polyspecific antiglobulin reagent confers no advantage over monospecific anti-IgG if plasma is used for antibody screening. However, it is important that screening cells having homozygous expression of *Jk*^{a} can be guaranteed by the supplier before a decision is taken to use anti-IgG in place of polyspecific antiglobulin reagent.

Immunoglobulin G-sensitized control red cells for the techniques above should be added to all negative tests to confirm the efficacy of the washing stage. In order to be fully effective, the level of IgG sensitization should be limited to that which gives a macroscopically negative result after the addition of 0.1% v/v serum in saline to the antiglobulin reagent.

8.3 Solutions

For phosphate-buffered saline (PBS), normal saline and LISS solutions, reference should be made to the *Guidelines for the Blood Transfusion Services in the United Kingdom* (Department of Health, 1996).

8.3.1 Ethylenediaminetetra-acetic acid for diluents

For the stock solution, prepare a 0.1 mol/l solution of EDTA (dipotassium salt) in distilled water; adjust the pH to 7.0, using 5 mol/l sodium hydroxide (NaOH). For the working solution, mix one volume of stock solution with nine volumes of saline or LISS. Check the pH and adjust to 7.0, if necessary.

Appendix 10.1: Methods for the antiglobulin technique

	Technique used	
	LISS tube	NISS tube
Serum: cell suspension ratio*	2 : 2	4 : 1
Red-cell concentration	1.5–2%	2–3%
Incubation time (min)	15–60	45–90
No. of saline washes	4	4
Volume of antiglobulin reagent	70–100 µl	70–100 µl
Centrifugation time/speed	In-house validation or as recommended by the manufacturer	
Reading method	Tip and roll	Tip and roll

* Total volume of serum should not exceed 200 µl. It may be helpful to use a reading aid, such as a hand lens, microscope or concave mirror, to assist in the interpretation of test results obtained in liquid-phase tube and microplate methods.

Appendix 10.2: Minimum recommendations for computer issue without a serological cross-match

Computer systems should not be considered for detecting an ABO mismatch unless the consultant responsible for the blood transfusion laboratory has ensured that the following minimum recommendations are met.

1 An automated system for ABO and Rh D grouping and antibody screening, including positive sample identification and electronic data transfer of results, is in place.

2 The antibody screening procedure conforms to the recommendations in Section 5.

3 The patient's plasma/serum does not or has not been known to contain clinically significant red-cell alloantibodies.

4 Computer software is validated to ensure that the criteria in **5** are met.

5 The release of ABO-incompatible blood must be prevented by conformation of the system to the following requirements.

(a) The issue of blood is not allowed if there is only one ABO and Rh D group on file.

(b) The issue of blood is not allowed if the current blood group does not match the historical record on file.

(c) The historical results of ABO, Rh D and antibody screening must not be displayed when manual entry of current results is made.

(d) The system must not permit the reservation and release of red-cell units that are ABO-incompatible with the ABO group of the patient.

6 The laboratory must assure the validity of the ABO and Rh D group of the donor blood. This will require written verification from the supplying blood transfusion centre or confirmatory testing within the hospital laboratory.

References

BCSH (1991a) Hospital blood bank documentation and procedures. In Roberts B. (ed.) *Standard Haematology Practice*, pp. 128–138. Blackwell Scientific Publications, Oxford.

BCSH (1991b) Compatibility testing in hospital blood banks. In Roberts B. (ed.) *Standard Haematology Practice*, pp. 150–163. Blackwell Scientific Publications, Oxford.

BCSH (1991c) Microplate techniques in liquid phase blood grouping and antibody screening. In Roberts B. (ed.) *Standard Haematology Practice*, pp. 164–188. Blackwell Scientific Publications, Oxford.

BCSH (1994) Guidelines for administration of blood products: transfusion of infants and neonates. *Transfusion Medicine* **4**, 63–69.

BCSH (1995) Guidelines for evaluation, validation and implementation of new techniques for blood grouping, antibody screening and crossmatching. *Transfusion Medicine* **5**, 145–150.

BCSH (1996) Guidelines on gamma irradiation of blood components for the prevention of transfusion-associated graft-versus-host disease. *Transfusion Medicine* **6**, 261–271.

Branch D.R. & Petz L.D. (1982) A new reagent (ZZAP) having multiple applications in immunohematology. *American Journal of Clinical Pathology* **78**, 161–167.

Department of Health (1996) *Guidelines for the Blood Transfusion Services in the United Kingdom*. HMSO, London.

Edwards J.M., Moulds J.J. & Judd W.J. (1982) Chloroquine dissociation of antigen–antibody complexes: a new technique for typing red blood cells with a positive direct antiglobulin test. *Transfusion* **22**, 59–61.

Judd W.J., Steiner E.A., O'Donnell D.B. & Oberman H.A. (1988) Discrepancies in reverse ABO typing due to prozone: how safe is the immediate-spin crossmatch? *Transfusion* **28**, 334–338.

Mollison P.L., Engelfriet C.O. & Contreras M. (1997) *Blood Transfusion in Clinical Medicine*, 10th edn. Blackwell Science, Oxford.

Ness P.M. (1994) To match or not to match: the question for chronically transfused patients with sickle cell anaemia. *Transfusion* **34**, 558–560.

Phillips P.K., Voak D., Whitton C.M., Downie D.M., Bebbington C. & Campbell G. (1993) BCSH–NIBSC anti-D reference reagent for antiglobulin tests: the in-house assessment of red cell washing centrifuges and of operator variability in the detection of weak, macroscopic agglutination. *Transfusion Medicine* **3**, 143–148.

Sazama K. (1990) Reports of 355 transfusion-associated deaths: 1976 through 1985. *Transfusion* **30**, 583–590.

Scott M., Voak D., Phillips P.K., Hoppe P.A. & Kochman S.A. (1994) Review of the problems involved in using enzymes in blood group serology – provision of freeze dried ICSH/ISBT protease enzyme and anti-D reference standards. *Vox Sanguinis* **67**, 89–98.

Voak D. (1992) Validation of new technology for antibody detection by antiglobulin tests. *Transfusion Medicine* **2**, 177–179.

Voak D., Downie D.M., Moore B.P.L., Ford D.S., Engelfriet C.P. & Case J. (1988) Replicate tests for the detection and correction of errors in anti-human globulin (AHG) tests: optimum conditions and quality control. *Haematologia* **21**, 3–16.

11 Recommendations for Evaluation, Validation and Implementation of New Techniques for Blood Grouping, Antibody Screening and Cross-matching
Prepared by the Blood Transfusion Task Force

1 Introduction

Several new systems and technologies for blood typing, antibody screening and compatibility testing have recently become available to transfusion laboratories. These systems are no longer dependent on agglutination of red cells in suspension as the assay signal, instead utilizing, for example, the pattern of red cells in a matrix after centrifugation, the pattern of red cells adhering to a plastic microwell, the particle-size analysis of red cells as they pass sensors during centrifugation or the absorbance of a chromogenic enzyme substrate. The methodologies employed and technical considerations for optimal performance with these systems can be widely divergent from those in conventional haemagglutination assays.

Laboratories look to new techniques to help improve aspects of performance, such as turn-round times, or to cope with increased workloads in the absence of a corresponding increase in resources. These new techniques must be shown to be better than, or at least as good as, existing techniques when they are in routine use. The problem, therefore, is how to evaluate a new methodology and what testing is required to validate it before introducing it into routine use.

Laboratories may use different approaches to evaluate new technology systems. For example, various contradictory publications on the relative sensitivity of the gel test for antibody detection have appeared as a result of different laboratories' evaluations (Bromilow et al., 1991; Voak et al., 1991; Phillips et al., 1992). It is difficult to compare the results reported by the different laboratories, as different approaches and techniques have been used for the evaluations (Voak, 1992). This chapter proposes guidelines for such evaluations. It is hoped that, if all laboratories follow these guidelines, future results of evaluations reported by different laboratories will be more reasonably comparable.

It should be the responsibility of any reagent/kit manufacturer to have carried out sufficient field trials on an *in vitro* diagnostic product to ensure that their product at least meets minimum requirements before marketing that product. In the USA, manufacturers of *in vitro* diagnostic reagents and kits have to satisfy the Food and Drug Administration (FDA) of the product's quality and efficacy before they are licensed to sell the product to

Reprinted with permission from *Transfusion Medicine*, 1995, **5**, 145–150.

US laboratories for routine use. A laboratory in the USA buying an FDA-licensed product can therefore have confidence that the product meets FDA requirements. However, FDA-licensed manufacturers do not need to meet FDA requirements for US-manufactured products sold outside the USA. In the UK, there are currently no regulations, procedures or guidelines (except for the UK Blood Transfusion Service (BTS) guidelines referred to in the next paragraph) in force that define the field-trial procedures and minimum requirements a manufacturer should meet, other than general laws and regulations relating to product liability, electrical safety, etc. The Medical Devices Directorate of the Department of Health has funded (via the British Committee for Standards in Haematology (BCSH)) an evaluation of new techniques for antibody detection in compatibility tests (Voak *et al.*, 1995); there is also currently a draft European Community directive relating to the future regulation of *in vitro* diagnostic medical devices, which is likely to come into operation in January 2000. Although most *in vitro* diagnostic devices would be covered by self-certification, the current proposal is that blood-grouping reagents ABO Rh (CčD, Eč) and Kell reagent products, as well as those for the detection of human immunodeficiency virus (HIV), hepatitis B and C, should be in the stricter category (Annex 2, list A), which will require third-party (independent) validation. However, there is currently no regulatory procedure in force in the UK. Without such regulation, manufacturers may also change the specification of their products, without validating this change by appropriate field trials or necessarily notifying their customers.

Guidelines for the UK BTS (1996) give the specifications, specificity and potency requirements for reagents produced by and for use within the UK BTS. The BCSH has produced guidelines (BCSH, 1991a, b) for hospital blood banks, including requirements for reagents used in routine testing. Both the above sets of guidelines are primarily concerned with the production and use of conventional liquid-phase reagents and techniques. These guidelines are intended to supplement the above with regard to specifications, quality control and validation of new technology systems.

These guidelines have been written to advise laboratories how to evaluate and validate a new system for routine use. They are not intended to substitute for the rigorous evaluation and clinical trials that a manufacturer should undertake in the development of a product. Laboratories considering the use of a new system should assure themselves that the manufacturer's trials and validations have been adequately undertaken. Manufacturers should be able to provide details of their evaluations, field trials and previous evaluations by other independent laboratories.

Evaluation and validation of new techniques by user laboratories is important to protect the interests of both the user laboratories and the patients they are serving. Not all laboratories will find it necessary to undertake full evaluations if suitable evaluations have already been carried out by other laboratories. They should use these guidelines to check that the evaluations that have been carried out are thorough and cover all aspects relating to their own laboratory's work. In addition to evaluation, it is recommended that all user laboratories should validate a new system for routine use by running it in parallel with the existing system of a minimum of 1 week's routine work.

2 General guidelines on evaluation procedures

Where a new system is being evaluated, the workers concerned should spend some time familiarizing themselves with the new system and identifying which parts of the procedure are most critical, e.g. the importance of mixing in microtube techniques, delay prior to mixing or the type of washing/centrifugation used in solid-phase systems and how they should be optimally performed. The manufacturer should include with every reagent/kit full instructions based around description, principle of test, specification, test procedure, limitations, quality control and health and safety information. Ideally, training should be given by the manufacturer, to make sure that the system being evaluated is being correctly used.

It is vital that the manufacturer's instructions are carefully followed. If a kit is being evaluated, all the component parts should be from one kit – reagents or components must not be substituted from other kits (even other kits from the same manufacturer) or in-house stocks. What seems a reasonable substitute reagent to the worker may not be if the manufacturer has used a specially modified reagent. A manufacturer may adjust the composition of the components of any one batch of a kit, so that the overall performance of the kit is equivalent to a previous batch; hence the performance of individual components of a kit may vary from batch to batch. No in-house modifications, such as diluting reagents, should be made, as any such amendment may invalidate the manufacturer's warranty and have product-liability implications.

In all cases, the performance of a new system should be compared with the current in-house system, using a range of samples and procedures designed to test for sensitivity, specificity (including freedom from false-positive reactions), reproducibility of results and robustness. Such test procedures are listed below in Sections 3, 4 and 5. Health and safety, legal and insurance implications, data capture security/efficiency and speed and ease of use should also be monitored and recorded. The staff skill level required to operate the system effectively should also be taken into consideration and reproducibility evaluated objectively by staff performing blind replicate tests on selected samples (Voak *et al.*, 1988). Overall cost-effectiveness should be assessed.

All samples which give rise to reproducible discrepant results between test systems should be investigated further and, if possible, samples should be referred to the manufacturer of the system under evaluation and an independent reference laboratory.

3 Evaluation of ABO and Rh D cell-grouping systems

Specific cells should be selected for testing to cover each category listed below which falls within the range of samples normally tested by the evaluating laboratory. Each category should include positive and negative samples for each specificity under test. For example, if samples coming to the laboratory are collected into different anticoagulants and/or supplied as clotted samples, the laboratory should test positive and negative cells for each specificity, collected in each of the relevant anticoagulants and without anticoagulant. If all samples received are always taken into one anticoagulant, assessment of different anticoagulants is not necessary. The concentration of cell suspensions used throughout should be assured.

All samples giving rise to discrepant results between the existing system and the new system under evaluation should be repeat-tested in both systems under the same conditions as originally tested to confirm the discrepancy, and then any repeatable discrepancy investigated further.

Types of red-cell samples to be considered in an evaluation are as follows.

1 Washed and unwashed red cells.

2 Red cells stored for different periods of time from venepuncture, to include donor cells close to expiry date.

3 Red cells stored in different storage media.

4 Red cells from blood collected into different anticoagulant solutions and/or from clotted samples.

5 Red cells from different patient groups, e.g. samples from neonates, geriatric patients, patients in different disease groups, haematology patients.

6 Red cells from persons from different ethnic groups.

7 Red cells negative for the antigen under test that have been sensitized with immunoglobulin G (IgG) antibody to give a strong positive direct antiglobulin test. (This is designed to see whether the system under test gives rise to false-positive reactions under these circumstances. The system under test may include control procedures to identify this phenomenon.)

8 Weak-phenotype red cells. For anti-A, this should be a minimum of three examples of A_2B cells (shown to be not H-deficient) and should also include three examples of a selected range of A_3 and A_x cells of known reactivity if the manufacturer claims detection of these weak phenotypes or if the laboratory currently expects to detect these.

For anti-B, this should be a minimum of three examples of A_1B cells.

For anti-D, this should be a minimum of three examples of R_1r cells and should also include three examples of $R_1^u r$ cells if the manufacturer claims detection of these weak phenotypes or if the laboratory currently expects to detect these.

Within a weak phenotype, a range of antigen-strength cells should be used, if possible, e.g. a high-, medium- and low-grade D^u. The weak-phenotype cells used should be well characterized or supplied by or checked by a reference laboratory. Procedures using thawed cells must not show lysis at the time of the test. Thawed cells showing lysis must be rewashed before use and suspended in 1–2% bovine serum albumin (BSA).

The robustness of a new system can be challenged by using the minimum and maximum requirements (e.g. incubation times and temperatures) suggested by the manufacturer. Blind replicate testing of weak-phenotype cells will give a good indication of the reproducibility of results obtained. If this is undertaken by staff representing the different skill levels within the laboratory, this will provide a further indicator of the robustness and reproducibility of the system.

4 Evaluation of antibody screening systems

Titration studies should be undertaken with at least one IgG anti-D, one IgG anti-Kell and one IgG anti-Fy^a. These should be weak, single-donor antibodies or, if available, national pooled standards for this purpose. The antibodies should have a macroscopic 1 + end-point titre of between 1/16 and 1/32 in the normal-ionic-strength saline (NISS) or low-ionic-strength saline (LISS) spin antiglobulin test, testing the anti-D with a pool of cells from four R$_1$r samples (or a pool of 10 random Rh D-positive donors), the anti-K with Kk cells and the anti-Fy^a with Fy(a + b+) cells. This will given an estimate of sensitivity and freedom from prozone-type effects.

Detection of a panel of weak clinically significant antibodies should be assessed. The panel should cover most of the major blood-group systems and contain examples of at least two specificities from each system. For the Rh system, the minimum of D, c and E specificities should be covered.

Assessments for false-positive reactions should be made with fresh ABO-compatible sera. Further samples should be tested which are known to contain antibodies that the laboratory does not consider clinically significant and does not wish to detect, e.g. cold-reactive antibodies, enzyme-only antibodies.

Specific weak-positive and inert sera should also be selected for testing, to cover each category listed below which falls within the range of samples normally tested and practice normally used by the evaluating laboratory.

1 Serum and plasma samples.
2 Samples separated and stored for various lengths of time at different temperatures after venepuncture.
3 Samples produced from whole blood by different methods, e.g. separated from clot.
4 Samples from different patient groups, e.g. neonatal samples, geriatric samples, disease groups, haematology patients.

Any samples giving rise to significantly discrepant results between the existing system and the new system under evaluation should be repeat-tested in both systems.

The robustness of a new system can be challenged by using the minimum and maximum requirements (e.g. incubation times and temperatures) suggested by the manufacturer. Blind replicate testing with known weak antibodies (giving + to + + reactions in an antiglobulin test) and inert sera will give a good indication of the reproducibility of results obtained. If this is undertaken by staff representing the different skill levels within the laboratory, this will provide a further indicator of the robustness and reproducibility of the system. Known reference materials should be included where available, e.g. UK BCSH–National Institute for Biological Standards and Control (NIBSC) reference weak anti-D 91/608 (used at 1/8), available from NIBSC (Phillips *et al.*, 1993).

If the manufacturer recommends that screening cells from other sources can be used in their system, both the manufacturer's screening cells and the alternative source cells should be tested in parallel in the new system.

In all instances, the manufacturer of a system should state the minimum specification of the screening cells/membranes used, in terms of the zygosity within the major blood-group systems. Each batch should be accompanied by a package insert showing the specification of the screening cells/membranes used in that batch. If possible, a batch with the minimum-specification cells should be used for evaluation. This approach may not be possible with all new systems, particularly those where the screening cells are supplied as membranes already attached to a solid phase.

5 Evaluation of cross-matching systems

Cross-matching systems should be evaluated as above (Section 4), except that the red cells used should be selected to cover the range and type of red-cell samples normally tested and show heterozygous expression of each of the antigens corresponding to the antibody specificity of the serum samples being tested.

6 Documentation of evaluations

A 'Materials and methods' section should cover the following points.
1   The type of samples tested, and how many in each category.
2   The dates of testing.
3   The grade and competence (as assessed by objective blind replicate testing with 91/608 reference anti-D[10]) of the personnel undertaking the tests.
4   The details of all reagents used (including those made in-house) and, where relevant, their batch numbers and expiry dates.
5   Full details of the standard technique against which the new system has been compared.
6   Full details of variable conditions used, e.g. temperature and duration of incubation stages, rcf, acceleration/deceleration rates and duration of centrifugation stages.
7   Details of equipment used.
8   Details of the reading method used, including cut-off levels, where appropriate.
    A 'Results' section should record and tabulate all the data obtained, including reactions of positive and negative control samples.
    A 'Summary' section should tabulate the numbers of samples tested in each category and the number and type of discrepant results obtained.
    A 'Discussion' section should summarize and discuss the possible reasons for all repeatable discrepancies between the systems tested. Comments should be recorded on aspects such as the following.
1   User-friendliness.
2   Robustness.
3   Cost-effectiveness (including details of the cost-analysis method used).
4   Staff skill levels required.
5   Additional resources required.
6   Training implications.

7 Space implications.

8 Availability of new product/system.

9 Shelf-life of new product/system, including performance at the end of the stated shelf-life.

10 Suitability for different types of use (such as bulk processing of batched samples or one-off emergencies).

11 Availability of automation.

12 Security of data capture and handling.

13 Ease of maintenance of equipment.

14 Health and safety aspects, including electrical safety.

Any relevant weaknesses highlighted in an evaluation and any suggestions for improvements to a system should be notified to the manufacturers. If the manufacturer responds and supplies a modified version for retesting, this should be noted in the report.

Evaluations should be logged with the BCSH Evaluation Group and the Blood Bank Technology Special Interest Group of the British Blood Transfusion Society (BBTS). This latter group will undertake collation of reports and make them available on request. Publication rights of all data and reports remain with the authors, unless they have entered into a specific contract for the evaluation that decrees otherwise.

7 Validation

In addition to evaluation, a system should be validated by all laboratories for routine use by parallel testing of the equivalent of a minimum of 1 week's routine samples in the proposed new system and the existing system. Procedures and results should be fully documented as above.

If a laboratory can satisfy itself that sufficient evaluation of a new system has already been carried out in laboratories with a routine environment similar to its own, then the above validation can be carried out without the necessity for a full evaluation.

8 Implementation

Before implementing a new system into routine use, laboratories should ensure that all staff using the new system are fully trained and conversant with the critical procedures involved and that a standard operating procedure (SOP) is written. Blind replicate testing (Voak *et al.*, 1988), with critical samples at regular intervals, is essential to assess and monitor the performance of the new system and the staff operating it.

References

BCSH (1991a) Compatibility testing in hospital blood banks. In Roberts B. (ed.) *Standard Haematology Practice*, pp. 150–163. Blackwell Scientific Publications, Oxford.

BCSH (1991b) Microplate techniques in liquid-phase blood grouping and antibody screening. In Roberts B. (ed.) *Standard Haematology Practice*, pp. 164–188. Blackwell Scientific Publications, Oxford.

Bromilow K.E., Adams J., Hope J., Eggington J.A. & Duguid J.K.M. (1991) Evaluation of the ID-Gel test for anti-body screening and identification. *Transfusion Medicine* **1**, 159–161.

Phillips P.K., Whitton C.M. & Laven F. (1992) The use of the antiglobulin gel-test for antibody detection. *Transfusion Medicine* **2**, 111–114.

Phillips P.K., Voak D., Whitton C.M., Downie D.M., Bebbington C. & Campbell G. (1993) BCSH–NIBSC anti-D reference reagent for antiglobulin tests: the in-house assessment of red cell washing centrifuges and of operator variability in the detection of weak macroscopic agglutination. *Transfusion Medicine* **3**, 143–148.

UK BTS (1996) *Guidelines for the Blood Transfusion Services in the United Kingdom*, 3rd edn. HMSO, London.

Voak D. (1992) Validation of new technology for antibody detection by antiglobulin tests. *Transfusion Medicine* **2**, 177–179.

Voak D., Downie D.M., Moore B.P.L., Ford D.S., Engelfriet C.P. & Case J. (1988) Replicate tests for the detection and correction of errors in anti-human globulin (AHG) tests: optimum conditions and quality control. *Haematologia* **21**, 3–16.

Voak D., Downie D.M., Campbell G. & Tolliday B. (1991) Optimal specification of AHG and microplate IAT for antibody detection with greater sensitivity than the Diamed gel test. *Transfusion Medicine* **1** (Suppl. 2), 37.

Voak D., Phillips P.K., Scott M.L., Evans R.G. & Chapman J. (1996) *Evaluation of Six New Technology Kits for Antibody Detection*. Available from Department of Health, Medical Devices Directorate, Room 222, 14 Russell Square, London WC1B 5EP.

12 Guidelines on the Clinical Use of Leucocyte-depleted Blood Components
Prepared by the Blood Transfusion Task Force

Definition: Leucocyte-depleted blood components must contain $<5 \times 10^6$ leucocytes per unit (red cells) or adult therapeutic dose (platelets).

Practical aspects: To achieve residual leucocyte counts of $<5 \times 10^6$, leucocyte-depletion should be carried out under controlled conditions, ideally within 48 h from the collection of the donor unit. The preparation of leucocyte-depleted blood components should be subject to a quality monitoring programme designed to assure 100% compliance.

Indications for leucocyte-depleted blood components

RECOMMENDED

Febrile nonhaemolytic transfusion reactions (FNHTRs)

1   To prevent recurrent FNHTRs after red cell transfusions, buffy coat-depleted red cell concentrates should be used, if they are available, or alternatively red cell concentrates filtered at the bedside.

2   If FNHTRs continue despite these measures, leucocyte-depleted red cell concentrates should be used.

3   To prevent FNHTRs in patients likely to be dependent on long-term red cell support, the use of buffy-coat-depleted or bedside filtered red cell concentrates should be considered from the outset of transfusion support.

4   The routine use of pooled platelets derived from buffy coats is associated with a low incidence of FNHTRs. The use of platelet concentrates leucocyte-depleted prior to storage is recommended for patients with reactions despite the use of such components. Bedside filtration of platelet concentrates is not recommended for the prevention of FNHTRs associated with platelet transfusions.

Reducing graft rejection after haemopoietic cell transplantation: Patients with severe aplastic anaemia who are potential haemopoietic cell transplant recipients should receive leucocyte-depleted blood components from the beginning of transfusion support. The same might apply to patients with haemoglobinopathies, but more evidence is required before a definite recommendation can be made.

Prevention of transmission of viral infections by blood transfusion: Leucocyte-depletion of blood components is an effective alternative to the use of CMV-seronegative

Reprinted with permission from *Transfusion Medicine*, 1998, **8**, 59–71.

blood components for the prevention of transfusion-transmitted CMV infection to at risk patients.

Fetal/neonatal transfusions: Leucocyte-depleted blood components should be used for intrauterine transfusions and for all transfusions to infants below 1 year of age.

POSSIBLE

Platelet refractoriness: There is currently no convincing evidence that routine leucocyte-depletion of blood components produces clinical benefits for patients receiving multiple platelet transfusions, although HLA alloimmunization and platelet refractoriness are reduced.

Kidney transplants: Pretransplant blood transfusion may confer some benefit to renal transplant recipients, although some patients will become alloimmunized leading to difficulties in the selection of donor kidneys. Consideration should be given to the leucocyte-depletion of transfusions to renal transplant patients to prevent HLA alloimmunization unless they are part of a deliberate pretransplant immunosuppression protocol.

Immunomodulation: There is insufficient evidence to recommend the routine use of leucocyte-depleted blood components for surgical patients for the prevention of either post-operative infection or tumour recurrence.

Progression of HIV infection: There is insufficient evidence to recommend the use of leucocyte-depleted blood components for reducing the progression of HIV infection.

NON-INDICATIONS. A significant number of recipients of blood components receive a limited number of transfusions over a short period of time, e.g. most general medical and surgical patients. Leucocyte-depletion of blood components is not indicated for these recipients unless there is an additional acceptable indication discussed in one of the other sections in this guideline. Prevention of transfusion-associated graft-vs.-host disease (TA-GvHD) is not an indication for leucocyte-depleted blood components. Gamma-irradiation of blood components is the standard method for avoiding TA-GvHD. There is no need to leucocyte-deplete non-cellular blood components such as fresh frozen plasma, cryoprecipitate and blood products prepared from pooled plasma.

1 Introduction

The presence of leucocytes in blood components is responsible for many of the complications associated with blood transfusion (Bordin *et al.*, 1994). Patients receiving standard red cell and platelet concentrates receive large numbers of allogeneic leucocytes, which are transfused without any intention of producing clinical benefit. There has been considerable interest in the removal of leucocytes from blood components, and this guideline is primarily intended to provide advice regarding the clinical indications for leucocyte-depleted red cell and platelet concentrates.

It is important to define what is meant by leucocyte-depletion. Some confusion is caused by the use of rather meaningless terms such as 'leuco-reduced', 'leuco-poor' and even 'leuco-free'. 'Leucocyte-depleted' is the accepted term for red cell and platelet concentrates that have been produced by technologies designed to yield low levels of leucocytes, and it has been accurately defined by national and international working groups. A

Table 12.1 Specifications of red cell and platelet components (derived from UK BTS/NIBSC, 1997)

	Red cells		
	Red cells/red cells in OAS*	Red cells in OAS, buffy coat-removed	Red cells/red cells in OAS, leucocyte-depleted
Vol. (mL)	$280 \pm 60/350 \pm 70$	280 ± 60	Locally specified volume ranges†
Hct	$0.55-0.75/0.50-0.70$	$0.50-0.70$	$0.55-0.75/0.50-0.70$
WBC per unit	$>2 \times 10^9$	$<1.2 \times 10^9*$	$<5 \times 10^6$

	Platelets			
	Derived from platelet-rich plasma (PRP)	Platelets, pooled, buffy coat-derived (BCD)	Apheresis	Leucocyte-depleted‡
Donors/adult dose	5	4	1	4 or 1
Vol. (mL)	Locally defined	Locally defined	Locally defined	Locally defined
Platelets ($\times 10^{11}$)	>2.75	>2.4	>2.4	>2.4
WBC/dose	$<10^9$	$<10^8*$	$<0.8 \times 10^9*$	$<5 \times 10^6$

* The leucocyte levels for buffy coat-removed red cells and both BCD and apheresis platelets are often lower than shown. Refer to your supplying blood centre for details.

† Leucocyte-depletion by filtration generally results in the loss of 20–30 mL red cells.

‡ Can be produced from PRP, BCD or apheresis platelets.

OAS, optimal additive solution (SAG-M or equivalent); Hct, haematocrit; WBC, white blood cell count.

leucocyte-depleted red cell concentrate is one containing $<5 \times 10^6$ leucocytes per unit, and an adult dose of leucocyte-depleted platelets is one containing $<5 \times 10^6$ leucocytes (UK BTS/NIBSC, 1997).

The situation is further complicated by the increasing introduction in the UK of component processing involving removal of the buffy coat to yield red cell concentrates and pooled platelet concentrates. These components both contain numbers of leucocytes intermediate between standard and leucocyte-depleted components, and are useful in clinical situations where reduced leucocyte levels but not 'true' leucocyte-depletion is required. The leucocyte levels in the different components are shown in Table 12.1.

Definition: leucocyte-depleted blood components must contain $<5 \times 10^6$ leucocytes per unit (red cells) or adult therapeutic dose (platelets).

2 Practical aspects of leucocyte-depletion of blood components

2.1 Methods

Various techniques have been used for removing leucocytes from blood components, including centrifugation and freeze/thawing, but filtration has been and currently remains the most commonly used technique for leucocyte-depletion of blood components. Apheresis technology, which provides leucocyte-depleted platelet concentrates without any need for filtration or further processing, is now available.

Blood filters have developed in three distinct phases or generations. First generation filters are 170–240 µm screens, which are part of all red cell transfusion administration sets for the removal of large clots and particulate debris. Second generation 40-µm filters were designed to remove microaggregates of fibrin, platelets and leucocytes from red cell concentrates. These filters reduce the number of leucocytes by one order of magnitude (or log) to $5–10 \times 10^8$ per unit. Third generation filters were designed specifically for the removal of 'free' leucocytes. They retain both microaggregates and free cells; see the review by Dzik (1993) for the mechanisms of leucocyte removal by these filters and their design. The number of leucocytes in red cell and platelet concentrates can be reduced by three orders of magnitude (or 3 logs) to less than 5×10^6 per unit using third generation filters, and new filters producing even greater leucocyte-depletion are already in routine use.

Filtration can be carried out: (i) at the bedside during the transfusion; or (ii) in the components processing laboratory. The main issues determining which is preferable are the timing of leucocyte-depletion in relation to the biological changes of storage and the ability to guarantee quality assurance.

2.2 Timing of leucocyte-depletion

Leucocyte-depletion within a relatively short time after collection has the advantage that leucocytes are eliminated before they release cytokines, fragments of cell membrane and possibly intracellular viruses, which may not be removed by filtration carried out just prior to transfusion. A relationship has been shown between the age of platelet concentrates and the level of cytokines, such as interleukin-1 and 6 and tumour necrosis factor, and the quantity of leucocyte fragments. Cytokines have been implicated in the pathogenesis of febrile non-haemolytic transfusion reactions (FNHTRs), particularly after platelet transfusions (see Section 3.1), and there is experimental evidence that leucocyte fragments may play a role in primary human leucocyte antigen (HLA) alloimmunization (Blajchman *et al.*, 1992).

Standardized procedures are necessary for optimal performance of the filters, but it is difficult to ensure this at the bedside and laboratory-based methods are now favoured (Perkins, 1993; Popovsky, 1996). For maximum confidence in the consistency of the process, filtration carried out as part of component processing offers the possibility of quality monitoring and of control of the age of the product at the time of filtration.

Filtration is usually performed within 48 h of the collection of the donor unit, but the optimal timing should be validated for each filter. It is sometimes necessary to filter blood that has been stored for a longer period just prior to its issue for transfusion, e.g. when selected phenotype units are required.

It has been suggested that leucocyte-depletion should be carried out 6–8 h after collection of blood, to allow phagocytosis of any bacteria present in the red cell or platelet concentrate. However, there is no evidence that concentrates filtered earlier than this or apheresis units prepared as leucocyte-depleted have an increased risk of bacterial contamination. Appropriate microbiological monitoring should be carried out (UK BTS/NIBSC, 1997).

2.3 Quality assurance

The preparation of leucocyte-depleted blood components should be subject to quality assurance, including adequate training of staff and maintenance of standard operating procedures that control the age of the component and the temperature and duration of filtration.

Quality control to ensure adequate leucocyte-depletion can be carried out by measuring leucocyte counts on every concentrate prior to release for transfusion, but this is labour-intensive. It is equally acceptable to use statistical process control to ensure that the leucocyte-depletion procedure remains within pre-determined limits, set after initial validation of each filter or other technology (Dumont *et al.*, 1996). An effective quality assurance programme has not yet been devised to demonstrate the reliable performance of bedside filtration in achieving residual leucocyte levels of $<5 \times 10^6$.

Methods which may be used for counting residual leucocytes in leucocyte-depleted blood components are flow cytometry and large volume microscopic chambers, such as the Nageotte chamber (Rebulla & Dzik, 1994). Automated blood cell counters do not accurately estimate the low levels of leucocytes present in leucocyte-depleted blood components, but can provide the necessary quality control for buffy coat-depleted red cell concentrates.

2.4 Labelling and storage

Red cell and platelet concentrates may be labelled as 'leucocyte-depleted' when the leucocyte count has been determined to be $<5 \times 10^6$ by one of the methods discussed above. At present, a unit labelled as 'leucocyte-depleted' does not indicate the method used for leucocyte-depletion or when it was carried out in relation to the time of donation.

The shelf-life and storage characteristics of leucocyte-depleted blood components do not differ from standard preparations of the same component, provided that leucocyte-depletion was carried out as a 'closed' procedure, either with an integral filter or with a filter attached using a sterile connecting device.

Recommendations: to achieve residual leucocyte counts of $<5 \times 10^6$, leucocyte-depletion should be carried out under controlled conditions, ideally within 48 h of the collection of the donor unit. A quality monitoring programme should be used to confirm, either by counting of individual concentrates or by statistical methods, that each concentrate contains $<5 \times 10^6$ leucocytes.

3 Indications for leucocyte-depleted blood components

3.1 Febrile non-haemolytic transfusion reactions

Febrile non-haemolytic transfusion reactions (FNHTRs) have been reported to occur with an incidence of 6.8% after red cell and 37.5% after platelet transfusions (Heddle *et al.*, 1993). However, the pathogenesis of FNHTRs following red cell and platelet transfusions is different, and different strategies for prevention are appropriate.

3.1.1 Associated with red cell transfusions

Human leucocyte antigen (HLA) alloimmunization is probably the major cause of severe FNHTR to red cells. However, FNHTRs after red cell transfusions are not always due to HLA antibodies, and reactions do not always recur. It is only considered necessary to use red cell concentrates with reduced levels of leucocytes for patients having recurrent (i.e. two or more consecutive) FNHTRs (Consensus Conference, 1993).

Leucocyte-depletion to $<5 \times 10^6$ leucocytes per unit is not usually necessary to prevent FNHTRs; a reduction in the number of leucocytes to 5×10^8 leucocytes per unit is sufficient in most cases. This can be achieved most cost-effectively using buffy coat-depleted red cell concentrates, if they are available, or by filtration at the bedside. Leucocyte-depleted blood components may be reserved for patients in whom FNHTRs persist despite the use of buffy coat-depleted red cell concentrates or bedside filtration. Microaggregate (40 μm) filtration, sometimes combined with cooling and centrifugation of the blood prior to filtration, can also prevent FNHTRs, but other methods for the prevention of FNHTRs have superseded this technique and it is not recommended.

Leucocyte-depleted red cell concentrates are effective in the prevention of FNHTRs in patients dependent on long-term transfusion support, e.g. patients with β-thalassaemia major (Sirchia & Rebulla, 1994). It could be argued that the development of FNHTRs could be awaited before switching to leucocyte-depleted red cell concentrates, but it is generally agreed that patients requiring long-term red cell support should receive red cell concentrates with leucocyte levels $<5 \times 10^8$ to prevent FNHTRs (Consensus Conference, 1993). This level of leucocyte-reduction can generally be achieved with buffy coat-depleted red cell concentrates. The benefits are best documented for patients with β-thalassaemia major, but other patient groups requiring long-term red cell support, such as those with chronic aplastic anaemia, myelodysplasia, sickle cell disease and the anaemia of chronic renal failure (unresponsive to treatment with recombinant erythropoietin), may also benefit (Consensus Conference, 1993; see Sections 3.7.1 and 3.7.4).

3.1.2 Associated with platelet transfusions

There is increasing evidence that the major cause of FNHTRs after platelet transfusions is the presence of pyrogenic cytokines released from leucocytes during the 5 days of platelet storage (Muylle *et al.*, 1993). A role for such cytokines or other mediators is supported by the observation that most FNHTRs after platelet transfusions are caused by the transfused plasma (Heddle *et al.*, 1994).

FNHTRs after platelet transfusions are not reliably prevented by bedside filtration of platelet concentrates, because of cytokine release during storage (Goodnough *et al.*, 1993). Increases in cytokine levels during storage have not been found in platelet concentrates prepared from pooled buffy coats, in concentrates prepared from platelet-rich plasma and leucocyte-depleted before storage or in concentrates prepared using modern apheresis technology to contain a low level of leucocytes (Muylle & Peetermans, 1994; Wadhwa *et al.*, 1996).

The routine use of pooled platelets derived from buffy coats is associated with a low rate (3.8%) of FNHTRs (Anderson *et al.*, 1997). For patients having reactions despite the use of this product, the transfusion of platelet concentrates leucocyte-depleted prior to storage is recommended.

Recommendations:

1 For the prevention of recurrent FNHTRs after red cell transfusions, the use of buffy coat-depleted red cell concentrates is recommended, if they are available, or bedside filtered red cell concentrates, if they are not.

2 For patients who continue to have FNHTRs after red cell transfusions despite the use of buffy coat-depleted or bedside filtered red cell concentrates, leucocyte depletion of red cell concentrates to $<5 \times 10^6$ leucocytes per unit is recommended.

3 For patients who are likely to be dependent on long-term red cell support, the use of buffy coat-depleted or bedside filtered red cell concentrates should be considered from the outset of transfusion support, for the prevention of FNHTRs.

4 The routine use of pooled platelets derived from buffy coats is associated with a low rate of FNHTRs. The use of platelet concentrates leucocyte-depleted prior to storage is recommended for patients with reactions despite the use of such components. Bedside filtration of platelet concentrates is not recommended for the prevention of FNHTRs associated with platelet transfusions.

3.2 Platelet refractoriness

3.2.1 Definition

Platelet refractoriness is the repeated failure to obtain satisfactory responses to platelet transfusions. It is a common problem in patients receiving multiple transfusions (Slichter, 1990). Various methods are used to assess responses to prophylactic platelet transfusions (BCSH, 1992). In practice, an increase in the patient's platelet count of less than $20 \times 10^9/l$ at 20–24 h after the transfusion is often used as a simple measure of a poor response (BCSH, 1992).

3.2.2 Causes

Many causes of platelet refractoriness have been described, and they can be subdivided into immune mechanisms, most importantly HLA alloimmunization, and non-immune platelet consumption associated with clinical factors, such as fever and/or septicaemia, bleeding, disseminated intravascular coagulation and splenomegaly (Slichter, 1990).

Recent evidence suggests that non-immune platelet consumption may be the most frequent mechanism of platelet refractoriness (Doughty *et al.*, 1994). However, immune-mediated platelet destruction remains an important and potentially more readily preventable cause, but it follows from these observations that the prevention of HLA alloimmunization will not eliminate platelet refractoriness.

The precise mechanism of HLA alloimmunization remains uncertain. It was postulated that primary HLA alloimmunization was only initiated by intact cells expressing both HLA class I and class II antigens. Such cells include lymphocytes and antigen-presenting cells. Platelets only express HLA class I antigens, providing the rationale for the use of leucocyte-depleted blood components for the prevention of HLA alloimunization and platelet refractoriness.

3.2.3 Prevention

Leucocyte-depletion of blood components
The development of HLA alloimmunization is dependent on the dose of leucocytes transfused, with the critical level being about 5×10^6 per transfusion (Fisher *et al.*, 1985). The risk of HLA alloimmunization has also been shown to be related to the patient's previous history of blood transfusions and pregnancies. A report of patients with bone marrow failure, mostly with haematological malignancies, supported with red cell and platelet concentrates leucocyte-depleted before storage found a very low level of HLA alloimmunization (3%) in patients with a negative history of previous transfusions or pregnancies, in comparison with a level of 31% in patients who had been previously transfused or pregnant (Novotny *et al.*, 1995).

There is controversy concerning the effectiveness of leucocyte-depletion of blood components for the prevention of HLA alloimmunization in patients who may have been sensitized by previous transfusions or pregnancies. In one study, the incidence of HLA immunization in patients with a history of previous pregnancies or transfusions was not reduced by leucocyte-depletion of blood components (Sintnicolaas *et al.*, 1995). It is possible that, in presensitized patients, the threshold for a secondary immune response may be considerably lower than 5×10^6 leucocytes and only achieved by a much greater degree of leucocyte depletion, but even this may not be sufficient, as it is possible that recipient memory B cells may be activated by the HLA class I antigens present on platelets (Claas *et al.*, 1981). However, in contrast to the study of Sintnicolaas *et al.* (1995), the Trial to Reduce Alloimmunization to Platelets (TRAP) Study Group (1997) found that leucocyte-depletion of blood components resulted in a reduction in HLA alloimmunization in previously pregnant women from 62% to 32%.

Trials comparing leucocyte-depleted against standard blood components for the prevention of HLA alloimmunization and platelet refractoriness have usually enrolled small numbers of patients. Three of the five prospective randomized controlled studies failed to show a statistically significant reduction in alloimmunization or platelet refractoriness (reviewed by Heddle, 1994). Moreover, these measures are often taken as surrogate markers for presumed clinical benefits, which remain unproved. Further prospective controlled trials are required to compare costs and clinical outcome in patients who receive leucocyte-depleted vs. standard products. Positive outcomes would include reduced morbidity and mortality due to clinical bleeding, reduced use of red cell and platelet concentrates and fewer patients requiring HLA-matched or crossmatch-compatible platelet transfusions. The main negative factor is the cost of providing leucocyte-depleted blood components.

A retrospective study of patients with acute leukaemia suggested that leucocyte-depletion of blood components had a beneficial effect on haemopoietic recovery after chemotherapy, use of blood components, occurrence of serious infections and relapse-free survival (Oksanen & Elonen, 1993), but these effects have not been found by others (Copplestone *et al.*, 1995). A cost-effectiveness analysis suggested that the use of leucocyte-depleted blood components would not increase the cost of transfusion support in patients with acute leukaemia (Balducci *et al.*, 1993), but the assumptions on which this conclusion was based were criticized (Perkins, 1993).

These studies emphasize the need for large randomized controlled studies of the benefits of prevention of platelet refractoriness by leucocyte-depletion of blood components and its cost-effectiveness. In the USA, the large multicentre TRAP study (TRAP Study Group, 1997) compared the incidence of platelet refractoriness due to HLA alloimmunization in a control group receiving pooled platelet-rich plasma (PRP)-derived platelet concentrates and three other groups of patients with acute myeloblastic leukaemia, given: (i) pooled PRP-derived platelet concentrates irradiated with ultraviolet-B light; (ii) leucocyte-depleted, pooled PRP-derived platelet concentrates; and (iii) leucocyte-depleted apheresis platelet concentrates during remission induction therapy. The study showed a significant reduction in HLA alloimmunization and platelet refractoriness in the three treatment groups compared with the control group. However, the incidence of major bleeding was <1% in all groups, and the study failed to demonstrate any clear clinical benefits in the treatment groups.

Irradiation of platelet concentrates with ultraviolet-B light
Available evidence suggests that inactivation of specialized, potent, antigen-presenting cells, such as dendritic cells, by irradiation with ultraviolet-B light may prevent recipient alloimmunization (Pamphilon & Blundell, 1992). In two recent clinical transfusion studies using platelet concentrates irradiated with ultraviolet-B light, alloimmunization was reduced, but the reduction was not statistically significant (Andreu *et al.*, 1993; Blundell *et al.*, 1996). The TRAP Study Group (1997) demonstrated a significant reduction in HLA alloimmunization and platelet refractoriness compared with the control group, but there was no clear clinical benefit.

Recommendation: there is currently no convincing evidence that routine leucocyte-depletion of blood components produces clinical benefits for patients receiving multiple platelet transfusions, although HLA alloimmunization and platelet refractoriness may be reduced.

3.3 Prevention of transmission of viral infections by blood transfusion

3.3.1 Cytomegalovirus
Transfusion-transmitted cytomegalovirus (CMV) infection may cause significant morbidity and mortality in immunocompromised CMV-seronegative patients. The use of blood components from CMV-seronegative donors has been the standard method for the prevention of

transmission of CMV by blood transfusion (see reviews by Sayers *et al.*, 1992; Hillyer *et al.*, 1994; Goldman & Delage, 1995). Patients for whom the risk of transfusion-transmitted CMV infection is well established include CMV-seronegative pregnant women, premature infants (<1.2 kg) born to CMV-seronegative women, CMV-seronegative recipients of allogeneic bone-marrow transplants from CMV-seronegative donors and CMV-seronegative patients with the acquired immunodeficiency syndrome (Sayers *et al.*, 1992).

The use of CMV-seronegative blood components has been shown to reduce the incidence of CMV infection in at risk groups to a level of about 1–3%, but transfusion-transmitted CMV infection is not completely prevented (Hillyer *et al.*, 1994; Goldman & Delage, 1995). This incomplete prevention of transmission of CMV may be due to the occasional failure to detect low level antibodies, the loss of antibodies in previously infected donors and the transfusion of components prepared from recently infected donors.

Cytomegalovirus (CMV) is transmitted by leucocytes, and there has been interest in the potential for leucocyte-depletion of blood components to prevent CMV transmission. A number of studies found that leucocyte-depletion of blood components was successful in preventing transfusion-transmitted CMV infection in neonates, acute leukaemia and bone marrow transplant patients (Hillyer *et al.*, 1994; Goldman & Delage, 1995). Furthermore, a recent prospective randomized study found that leucocyte-depletion using bedside filtration was as effective as the use of CMV-seronegative blood components in bone marrow transplant patients (Bowden *et al.*, 1995). However, in view of concerns about the quality control of leucocyte-depletion carried out by bedside filtration, blood components leucocyte-depleted under controlled, validated conditions are to be recommended in preference to bedside filtration as a substitute for CMV-seronegative blood components.

Recommendations: leucocyte-depletion of blood components is an effective alternative to the use of CMV-seronegative blood components for the prevention of transfusion-transmitted CMV infection to at risk patients. Whether leucocyte-depleted or CMV-seronegative blood components are used in individual patients depends on factors such as the cost and availability of each type of blood component and whether leucocyte-depleted blood components will be used anyway to prevent another complication of blood transfusion.

3.3.2 Human T-cell leukaemia/lymphoma virus types I and II
Human T-cell leukaemia/lymphoma virus types I and II (HTLV-I and II) target T lymphocytes and are solely transmitted by cellular blood components (reviewed by Sandler *et al.*, 1991). The minimum infective dose of lymphocytes is unknown, but there are epidemiological and experimental data to suggest that it might be very low. There is no clinical or laboratory evidence that leucocyte-depletion of blood components to currently achievable levels will significantly protect against HTLV infection.

3.3.3 Other viral infections
Leucocyte-depletion of blood components is not an option for preventing transmission of viruses present in plasma, including human immunodeficiency virus (HIV) 1 and 2, hepatitis B and C and parvovirus B19.

3.4 Immunomodulation

Ever since observations were made of the favourable effect of transfusion on survival of subsequent renal allografts, the basis of transfusion-induced immunomodulation has been the subject of debate. Many investigators have attempted to examine the influence of transfusion on putative clinical effects of immunomodulation, such as postoperative infection and tumour recurrence, but the findings have been conflicting. It has often been assumed that allogeneic leucocytes are required for this effect, but there are very few studies in which leucocyte-depleted blood has been formally compared with standard components.

3.4.1 Postoperative infection

In a study of colorectal cancer patients, the postoperative infection rate was increased in patients receiving whole blood transfusions compared with non-transfused patients, but patients receiving leucocyte-depleted red cell concentrates had the same incidence of infection as non-transfused patients (Jensen *et al.*, 1992). However, there were conflicting results from two randomized studies comparing postoperative infection rates in patients receiving leucocyte-depleted or buffy coat-depleted red cell concentrates; one study found no difference (Houbiers *et al.*, 1994) and one found a significantly lower incidence in the patients receiving leucocyte-depleted blood (Jensen *et al.*, 1996).

A recent analysis of trials in this area, albeit before publication of the study by Jensen *et al.* (1996), concluded that any transfusion effect on infection was small and that leucocyte depletion did not confer any convincing benefit over other components (Vamvakas, 1996). Further analysis, including the study of Jensen *et al.* (1996), agreed that no definite conclusion could be drawn at the present time (Blajchman, 1997).

3.4.2 Cancer recurrence

Retrospective observational studies of cancer patients are conflicting as to whether tumour-free survival is influenced by transfusion, with almost equal numbers for and against the hypothesis (Vamvakas & Moore, 1993). There was no difference in tumour-free survival when leucocyte-depleted and buffy coat-depleted red cell concentrates were compared in patients with colonic cancer (Houbiers *et al.*, 1994).

In acute myeloblastic leukaemia, an improved relapse-free survival was found in one study of patients receiving leucocyte-depleted blood components (Oksanen & Elonen, 1993), but other studies have not demonstrated such a beneficial effect (Copplestone *et al.*, 1995).

Recommendation: there is insufficient evidence to recommend the routine use of leucocyte-depleted blood components for surgical patients for the prevention of either postoperative infection or tumour recurrence.

3.5 Reactivation of latent viral infections

3.5.1 Cytomegalovirus

Herpes viruses, such as CMV, cause latent infection and may become reactivated after an immunological stimulus, such as transfusion or co-culture with allogeneic cells (Olding *et al.*, 1975). This may be relevant in pregnancy, where blood transfusion might reactivate maternal CMV infection, which could be transmitted to the fetus, with potentially serious clinical sequelae (Sayers *et al.*, 1992).

In addition to the use of CMV-seronegative or leucocyte-depleted blood components to prevent transmission of CMV to CMV-seronegative pregnant women (see Section 3.3.1), it could be argued that CMV-seropositive pregnant women should receive leucocyte-depleted blood components to prevent reactivation of latent CMV infection, although there are no published data suggesting that reactivation of CMV infection due to allogeneic transfusion is a major problem. One possible way of combining these two recommendations would be to use leucocyte-depleted blood components for all transfusions to women during pregnancy, and this would standardize transfusion practice for all women during pregnancy. An alternative standard approach, which is less expensive, is the use of CMV-seronegative blood components for all transfusions to pregnant women, both CMV-seronegative and CMV-seropositive.

Recommendation: leucocyte-depleted blood components may be used as an alternative to CMV-seronegative blood components to prevent transfusion-transmitted CMV infection to CMV-seronegative women during pregnancy. To standardize transfusion practice for all pregnant women, consideration could be given to the use of leucocyte-depleted blood components or CMV-seronegative blood components for all transfusions in pregnancy.

3.5.2 Human immunodeficiency virus

Increased HIV secretion may be induced in HIV-infected cells *in vitro* by allogeneic leucocytes but not by red cells, platelets or plasma (Busch *et al.*, 1992). Two retrospective studies provided evidence that transfused patients with HIV infection have a worse outcome than non-transfused patients (Vamvakas & Kaplan, 1993; Sloand *et al.*, 1994). While some centres already use leucocyte-depleted blood components to avoid any possible additive immunosuppressive effect of transfusion in patients with HIV infection, further evidence from prospective studies is needed before a definite recommendation can be made. A multicentre randomized trial of standard and leucocyte-depleted blood components in HIV-infected patients is in progress in the USA – the Viral Activation Transfusion Study (VATS) (Busch *et al.*, 1996).

Recommendation: in patients with HIV infection, there is insufficient evidence to recommend the use of leucocyte-depleted blood components for the prevention of the reactivation of CMV infection or the progression of HIV infection.

3.6 Avoidance of sensitization to transplantation antigens in potential transplant recipients

Sensitization to transplantation antigens by preceding blood transfusions has been shown to have an adverse effect in patients with aplastic anaemia undergoing bone marrow transplantation and in renal transplant patients. Sensitization to transplantation antigens can potentially be prevented by leucocyte-depletion of pretransplant transfusions, and this issue will be discussed in the following section on the use of leucocyte-depleted blood components in specific patient groups.

3.7 Use of leucocyte-depleted blood components in some specific patient groups not already considered

3.7.1 Severe aplastic anaemia

Preceding blood transfusions have been found to increase the risk of graft rejection in patients with aplastic anaemia (Anasetti *et al.*, 1986). This led to the practice of avoiding pretransplant transfusions, particularly from the marrow donor and other family members. Studies in an animal model showed that leucocyte depletion of pretransplant transfusions significantly reduced the incidence of graft rejection (Storb *et al.*, 1979), although these results have not been confirmed in human studies.

Recommendation: patients with severe aplastic anaemia who are potential haemopoietic cell transplant recipients should receive leucocyte-depleted blood components from the beginning of transfusion support to minimize the risk of graft rejection.

3.7.2 Haemopoietic cell transplantation for patients with haematological malignancies

Graft rejection following haemopoietic cell transplantation is less of a problem in patients with haematological malignancies, compared with those with aplastic anaemia. There is no evidence that prevention of sensitization to transplantation antigens is important in patients with acute leukaemia who are potential recipients of allogeneic transplants, although it has been recommended that family member transfusions are avoided (Slichter, 1988).

Recommendation: leucocyte-depleted blood components are not indicated for patients undergoing transplantation for haematological malignancies, other than as a substitute for CMV-seronegative blood components for patients who are CMV-seronegative and who are potential recipients of an allogeneic transplant.

3.7.3 Haemoglobinopathies

Patients with β-thalassaemia major and patients with sickle cell anaemia requiring long-term transfusion support should receive leucocyte-depleted blood components to prevent FNHTRs (see Section 3.1). A recent study found allograft rejection in 4/22 patients undergoing bone marrow transplantation for sickle cell disease (Walters *et al.*, 1996). This high level of graft rejection could be due to transfusion-induced alloimmunization, which could potentially be prevented by leucocyte-depletion of pretransplant transfusions, as in aplastic anaemia.

Recommendation: buffy coat-depleted or bedside filtered red cell concentrates are recommended for the prevention of FNHTRs in patients with haemoglobinopathies requiring long-term transfusion support. Consideration could be given to the use of leucocyte-depleted blood components for patients with sickle cell disease or β-thalassaemia major who are potential candidates for haemopoietic cell transplantation to reduce the risk of graft rejection.

3.7.4 Solid organ transplant recipients

Kidney transplants

A number of factors affect graft survival, including the underlying renal disease, the age, sex and race of the patient, the immunosuppressive drug regimen employed, the degree of HLA mismatching and the use of pretransplant blood transfusions (Blajchman & Singal, 1989). Opelz *et al.* (1973) reported that graft survival was better in transfused patients, irrespective of matching for HLA-A, B or DR antigens. The mechanism of the 'transfusion effect' was poorly understood, but it seemed to be due to transfused leucocytes.

The transfusion effect became less apparent following the introduction of cyclosporin for postgraft immunosuppression and improved patient management in the 1980s, although multicentre studies continue to show that transfused patients have a better outcome than non-transfused patients (Opelz *et al.*, 1997). However, many centres have switched their attention to the prevention of HLA alloimmunization caused by pretransplant transfusions, by using recombinant erythropoietin to avoid the need for transfusions and by the use of leucocyte-depleted blood components if transfusions are necessary. One attempt to preserve the immunosuppressive effect of transfusion without causing alloimmunization has involved careful selection of the donor of the transfused blood so that there is a common HLA haplotype or shared HLA-DR and HLA-B antigens (Lagaaij *et al.*, 1989; van Twuyver *et al.*, 1991).

Recommendation: pretransplant blood transfusion may confer some benefit to renal transplant recipients, although some patients will become alloimmunized, leading to difficulties in the selection of donor kidneys. Consideration should be given to the leucocyte-depletion of transfusions to renal transplant patients to prevent HLA alloimmunization, unless they are part of a deliberate pretransplant immunosuppression protocol. The additional advantage of the routine use of leucocyte-depleted blood components is that there is no need to provide CMV-seronegative blood components for CMV-seronegative patients whose kidney donors are also CMV-seronegative.

Liver transplants

Unlike allogeneic haemopoietic cell or renal transplantation, liver transplantation does not appear to require HLA matching or lymphocyte cross matching before transplantation

(Nusbacher, 1991), although there have been recent reports of a poorer outcome with positive lymphocyte cross matches (Takaya *et al.*, 1992; Katz *et al.*, 1994).

Recommendation: leucocyte-depleted blood components are not indicated, apart from as a substitute for CMV-seronegative blood components for CMV-seronegative patients whose donors are also CMV-seronegative.

Heart transplants

Graft survival is significantly influenced by HLA compatibility (Opelz & Wujciak, 1994). Evidence is increasing in support of prospective HLA matching, including lymphocyte cross matching in sensitized patients, in order to select well-matched recipients for cardiac transplantation (Morris, 1994). There is no information about the possible benefit of preventing HLA alloimmunization by leucocyte-depletion of pretransplant transfusions.

Recommendation: leucocyte-depleted blood components are not indicated, apart from as a substitute for CMV-seronegative blood components for CMV-seronegative patients whose donors are also CMV-seronegative.

3.7.5 Fetal/neonatal transfusions

Fetal/neonatal transfusions often consist of relatively fresh blood, containing viable leucocytes. There is consequently a high risk of transmission of leucocyte-associated viruses, such as CMV, which was considered in the British Committee for Standards in Haematology (BCSH) recommendations on the transfusion of infants and neonates (BCSH, 1994). There is also a theoretical risk of immunosuppression, for which the fetus/neonate may be at particular risk because of physiological immune incompetence, and HLA alloimmunization, which can occur in multiply transfused infants. The presence of fresh, viable lymphocytes may cause TA-GvHD, which can be prevented by gamma-irradiation of blood components, according to BCSH recommendations (BCSH, 1996).

Intrauterine transfusion of cellular blood components was included in the recommended indications for leucocyte-depletion of blood components (Consensus Conference, 1993), on the grounds of the potential long-term benefits and the limited costs of such a recommendation. The same approach could be taken for transfusions of both red cell and platelet concentrates to neonates. While it could be argued that definitive proof of benefit should be awaited in the perinatal group of patients, the potential to avoid theoretical long-term sequelae already exists, without a great increase in costs. Another working party recommended that leucocyte-depleted blood components should be used for infants below 3 months of age (Danish Society of Clinical Immunology, 1996), and the Department of Health has recently recommended that all transfusions to neonates and infants under 1 year of age should be leucocyte-depleted.

Recommendations: leucocyte-depleted blood components should be used for intrauterine transfusions and for all transfusions to infants below 1 year of age.

4 Non-indications for leucocyte-depleted blood components

1   A significant number of recipients of blood components receive a limited number of transfusions over a short period of time. These recipients include a large proportion of surgical patients, as well as medical and other groups of patients. Leucocyte-depletion of blood components is not appropriate in these recipients, unless there is an additional acceptable indication discussed in one of the previous sections in this guideline.

2   Prevention of TA-GvHD is not an indication for leucocyte-depleted blood components. Gamma-irradiation of blood components is the standard method for avoiding TA-GvHD (BCSH, 1996).

3   Transfusion-related acute lung injury (TRALI) is a rare complication of blood transfusion, in which the patient has a severe reaction, characterized by chills, fever, cough and dyspnoea (Popovsky *et al.*, 1992). The chest X-ray shows perihilar and lower-lobe nodular shadowing. It is believed to be due to preformed leucocyte antibodies in the plasma of the donors, most of whom are multiparous. Leucocyte-depletion of blood components would not be expected to prevent TRALI.

4   Fresh frozen plasma, cryoprecipitate and blood products prepared from pooled plasma are prepared to ensure minimum cellular contamination and are virtually free of cellular material. There is no indication to leucocyte-deplete these blood components and products.

5 Variant Creutzfeldt–Jakob disease

Classical Creutzfeldt–Jakob disease (CJD) is a rare disease with an annual incidence of approximately one case/million population. Most cases are spontaneous or familial, with iatrogenic cases associated with the use of pituitary-derived hormones, transplants of dura mater or cornea or contaminated neurosurgical instruments. There is no epidemiological evidence that classical CJD can be transmitted via blood components. However, individuals at particular risk of classical CJD are excluded from blood donation.

    Variant CJD (vCJD) was first identified in 1996, and is thought to have arisen from the ingestion of beef products contaminated with the agent responsible for bovine spongiform encephalopathy (BSE) in cattle. Over 20 cases have been identified to date, and they are clinically distinct from classical CJD. For example, the abnormal prion-related protein can be found in the tonsils and the spleen of patients with vCJD, but not in those with classical CJD. This raises the theoretical possibility that circulating lymphocytes might harbour the agent responsible for vCJD, leading to concerns that the disease could be transmitted via blood transfusion. Recent data have also highlighted the role of lymphocytes in the transport of the abnormal prion protein to the nervous system. However, no data are available on the likely transmissibility of vCJD by blood transfusion.

    At the time of production of these guidelines, a risk assessment of vCJD in relation to transfusion is ongoing at Department of Health level. This includes consideration of the possible benefits of leucocyte-depletion of all blood components (including plasma for fractionation). Until this exercise is completed or until new scientific data become available, the Blood Transfusion Task Force considers that these guidelines represent the current state of knowledge regarding the overall clinical benefits of leucocyte-depletion of blood components.

References

Anasetti C., Doney K.C., Storb R. *et al.* (1986) Marrow transplantation for severe aplastic anaemia: long-term outcome in fifty 'untransfused' patients. *Annals of Internal Medicine* **104**, 461–466.

Anderson N.A., Gray S., Copplestone J.A. *et al.* (1997) A prospective randomized study of three types of platelet concentrates in patients with haematological malignancy: corrected platelet count increments and frequency of nonhaemolytic transfusion reactions. *Transfusion Medicine* **6**, 33–39.

Andreu G., Norol F., Schooneman F. *et al.* (1993) Prevention of HLA alloimmunisation using UV-B irradiated platelet concentrates (PC): results of a prospective randomised clinical trial. *Transfusion* **33** (Suppl.), 73S.

Balducci L., Benson K., Lyman G.H. *et al.* (1993) Cost-effectiveness of white cell-reduction filters in treatment of adult acute myelogenous leukemia. *Transfusion* **33**, 665–670.

BCSH (1992) Guidelines for platelet transfusions. *Transfusion Medicine* **2**, 311–318.

BCSH (1994) Guidelines for administration of blood products: transfusion of infants and neonates. *Transfusion Medicine* **4**, 63–69.

BCSH (1996) Guidelines on gamma irradiation of blood components for the prevention of transfusion-associated graft-versus-host disease. *Transfusion Medicine* **6**, 261–271.

Blajchman M.A. (1997) Allogeneic blood transfusions, immunomodulation, and post-operative bacterial infection: do we have the answers yet? *Transfusion* **37**, 121–125.

Blajchman M.A. & Singal D.P. (1989) The role of red blood cell antigens, histocompatibility antigens, and blood transfusions on renal allograft survival. *Transfusion Medicine Reviews* **3**, 171–179.

Blajchman M.A., Bardossy L., Carmen R.A., Goldman M., Heddle N.M. & Singal D.P. (1992) An animal model of allogeneic donor platelet refractoriness: the effect of time of leukocyte depletion. *Blood* **79**, 1371–1375.

Blundell E.L., Pamphilon D.H., Fraser I.D. *et al.* (1996) A prospective, randomized study of the use of platelet concentrates irradiated with ultraviolet-B light in patients with haematologic malignancy. *Transfusion* **36**, 296–302.

Bordin J.O., Heddle N.M. & Blajchman M.A. (1994) Biologic effects of leukocytes present in transfused cellular blood products. *Blood* **84**, 1703–1721.

Bowden R.A., Slichter S.J., Sayers M. *et al.* (1995) A comparison of filtered leucokyte-reduced and cytomegalovirus negative blood products for the prevention of transfusion-associated CMV infection after marrow transplant. *Blood* **86**, 3598–3603.

Busch M.P., Lee T.-H. & Heitman J. (1992) Allogeneic leukocytes but not therapeutic blood elements induce reactivation and dissemination of latent human immunodeficiency virus type 1 infection: implications for transfusion support of infection patients. *Blood* **80**, 2128–2135.

Busch M.P., Collier A., Gernsheimer T. *et al.* (1996) The Viral Activation Transfusion Study (VATS): rationale, objectives, and design overview. *Transfusion* **36**, 854–859.

Claas F.H.J., Smeenk R.J.T., Schmidt R., van Steenbrugge J.G. & Eernisse J.G. (1981) Alloimmunization against the MHC antigens after platelet transfusions is due to contaminating leucocytes in the platelet suspension. *Experimental Haematology* **9**, 84–89.

Consensus Conference (1993) *Leucocyte Depletion of Blood and Blood Components.* Royal College of Physicians, Edinburgh.

Copplestone J.A., Williamson P., Norfolk, D.R., Morgenstern G.R., Wimperis J.Z. & Williamson L.M. (1995) Wider benefits of leukodepletion of blood products. *Blood* **86**, 409–410.

Danish Society of Clinical Immunology (1996) Danish recommendations for the transfusion of leukocyte-depleted blood components. *Vox Sanguinis* **70**, 185–186.

Doughty H.A., Murphy M.F., Metcalfe P., Rohatiner A.Z.S., Lister T.A. & Waters A.H. (1994) Relative importance of immune and non-immune causes of platelet refractoriness. *Vox Sanguinis* **66**, 200–205.

Dumont L., Dzik W.H., Rebulla P., Brandwein H. & the members of the BEST Working Party of the ISBT (1996) Practical guidelines for process validation and process control of white cell-reduced blood components: report of the Biomedical Excellence for Safer Transfusion (BEST) Working Party of the International Society of Blood Transfusion. *Transfusion* **36**, 11–20.

Dzik S. (1993) Leukodepletion blood filters: filter design and mechanisms of leukocyte removal. *Transfusion Medicine Reviews* **7**, 65–77.

Fisher M., Chapman J.K., Ting A. & Morris P.J. (1985) Alloimmunisation to HLA antigens following transfusion with leucocyte-poor and purified platelet suspensions. *Vox Sanguinis* **49**, 331–335.

Goldman M. & Delage G. (1995) The role of leukodepletion in the control of transfusion-transmitted disease. *Transfusion Medicine Reviews* **9**, 9–19.

Goodnough L.T., Riddell J., Lazarus H. *et al.* (1993) Prevalence of platelet transfusion reactions before and after implementation of leukocyte-depleted platelet concentrates by filtration. *Vox Sanguinis* **65**, 103–107.

Heddle N.M. (1994) The efficacy of leukodepletion to improve platelet transfusion response: a critical appraisal of clinical studies. *Transfusion Medicine Reviews* **8**, 15–29.

Heddle N.M., Klama L.N., Griffith L., Roberts R., Shukla G. & Kelton J.G. (1993) A prospective study to identify the risk factors associated with acute reactions to platelet and red cell transfusions. *Transfusion* **33**, 794–797.

Heddle N.M., Klama L., Singer J. *et al.* (1994) The role of plasma from platelet concentrates in transfusion reactions. *New England Journal of Medicine* **331**, 625–628.

Hillyer C.D., Emmens R.K., Zago-Novaretti M. & Berkman E.M. (1994) Methods for the reduction of transfusion-transmitted cytomegalovirus infection: filtration versus the use of seronegative donor units. *Transfusion* **34**, 929–934.

Houbiers J.G., Brand A., van de Watering L.M.G. *et al.* (1994) Randomised controlled trial comparing transfusion of leucocyte-depleted or buffy-coat-depleted blood in surgery for colorectal cancer. *Lancet* **344**, 573–578.

Jensen L.S., Andersen A.J., Christiansen P.M. *et al.* (1992) Postoperative infection and natural killer function following blood transfusion in patients undergoing elective colorectal surgery. *British Journal of Surgery* **79**, 513–516.

Jensen L.S., Kissmeyer-Nielsen P., Wolff B. & Qvist N. (1996) Randomised comparison of leucocyte-depleted versus buffy-coat-poor blood transfusion after colorectal surgery. *Lancet* **348**, 841–845.

Katz S.M., Kimball P.M., Ozaki C. *et al.* (1994) Positive pre-transplant crossmatches predict early graft loss in liver allograft recipients. *Transplantation* **57**, 616–620.

Lagaaij E.L., Hennemann P.H., Ruigrok M. *et al.* (1989) Effect of one HLA-DR antigen-matched and completely HLA-DR mismatched blood transfusions on survival of heart and kidney allografts. *New England Journal of Medicine* **321**, 701–705.

Morris P.J. (1994) HLA matching and cardiac transplantation. *New England Journal of Medicine* **330**, 857–858.

Muylle L. & Peetermans M.E. (1994) Effect of prestorage leukocyte removal on the cytokine levels in stored platelet concentrates. *Vox Sanguinis* **66**, 14–17.

Muylle L., Joos M., Wouters E., de Bock R. & Peetermans M.E. (1993) Increased tumour necrosis factor alpha (TNF-alpha), interleukin 1, and interleukin 6 (IL-6) levels in the plasma of stored platelet concentrates: relationship between TNF-alpha and IL-6 levels and febrile transfusion reactions. *Transfusion* **33**, 195–199.

Novotny V.M.J., van Doorn R., Witvliet M.D., Claas F.H.J. & Brand A. (1995) Occurrence of allogeneic HLA and non-HLA antibodies after transfusion of prestorage filtered platelets and red blood cells: a prospective study. *Blood* **85**, 1736–1741.

Nusbacher J. (1991) Blood transfusion support in liver transplantation. *Transfusion Medicine Reviews* **3**, 207–213.

Oksanen K. & Elonen E. (1993) Impact of leucocyte-depleted blood components on the haematological recovery and prognosis of patients with acute myeloid leukaemia. *British Journal of Haematology* **84**, 639–647.

Olding L.B., Jensen F.C. & Oldstone M.B.A. (1975) Pathogenesis of cytomegalovirus infection: activation of virus from bone marrow derived lymphocytes by *in vivo* allogeneic interaction. *Journal of Experimental Medicine* **141**, 561–572.

Opelz G. & Wujciak T. (1994) The influence of HLA compatibility on graft survival after heart transplantation. *New England Journal of Medicine* **330**, 816–819.

Opelz G., Sengar D.P.S., Mickey M.R. & Terasaki P.I. (1973) The effect of a blood transfusion on subsequent kidney transplantation. *Transplantation Proceedings* **5**, 253–259.

Opelz G., Vanrenterghem Y., Kirste G. *et al.* (1997) Prospective evaluation of pretransplant blood transfusions in cadaver kidney recipients. *Transplantation* **63**, 964–967.

Pamphilon D.H. & Blundell E.L. (1992) Ultraviolet-B irradiation of platelet concentrates: a strategy to reduce transfusion recipient allosensitisation. *Seminars in Haematology* **29**, 113–121.

Perkins H.A. (1993) Is white cell reduction cost-effective? *Transfusion* **33**, 626–628.

Popovsky M.A. (1996) Quality of blood components filtered before storage and at the bedside: implications for transfusion practice. *Transfusion* **36**, 470–474.

Popovsky M.A., Chaplin H.C. & Moore S.B. (1992) Transfusion-related acute lung injury: a neglected, serious complication of hemotherapy. *Transfusion* **32**, 589–592.

Rebulla P. & Dzik W.H. (1994) Multicenter evaluation of methods for counting residual white cells in leukocyte-depleted red blood cells. *Vox Sanguinis* **66**, 25–32.

Sandler S.G., Fang C.T. & Williams A.E. (1991) Human T-cell lymphotrophic virus type I and II in transfusion medicine. *Transfusion Medicine Reviews* **5**, 93–107.

Sayers M.H., Anderson K.C., Goodnough L.T. *et al.* (1992) Reducing the risk for transfusion-transmitted cytomegalovirus infection. *Annals of Internal Medicine* **116**, 55–62.

Sintnicolaas K., van Marwijk Kooy M., van Prooijen H.G. *et al.* (1995) Leukocyte depletion of random single-donor platelet transfusions does not prevent secondary human leukocyte-alloimmunisation and refractoriness: a randomised prospective study. *Blood* **85**, 824–828.

Sirchia G. & Rebulla P. (1994) Leucocyte-depletion of red cells. In Lane T.A. & Myllyla G. (eds) *Leucocyte Depleted Blood Products*, pp. 6–17. Karger, Basle.

Slichter S.J. (1988) Transfusion and bone marrow transplantation. *Transfusion Medicine Reviews* **2**, 1–17.

Slichter S.J. (1990) Mechanisms and management of platelet refractoriness. In Nance S.J. (ed.) *Transfusion Medicine in the 1990s*, pp. 95–179. American Association of Blood Banks, Arlington, Virginia.

Sloand E., Kumar P., Klein H.G., Merritt S. & Sacher R. (1994) Transfusion of blood components to persons infected with human immunodeficiency virus type 1: relationship to opportunistic infection. *Transfusion* **34**, 48–53.

Storb R., Weiden P.L., Deeg H.J. *et al.* (1979) Rejection of marrow from DLA-identical canine littermates given transfusions before grafting: antigens involved are expressed on leukocytes and skin epithelial cells but not on platelets and red blood cells. *Blood* **54**, 477–484.

Takaya S., Bronsther O., Iwaki Y. *et al.* (1992) The adverse effect on liver transplantation of using positive cytotoxic crossmatch donors. *Transplantation* **53**, 400–406.

Trial to Reduce Alloimmunization to Platelets (TRAP) Study Group (1997) Leukocyte reduction and ultraviolet B irradiation of platelets to prevent alloimmunization and refractoriness to platelet transfusions. *New England Journal of Medicine* **337**, 1861–1869.

UK BTS/NIBSC Liaison Group (1997) *Guidelines for the Blood Transfusion Service*, 3rd edn. HMSO, London.

Vamvakas E.C. (1996) Transfusion-associated cancer recurrence and postoperative infection: meta-analysis of randomised, controlled clinical trials. *Transfusion* **36**, 175–186.

Vamvakas E. & Kaplan H.S. (1993) Early transfusion and length of survival in acquired immune deficiency syndrome: experience with a population receiving medical care at a public hospital. *Transfusion* **33**, 111–118.

Vamvakas E. & Moore S.B. (1993) Perioperative blood transfusion and colorectal cancer recurrence: a qualitative statistical overview and meta-analysis. *Transfusion* **33**, 754–765.

van Twuyver E., Mooijaart R.J.D., ten Berge I.J.M. *et al.* (1991) Pretransplantation blood transfusion revisited. *New England Journal of Medicine* **325**, 1210–1213.

Wadhwa M., Seghatchian M.J., Lubenko A. *et al.* (1996) Cytokine levels in platelet concentrates: quantitation by bioassays and immunoassays. *British Journal of Haematology* **93**, 225–234.

Walters M.C., Patience M., Leisenring W. *et al.* (1996) Bone marrow transplantation for sickle cell disease. *New England Journal of Medicine* **335**, 369–376.

13 Guidelines for Autologous Transfusion II: Perioperative Haemodilution and Cell Salvage
Prepared by the Blood Transfusion Task Force

1 Introduction

Part I of the Guidelines for Autologous Transfusion dealt with preoperative autologous donation and was published by the British Committee for Standards in Haematology (BCSH) Task Force in 1993. Part II deals with acute normovolaemic haemodilution (ANH) in the perioperative period and red-cell salvage procedures.

The purpose of all forms of autologous transfusion is to avoid the transfusion of allogeneic blood. This may be necessitated, for instance, by difficulty in obtaining compatible blood for a particular patient – for example, when the patient has a rare blood group or when multiple red-cell antibodies are present – but more commonly it is used as a general strategy for avoidance of the risks (infectious and immunological) of allogeneic transfusion. Autologous transfusion procedures are not usually acceptable to Jehovah's Witnesses, although some accept intraoperative cell salvage (see Section 3.1). The option must be discussed with patients individually.

In order to maximize the potential benefits, the various forms of autologous transfusion should be seen as complementary, and it is essential that an appropriate transfusion strategy should be developed for each individual patient's needs. Coordination of autologous transfusion procedures is of vital importance, with clear methods for communicating whether predeposited autologous blood is available, as it may be unnecessary to use additional autologous techniques in some patients. It must be remembered that the serious risks of allogeneic transfusion are lower in the UK than in many other countries, and that the procedures used for autologous transfusion of whatever type must be considered carefully so as to minimize potential adverse effects of the procedure itself. The decision to transfuse the autologous blood should be based on that particular patient's need for blood, rather than simply on its availability.

Specific consent for autologous transfusion procedures carried out in theatre is not considered to be necessary. Currently, this requirement is considered to be covered by generic surgical consent, although patients must be given full information about the proposed treat-

Reprinted with permission from *British Journal of Anaesthesia*, 1997, **6**, 768–771.

ment. The information sheet should state that it may be necessary to administer allogeneic blood in an emergency.

While these guidelines seek to deal with situations likely to be met in current clinical practice, it is recognized that exceptional circumstances may arise and that the final decision regarding the use of autologous transfusion rests with the consultant (or deputy) who undertakes the procedure.

2 Acute normovolaemic haemodilution

Acute normovolaemic haemodilution (ANH) is defined as the removal of blood from a patient immediately before operation, either before or shortly after induction of anaesthesia, and simultaneous replacement with an appropriate volume of crystalloid or colloid fluids, alone or in combination, such as to maintain the circulating volume.

The risks of haemodilution (i.e. of a low intraoperative haematocrit) can be minimized by limiting its extent (target haematocrit 25–30%); however, studies using mathematical modelling techniques suggest that savings in allogeneic blood use in such circumstances are likely to be small. Prospective controlled studies are needed to elucidate the effectiveness or otherwise of moderate ANH in reducing the need for allogeneic transfusion (Consensus Conference, 1996).

Extreme haemodilution (target haematocrit <20%) is likely to be more efficacious in reducing allogeneic transfusion requirements, but the risks are correspondingly greater. This procedure should be restricted to relatively healthy patients with a low risk of ischaemic heart disease and must be supervised by an expert anaesthetist using appropriate monitoring techniques.

A degree of haemodilution is inevitable in patients on cardiopulmonary bypass, unless a blood prime is used; this must be taken into account when additional haemodilution is undertaken.

Preoperative apheresis to obtain autologous platelets/fresh-frozen plasma (FFP)/red cells should currently be viewed as a research technique, the benefits of which are not proved. These techniques cannot yet be considered to have a place in routine practice.

Acute normovolaemic haemodilution may confer benefits other than those implied by the avoidance of allogeneic transfusion – for example, reduction in red-cell loss during operation (secondary to reduced haematocrit) and improved oxygen delivery (secondary to reduction in whole-blood viscosity). The availability of blood containing normal concentrations of coagulation factors and functioning platelets for transfusion at the end of the procedure is of theoretical benefit. There is no evidence that these factors confer measurable clinical benefit.

The decision to recommend ANH for an individual patient should lie with the anaesthetist and surgeon. The responsibility for the procedure itself normally lies with the anaesthetist. The involvement of the haematologist in charge of the blood bank is to be encouraged, both in developing transfusion strategies and in assisting with the production of standard operating procedures (SOPs). Where appropriate, the consultants in the local transfusion centre should be invited to assist in the training of staff and the production of SOPs.

2.1 Selection of patients

Acute normovolaemic haemodilution should only be considered when the potential blood loss is likely to be greater than 20% of blood volume. It should not be considered unless the preoperative haemoglobin concentration is >110 g/l. Although the risk of complications relating to unsuspected atheromatous disease, particularly silent myocardial ischaemia, increases with age, patients of any age may be considered for the procedure. Particular caution should be exercised in patients more than 45 years of age in the assessment of the risk of underlying ischaemic heart disease, and in patients with severe diseases of other systems.

Patients with severe myocardial disease of any cause – for example, moderate to severe left-ventricular impairment, unstable angina, severe aortic stenosis, critical left-main-stem disease or the equivalent – should only undergo haemodilution over and above that necessarily incurred during cardiopulmonary bypass with extreme caution.

Patients undergoing ANH need not be screened routinely for viral markers. Universal precautions to protect staff from the risks of virus transmission must always be observed. The used container and giving set must be disposed of in accordance with the hospital policy for the disposal of hazardous waste; the fate of all units must be documented.

2.2 Procedures

A suggested operating procedure is outlined in Appendix 13.1.

The safety of ANH depends on the maintenance of normovolaemia. In all patients, care must be taken to match the continuous replacement of volume with the removal of blood. In older patients and where cardiac disease may be suspected, additional care is necessary.

Appropriate blood-collection packs must be used to ensure a standard anticoagulant/ blood ratio. The approximate volume of blood to be removed (in litres) to achieve the desired haematocrit can be calculated using the following formula:

$$V = \text{EBV} \times (H_o - H_f / H_{av})$$

where V = volume to be removed, EBV = estimated blood volume (usually taken as 70 ml/kg body weight), H_o = initial haematocrit, H_f = desired haematocrit and H_{av} = average haematocrit (mean of H_o and H_f).

2.2.1 Labelling

All units must be labelled with the patient's name, hospital number and date of birth, the date and time of collection and the name of the person carrying out the procedure. The label must be clear, and should state 'UNTESTED BLOOD: FOR AUTOLOGOUS USE ONLY'. Preinfusion checks of identity are mandatory and should be equivalent to the hospital's standard procedures for administration of allogeneic blood.

2.2.2 Storage

Blood removed during haemodilution must remain with the patient and should not be removed to a blood refrigerator. It may be kept for up to 6 h at room temperature, preferably in an insulated box or other container to minimize temperature fluctuations. The container should be labelled with the patient's full details, with a warning that it must not be used for another patient.

2.2.3 Disposal

In general, all such blood should be used in theatre. If ANH blood is transported with the patient to a recovery area or ward, a written procedure should be in place to ensure that the blood is handled and administered to the patient according to the standards outlined in Sections 2.2.1 and 2.2.2 above. Blood from patients known to have markers for viral infections (human immunodeficiency virus (HIV), hepatitis B and C viruses (HBV, HCV)) must not be allowed to leave theatre unless the infusion has already commenced.

Any unused autologous blood is to be disposed of as hazardous waste, preferably in theatre; the fate of all units must be documented. These procedures should be included in a local SOP, which should also include instructions to ensure that no autologous blood is transferred to the general blood supply.

The number of units of blood and total volume removed from the patient must be recorded in the patient's case notes. Where allogeneic blood is given, the reasons must be documented clearly in the patient's notes.

Serious adverse events should be reported to the hospital transfusion committee and to any appropriate national reporting system.

Regular audit of procedures should be undertaken under the aegis of the hospital transfusion committee. Audit and comparison with allogeneic blood usage would be facilitated by the routine recording of autologous-blood use in theatre.

3 Red-cell salvage

The indications, contraindications, potential adverse effects and range of methods of red-cell salvage are described in Appendix 13.2.

A designated member of the consultant medical staff must be responsible for training and supervision of the staff carrying out cell-salvage procedures.

3.1 Selection of patients

Cell salvage is appropriate where there is a clean wound. The technique is applicable to open heart surgery, vascular surgery, total joint replacements, spinal surgery, liver transplantation, ruptured ectopic pregnancy and some neurosurgical procedures. Some Jehovah's Witnesses may accept transfusion of autologous cells salvaged by a continuous-circuit device; specific consent to the procedure should be sought in this instance.

3.2 Contraindications

Cell-salvage techniques should not be used in the presence of bacterial contamination of the operative field. Malignant disease has been considered a contraindication, but recent published work suggests that the risk of dissemination of malignant disease is minimal. Blood containing fat or amniotic fluid should not be salvaged, because of the risk of embolism and disseminated intravascular coagulation (DIC). Topical clotting agents, such as collagen, cellulose, gelatin and thrombin, and topical antibiotics or cleansing agents used in the operative field should not be aspirated into a cell-salvage device. Complications have been reported in patients with sickle-cell disease.

Patients undergoing cell salvage need not be screened routinely for viral markers. Universal precautions to protect staff from the risks of virus transmission must always be observed. The used container and giving set must be disposed of in accordance with the hospital policy for the disposal of hazardous waste.

All blood-salvage devices should be used in strict compliance with the manufacturers' instructions. The responsible consultant must ensure that a designated person is responsible for the maintenance of equipment, adherence to SOPs and documentation of all procedures.

Blood for reinfusion must be labelled according to the specifications given for ANH. Labelling, storage and disposal of salvaged blood must be in accordance with the standards outlined in Sections 2.2.1–2.2.3.

All cell-salvage procedures and volumes of blood reinfused must be recorded in the patient's case notes. Where allogeneic blood is given, the reasons must be clearly documented in the patient's notes.

Serious adverse events should be reported to the hospital transfusion committee and to any appropriate national reporting system.

Regular audit of procedures should be undertaken under the aegis of the hospital transfusion committee. Audit and comparison with allogeneic blood usage would be facilitated by the routine recording of autologous-blood use in theatre.

Appendix 13.1: Blood collection

The following points are important in collecting blood during preoperative haemodilution.

1 Blood may be collected into a single pack with CPDA-1 anticoagulant. (Licensed blood packs for collection of approximately 450 ml ± 10% or 250 ml ± 10% are available. Appropriate pack-size selection is important to maintain anticoagulant-to-blood ratios. Some manufacturers may make dedicated packs.)

2 A regularly calibrated balance should be used to measure the volume of blood drawn.

3 Skin should be cleaned thoroughly, using chlorhexidine (in alcohol) or equivalent.

4 The donor tubing should be clamped – for example, with non-toothed Spencer Wells forceps – before the guard is removed from the needle. The clamp should remain in place until after the venepuncture. This prevents air entering the bag and possibly contaminating the donation.

5 The blood pack should be labelled during donation. The label affixed to the blood pack should include the following information:

surname;

first names;

date of birth;

hospital number;

date and time of collection;

responsible medical officer;

and should state: 'UNTESTED BLOOD: FOR AUTOLOGOUS USE ONLY'.

6 The pack should be agitated gently throughout collection to mix the blood with the anticoagulant.

7 The bleed line should be sealed with clips or a heat sealer, both at its cut end and close to the pack.

Appendix 13.2: Indications, contraindications, potential adverse effects and methods of red cell salvage

Technique	Indications	Contraindications	Potential adverse effects	Comments
Acute normovolaemic haemodilution	Elective surgery with expected loss >20% TBV	Aortic stenosis, unstable angina, left-main-stem disease or equivalent, moderate to severe left-ventricular impairment	Requires adequate monitoring and maintenance of normovolaemia to prevent haemodynamic instability and possible myocardial ischaemia in susceptible patients	This is a widely available, low-cost option, with the potential advantage of a reduction in blood viscosity. Efficacy in reducing transfusion requirements has been questioned
Preoperative component collection (e.g. platelet-rich plasma)				Research technique. Controlled studies have so far failed to confirm efficacy
Red-cell salvage centrifugal processors	Elective and emergency surgery with expected loss >20% TBV	Bacterial contamination of wound; malignant disease; sickle-cell disease and sickle-cell trait are relative contraindications	In large volume losses, risk of dilutional coagulopathy. Preventable with component Rx. Training required for operator	Excellent long-standing safety record. Becomes increasingly cost-effective with large volume losses. Some Jehovah's Witnesses will accept this
Red-cell salvage haemofiltration processors	As above	As above	Relatively new technology. Training required for operator	Slower processing than centrifugal devices. Filter needs changing after two processing cycles

Continued p. 182

Appendix 13.2 (*Contd.*)

Technique	Indications	Contraindications	Potential adverse effects	Comments
Red-cell salvage single-reinfusion devices	As above	As above	Safety and efficacy to be demonstrated by larger studies. Worries concerning reinfusion of activated clotting factors, may increase risk of DIC	Simple and cheap for low volume losses
Red-cell salvage mediastinal reinfusion	Postoperative cardiac-surgical patients emergency/elective	Sickle-cell disease, bacterial contamination of wound	Worries concerning reinfusion of activated clotting factors, may increase risk of DIC	Unprocessed defibrinated blood transfused. Reduces banked blood requirements in patients with high mediastinal losses

TBV, total blood volume.

References

BCSH (1993) Guidelines for autologous transfusion, Part I: pre-operative autologous donation. *Transfusion Medicine* **3**, 307–316.
Consensus Conference on Autologous Transfusion (1996) Final consensus statement. *Transfusion* **36**, 667.

14 Guidelines on Gamma-irradiation of Blood Components for the Prevention of Transfusion-associated Graft-versus-host Disease
Prepared by the Blood Transfusion Task Force

1 Introduction and terms of reference

Transfusion-associated graft-versus-host disease (TA-GvHD) is a rare but usually fatal complication of transfusion. The American Association of Blood Banks survey of 1990 revealed 12 cases in the context of 13.8×10^6 non-irradiated components transfused (Anderson *et al.*, 1991). The risk associated with an individual transfusion depends on the number and viability of contaminating lymphocytes, the susceptibility of the patient's immune system to the engraftment and the degree of immunological (human leucocyte antigen (HLA)) disparity between donor and patient. There is relatively little scientific information in the literature on which to base guidelines for clinical practice and no precise estimates of TA-GvHD risk in different clinical settings. Gamma-irradiation of cellular blood components has been the mainstay of TA-GvHD prevention, but surveys of blood banks in both the USA and the UK have revealed wide variations among centres in irradiation dosage, clinical indications and quality control (Anderson *et al.*, 1991).

This guideline will therefore consider: (i) the frequency, clinical features and diagnosis of TA-GvHD in a variety of clinical settings, with recommendations of patient groups for whom prevention of TA-GvHD should be considered; (ii) prevention of TA-GvHD by gamma-irradiation of blood components and the components which should be so treated; (iii) the implications of gamma-irradiation for blood-component function, storage and labelling and any possible hazards to recipients of such components; and (iv) provision and quality control of equipment and dosimetry for the gamma-irradiation of blood components.

The document will not discuss ultraviolet irradiation of blood products as a means of preventing HLA alloimmunization, nor will therapy of TA-GvHD be considered.

2 Pathogenesis, clinical features and diagnosis of transfusion-associated graft-versus-host disease

2.1 Pathogenesis and clinical features
Transfusion-associated GvHD is a potential complication of transfusion of any blood

Reprinted with permission from *Transfusion Medicine*, 1996, **6**, 261–271.

component containing viable T lymphocytes where there is a degree of disparity in histocompatibility antigens between donor and patient. There appears to be a particular risk when donor and patient share an HLA haplotype, as occurs within families or in populations with restricted haplotypes. Under certain circumstances, these cells engraft and proliferate in the patient. Interaction between donor T lymphocytes and recipient cells carrying either class I or class II HLA antigens results in cellular damage, which may be natural killer (NK)-cell-mediated. Major target tissues include skin, thymus, gastrointestinal tract, liver, spleen and bone marrow. The risks of TA-GvHD are highest in recipients with immunodeficiency or immunosuppression, although TA-GvHD has not been described in patients infected with the human immunodeficiency virus (HIV). In immunocompetent individuals, sharing of an HLA haplotype with the donor appears to be a major contributory factor. Since the onset of clinical features is delayed for 1–2 weeks after transfusion, a high index of suspicion is necessary. The classical early features of fever, maculopapular skin rash, diarrhoea and hepatitis, with or without jaundice, may be attributed to other causes in immunosuppressed patients. Neonates may demonstrate early hepatosplenomegaly and lymphadenopathy, followed by lymphoid regression. Bone-marrow involvement produces severe hypoplasia, with profound pancytopenia. The symptoms and signs are particularly difficult to differentiate from primary infection in premature or congenitally immunodeficient neonates. The disease generally follows a downhill course, with death, usually due to infection, in >90% of cases (Sazama & Holland, 1993). A further rare complication, namely blood donor-mediated rejection of transplanted marrow, has also been reported in two cases.

2.2 Diagnosis and incidence

The most rapid way to make the diagnosis is by skin biopsy, although the histological features may be supportive rather than pathognomonic. It is therefore useful to have additional evidence of persistence of donor lymphocytes by cytogenetic or HLA analysis. Deoxyribonucleic acid (DNA) analysis by restriction fragment length polymorphism digestion, followed by radiolabelled DNA probes, allows identification of transfused cells from small-volume blood samples. However, their presence alone does not necessarily indicate TA-GvHD, since donor lymphocytes can persist for at least 1 week in adults, up to 6–8 weeks in neonates after exchange transfusion (ET) and for up to 2 years after intrauterine transfusion (IUT), without the development of TA-GvHD. Almost certainly, TA-GvHD is underdiagnosed, making it impossible to state with certainty the frequency and risk of the problem in any clinical situation, particularly since the indications for irradiated components are not consistent across the UK. In addition, the real incidence may change, as newer methods of blood-component production result in reduced lymphocyte contamination. It has also been suggested that some donors may be radio-resistant.

There is now a formal reporting system in the UK whereby cases of TA-GvHD can be collated. TA-GvHD is included in the complications reported to the Serious Hazards of Transfusion (SHOT) reporting scheme.

Recommendation: all cases of TA-GvHD should be notified to SHOT.

3 Prevention of transfusion-associated graft-versus-host disease

3.1 Techniques of lymphocyte disarmament

The 'threshold' dose of lymphocytes required for TA-GvHD in humans is unknown, but may depend on the recipient's ability to reject transfused lymphocytes. At least one case has been reported after transfusion of only 8×10^4 lymphocytes/kg. Successful prevention therefore depends either on physical removal of donor lymphocytes or on destruction of their proliferative capacity. Current filtration technology cannot consistently produce the levels of lymphocyte removal required, and at least one case of TA-GvHD has been seen after transfusion of filtered blood products. As filtration technology advances, however, this situation may change. The mainstay of prevention therefore continues to be gamma-irradiation to prevent lymphocyte proliferation, despite theoretical concerns about long-term carcinogenicity.

Recommendation: gamma-irradiation is currently the only recommended method for TA-GvHD prevention. Leucodepletion by current filtration technology is inadequate for this purpose.

3.2 Dose of gamma-radiation

Experience has revealed the importance of the selection of an effective dose of gamma-radiation, validation of the dose actually delivered throughout the irradiation field and some form of assurance that a given component has been irradiated. Initial work, based on abolition of mixed lymphocyte culture (MLC) reactions, suggested that a dose of 15 Gy was sufficient to inactivate lymphocyte responses. However, TA-GvHD has since been reported following components irradiated with 20 Gy. Techniques of residual T-lymphocyte growth detection have led to the recommendation of 25 Gy as the appropriate dose.

With commercial irradiators, the dose of gamma-radiation delivered can vary from the centre of the container to the periphery by up to 35% and along the central axis by up to 30%. Thus, it is important to specify whether the recommended dose is an average value or the minimum dose to any point of the container. In the USA, the Food and Drug Administration requires a central dose of 25 Gy and a minimum of 15 Gy to any other point in the container (J. Fratantoni, April 1993, pers. comm.). In the UK, a minimum of 25 Gy is recommended (NBTS/NIBSC, 1993). To ensure by dosimetry that this dose distribution is achieved, consultation with supporting physicists is recommended.

Recommendation: the minimum dose achieved in the irradiation field should be 25 Gy, with no part receiving >50 Gy.

3.3 Standard blood components which should be gamma-irradiated

Lymphocyte viability is retained in stored red cells for at least 3 weeks, and TA-GvHD has developed following transfusion of whole blood, red cells, platelets and granulocytes.

Fresh unfrozen plasma, containing only 10^4 lymphocytes/kg, has been implicated only in the context of congenital immunodeficiency and, in any case, is now never administered. Transfusion of granulocytes poses a particular risk, on account of both freshness and number of contaminating lymphocytes and the likelihood that the recipient is immuno-incompetent. Transfusion-associated GvHD has not been described following transfusion of frozen deglycerolized cells, which are, in any case, thoroughly washed free of leucocytes after thawing.

Transfusion-associated GvHD has not been described following transfusion of cryo-precipitate or fractionated plasma products, such as clotting-factor concentrates, albumin and intravenous immunoglobulin. Only one case has been ascribed to transfusion of fresh-frozen plasma, but this infant (with thymic hypoplasia) had already received several trans-fusions of red cells (albeit irradiated) and it is possible that these may have been the source of the viable lymphocytes. The likelihood of any lymphocytes surviving freezing and thaw-ing in the absence of a cryoprotectant and possessing intact proliferative potential appears remote and is only of potential significance in the context of congenital immunodeficiency.

Recommendation: for at-risk patients, all red-cell, platelet and granulocyte transfusions should be irradiated, except cryopreserved red cells after deglycerolization. It is not neces-sary to irradiate fresh-frozen plasma, cryoprecipitate or fractionated plasma products.

3.4 Donations from family members and human leucocyte antigen-selected donors

Because of the sharing of HLA haplotypes, donations from family members pose a parti-cular risk of TA-GvHD, especially when the recipient is a neonate, e.g. maternal platelets to treat perinatal alloimmune thrombocytopenia. Red cells, granulocytes and fresh plasma have all been implicated in TA-GvHD after transfusion from family members. There is an increased risk from donations from both first- and second-degree relatives, while consan-guineous relationships increase the risk (McMilin & Johnson, 1993).

Several cases of TA-GvHD have been reported from Japan, where fresh blood is not infrequently used and where common HLA haplotypes increase the chance of a transfusion recipient receiving blood from a haploidentical donor, often homozygous. Two additional cases were from family donations and one case had an HLA-haploidentical donor. These observations are of particular relevance for patients receiving HLA-selected platelet con-centrates from non-family members, because of refractoriness to random donor platelets. This would be expected to increase the risk of TA-GvHD, especially if the platelet donor is homozygous for one of the recipient's HLA haplotypes, since this is analogous to donations within families or within racial groups of limited genetic diversity. A case of TA-GvHD following transfusion of blood components from an unrelated HLA homozygous donor was recently reported. It does not appear to be common practice in the UK at present to irradiate platelets in this setting, other than for recipients of an allogeneic bone-marrow transplant (BMT). The risk from HLA-selected platelets where the donor is not homozy-gous is uncertain. However, many transfusion centres now specifically maintain panels of homozygous donors for refractory patients and, in practice, it is probably more reliable to recommend irradiation of all HLA-selected platelets, rather than risk the misallocation of some donations.

Recommendation: all transfusions from first- or second-degree relatives should be irradiated, even if the patient is immunocompetent. Likewise, all HLA-selected platelets should be irradiated, even if the patient is immunocompetent.

4 Manufacturing aspects

Undertaking the irradiation of blood components constitutes a manufacturing process. The responsible department is therefore expected to comply with relevant aspects of the *EC Guide to Good Manufacturing Practice* (Commission of the European Communities, 1992).

4.1 Effect of irradiation on blood components

The use of gamma-irradiation in the prevention of TA-GvHD aims to inactivate T lymphocytes while preserving the function of other blood cells.

4.1.1 Red cells

Recovery
There is evidence that gamma-irradiation results in reduced post-transfusion red-cell recovery, but only after prolonged storage. Red cells irradiated within 24 h of collection and subsequently stored for 28 days show a reduced 24-h recovery compared with non-irradiated controls, but still above the minimum acceptable 75%. It has also been suggested that red cells can be irradiated up to 14 days after collection and stored for at least a further 14 days. Loss of viability was the same whether the cells were irradiated on day 1 or day 14 (FDA, 1993). It is clear that many different combinations of pre- and post-irradiation storage times can still produce an acceptable red-cell component. Irradiation has no clinically significant effect on red-cell, pH, glucose consumption, adenosine triphosphate (ATP) and 2,3-diphosphoglycerate levels. Supernatant-free haemoglobin levels are increased.

Potassium
Gamma-irradiation of red cells increases the level of extracellular potassium. The potassium level in irradiated units is approximately twice that of non-irradiated controls, a ratio that persists throughout storage, although the rise in the first 24 h may be more than double that of non-irradiated controls. In considering the clinical significance of this, both the speed and volume of the transfusion, as well as the age of the blood, must be taken into account. Previous recommendations of a 1-day shelf-life for large-volume transfusion to neonates and a 4-day shelf-life to other patients may be overly prescriptive.

It has been calculated that 'top-up' transfusions, when given at standard flow rates, do not constitute a risk of hyperkalaemia, even when given to premature neonates. For example, red cells, even when stored for 14 days after irradiation, when given as a 10 ml/kg 'top-up' transfusion, will provide less than half the daily potassium requirements of 2 mmol/kg and the amount given (≈ 0.05 mmol/h) will be rapidly distributed throughout the total body water (Strauss, 1990).

In contrast, potassium load may become clinically important in rapid large-volume transfusions, such as exchange transfusion (ET) and, in particular, intrauterine transfusion (IUT). In the latter situation, infusion of large volumes of 90% haematocrit irradiated red cells may present the fetus with a total potassium influx of ≈ 9.3 mmol/l into a central vein, a procedure sometimes associated with otherwise unexplained bradycardias.

Similar considerations should apply to ET, large-volume transfusions via a central line to children and adults and where there is pre-existing hyperkalaemia. The routine removal of supernatant plasma and washing of irradiated red cells has been advocated, but is not considered necessary and such manipulation simply increases the risk of error and contamination.

Recommendation: blood may be irradiated at any time up to 14 days after collection and thereafter stored for a further 14 days from irradiation. Where the patient is at particular risk from hyperkalaemia, e.g. IUT or ET, it is recommended that red cells be transfused within 24 h of irradiation.

4.1.2 Platelets
Gamma-irradiation below 50 Gy has not been shown to produce significant clinical changes in platelet function.

Recommendation: platelets can be irradiated at any stage in their 5-day storage and can thereafter be stored up to their normal shelf-life of 5 days after collection.

4.1.3 Granulocytes
The evidence for irradiation damage to granulocyte function is conflicting, but, in any case, granulocyte products should be transfused as soon as possible after preparation.

Recommendation: granulocytes for all recipients should be irradiated as soon as possible after production and thereafter transfused with minimum delay.

4.2 Potential hazards of irradiation of blood components

4.2.1 Radiation-induced malignant change
Concern has been expressed at the potential for radiation-induced malignant change in nucleated cells capable of survival in the recipient. No such cases have been reported and it is likely that the dose of gamma-irradiation delivered to blood components significantly exceeds the lethal dose for such cells at high dose rates ($3-4$ Gy/min), resulting in complete cell death rather than transformation.

4.2.2 Reactivation of latent viruses

Gamma-irradiation can activate latent viruses and could theoretically result in transfusion-transmitted infection of the recipient. Again, no such cases have been reported and the doses routinely delivered are likely to exceed significantly those associated with such activation.

4.2.3 Leakage of plasticizer

Leakage of plasticizer is a theoretical risk for the recipients of large-volume transfusions of irradiated components and for neonates in particular. No increase in the rate of plasticizer leaching was found in one study of traditional polyvinyl chloride (PVC) bags, but the effect of irradiation on the multiplicity of new plastics and plasticizers needs to be determined.

Recommendation: irradiated components not used for the intended recipient can safely be returned to stock to be used for recipients who do not require irradiated components. The reduction in shelf-life must be observed.

4.3 Labelling and documentation requirements

Irradiated components must be identified by an approved overstick label. The label should be permanent and include the date of irradiation and any reduction in shelf-life. Approved bar-code labels should be used.

Labels that are sensitive to gamma-rays and change from 'NOT IRRADIATED' to 'IRRADIATED' are available and are considered a useful indicator of exposure to gamma-rays. The dose at which the label changes to 'IRRADIATED' must be marked on the label. As a minimum, a label should be included with every batch. However, it is not necessary to attach a label to every pack in a batch, provided that the irradiation procedure follows a validated, documented and well-controlled system of work that is integrated to component labelling and release mechanisms and permits retrospective audit of each stage of the irradiation process. Clear physical separation of non-irradiated and irradiated units is essential. In practice, the presence of a radiation-sensitive label on every pack will be of reassurance to staff subsequently handling the product. Batch control can also be performed, using thermoluminescent dosimeters. The use of radiation-sensitive labels does not replace the need for regular and precise dosimetry.

There should be a permanent record of all units irradiated. This should include details of irradiation batch and donation numbers, component type, the site of irradiation and when irradiation was performed and by whom.

Recommendation: all irradiated units should be labelled as such, using an approved bar-code label. Each batch of one or more units should be monitored, using a radiation-sensitive device, and should be permanently recorded, manually or by computer.

5 Equipment, dosimetry and maintenance

Laboratories performing irradiation of blood components must work to a clearly defined specification and are strongly recommended to work closely with a medical physicist. The collaboration starts with the initial delivery and installation procedures and continues with the required in-house validation of the defined irradiation procedure, followed by regular monitoring of blood-unit dosimetry and the laboratory environment.

A set of technical guidelines is provided in Appendix 14.1. These have been written for dedicated blood-irradiation machines, an approach which is encouraged. If the irradiations are done on a radiotherapy machine, these guidelines should be shown to the radiotherapy physicist who will draw up an equivalent protocol.

6 Clinical indications for gamma-irradiated blood components

Many patients who will require irradiated products are treated by a 'shared care' approach, involving more than one hospital. To reduce the likelihood of non-irradiated products being given inadvertently, it is suggested that patients be issued with a laminated card, like a blood-group card, to indicate the need for irradiated products.

7 Paediatric practice

The newborn may be at particular risk of TA-GvHD, either because of possible physiological immune incompetence or because of an underlying congenital T-cell immunodeficiency. There is indirect clinical evidence that neonates may not be able to reject transfused allogeneic lymphocytes and that transfusion, at least in large volumes, may result in either immunological tolerance or further immune suppression. Normal circulating donor lymphocytes have been found 6–8 weeks after routine ET and maternal cells have been detected after IUT for haemolytic disease of the newborn (HDN) 2–4 years after transfusion in otherwise healthy newborns. The majority of cases of TA-GvHD reported in apparently immune-competent infants have occurred in the setting of IUT followed by ET, suggesting transfusion-induced tolerance or immune suppression. Also, neonates who have had an ET with fresh blood will not reject a skin homograft from the same donor.

7.1 Categories of neonates at risk of transfusion-associated graft-versus-host disease

Two surveys of current practice in the USA have revealed wide differences in neonatal practice (Sanders & Graeber, 1990; Anderson *et al.*, 1991).

7.1.1 Intrauterine and exchange transfusions

Intrauterine transfusion alone
Despite the lack of reported cases of TA-GvHD following IUT alone from unrelated donors, it is difficult not to recommend irradiation in this setting, combining as it does a large-volume transfusion of fresh blood with a recipient of considerable immaturity. The

absence of reported cases may represent a combination of the rarity of the disorder, under-diagnosis and/or the already established practice of irradiation in this situation. However, irradiation alone will not prevent the possible immunomodulatory effects of contaminating leucocytes, prevention of which would also require leucodepletion (Royal College of Physicians of Edinburgh, 1993).

Intrauterine transfusion and subsequent exchange transfusion
The majority of TA-GvHD in apparently immunocompetent infants have been reported in the setting of ET following IUT for HDN in preterm and term infants. Although reports are scarce, the published evidence supported irradiation of blood for IUT and any subsequent ET such babies may receive (Parkman *et al.*, 1974).

Exchange transfusion alone
Only two cases of TA-GvHD have been reported following ET alone, one in a preterm infant and one in a term infant, but in the latter an immune defect could not be excluded. Therefore, the argument for irradiation of blood for ET in either preterm or term infants is not compelling at the present time. However, like IUT, ET represents a large-volume transfusion of relatively fresh blood. Thus, while irradiation may represent the counsel of perfection, particularly for premature neonates, the risks of TA-GvHD must be balanced against those of any delay in transfusion while irradiation is performed.

Recommendation: all blood for IUT should be irradiated. It is essential to irradiate blood for ET if there has been a previous IUT or if the donation comes from a first- or second-degree relative. For other ET cases, irradiation is recommended provided this does not unduly delay transfusion. For IUT and ET, blood should be transfused within 24 h of irradiation and, in any case, at 5 days or less from collection.

7.1.2 Top-up transfusion

Preterm infants
The preterm infant is commonly multiply transfused and yet there are only two case reports of TA-GvHD, one following three transfusions from an unrelated donor and one following a single transfusion. While the risk appears small, the scenario of repeated donations from a single donor is increasing, since blood donations are now often divided into many aliquots dedicated to a single neonate in an attempt to reduce donor exposure.

Term infants
With increasing gestational age, the ability of transfusions to induce tolerance decreases and the term or near-term infant seems capable of responding appropriately to transfused cells. Even in the setting of multiple transfusions associated with extracorporeal membrane oxygenation (ECMO), there has been only one case of TA-GvHD and therefore these infants appear not to be at risk.

Recommendation: there is no necessity to irradiate blood for routine top-up transfusions of premature or term infants unless either there has been a previous IUT or the blood has come from a first- or second-degree relative, in which case the blood should be irradiated.

7.1.3 Platelet transfusions

There have been no reported cases of TA-GvHD following platelet transfusion alone, but, since platelets are also contaminated with small numbers of lymphocytes, the recommendations for red-cell transfusion should also apply to platelets.

Recommendation: irradiation should be performed on platelets transfused in utero *to treat alloimmune thrombocytopenia and on platelet transfusions given after birth to infants who have received either red cells or platelets* in utero. *However, there is no need to irradiate other platelet transfusions for preterm or term infants, unless they have come from first- or second-degree relatives.*

7.1.4 Granulocyte transfusions

As with platelets, there have been no cases of TA-GvHD clearly attributed to granulocytes. However, since these products are heavily lymphocyte-contaminated, transfused extremely fresh and prescribed for infants who are already severely ill, it would be reasonable to irradiate all granulocyte transfusions.

Recommendation: all granulocyte transfusions should be irradiated for babies of any age and transfused as soon as possible after irradiation.

7.2 Cardiac surgery

There have been no published reports to date of TA-GvHD occurring in immunocompetent neonates undergoing cardiopulmonary bypass surgery or any other surgical procedure. However, there is an unreported case of TA-GvHD following cardiac surgery in an infant with Di George syndrome in association with a second congenital malformation of the head or neck and a heart defect (Dr Sheela Amin, Harefield Hospital, Middlesex, pers. comm.). There needs to be a high index of suspicion concerning coexisting cardiac defects and immunodeficiency. Dysmorphic features, anomalies of ear, lip or palate, hypocalcaemia and absolute lymphopenia ($<2 \times 10^9$/l) are all suggestive of an immunodeficiency syndrome. If in doubt, blood should be irradiated until a definitive diagnosis is made. If Di George syndrome is confirmed, then irradiated products are essential.

Recommendation: there is no need to irradiate red cells or platelets for infants undergoing cardiac surgery unless clinical or laboratory features suggest coexisting immunodeficiency.

7.3 Congenital immunodeficiencies in infants and children

To date, TA-GvHD has been reported in children with a number of congenital immunodeficiencies (Table 14.1). These immunodeficiency states have in common a defect of

Table 14.1 Congenital immunodeficiency states with predominant defect of cell-mediated immunity

In which TA-GvHD has been reported:
  SCID, not otherwise classified
  SCID, with dwarfism
  3rd and 4th arch/pouch syndrome (Di George)
  Wiskott–Aldrich syndrome
  Purine nucleoside phosphorylase deficiency
  Cell-mediated immunodeficiency, not otherwise classified
  Reticular dysgenesis
In which TA-GvHD has not been reported:
  Adenosine deaminase deficiency
  MHC class I deficiency
  MHC class II deficiency
  Leucocyte adhesion deficiency
  Immunodeficiency with eosinophilia (Omenn's syndrome)
  Ataxia telangiectasia
  Chronic mucocutaneous candidiasis

MHC, major histocompatibility complex; SCID, severe combined immunodeficiency; TA-GvHD, transfusion-associated graft-versus-host disease.

T-cell function, with many also manifesting B-cell defects. The occurrence of TA-GvHD in this patient group following transfusions of fresh plasma containing very few lymphocytes suggests that the degree of immunodeficiency is critical in determining susceptibility.

A number of other congenital disorders whose features include a clinically significant degree of T-cell dysfunction are recognized (Table 14.1) but have not been reported in association with TA-GvHD. With the exception of chronic mucocutaneous candidiasis (CMC), the immunological features of these diseases are very similar and these patients may therefore also be at risk of TA-GvHD. In CMC, the lymphocyte response to allogeneic cells appears intact and it is unlikely that these patients would develop TA-GvHD. However, as there is no clear laboratory parameter which will distinguish those who are certainly at risk of GvHD from those who are not, products should be irradiated from the time an immune disorder is suspected. In the newborn infant, the presenting features of immunodeficiency syndromes may be unrelated to the immune defect (e.g. cardiac disease, hypocalcaemia, thrombocytopenia, eczema) and a high index of suspicion is required, particularly in infants less than 6 months old with recurrent chest infections. Confusion may arise, as similar clinical features may be present in such patients, due to acute or chronic infection, and these may be difficult to distinguish from GvHD, even at a histological level. Human leucocyte antigen typing of lymphocytes is advised whenever TA-GvHD is suspected.

There have been no reports of TA-GvHD occurring in patients with isolated defects of humoral immunity.

Recommendation: it is recommended that all the immunological deficiency states outlined in Table 14.1, with the exception of CMC, should be considered as indications for

irradiation of cellular blood products. Once a diagnosis of immunodeficiency is suspected, irradiated products should be given while further diagnostic tests are being undertaken.

7.4 Acquired immunodeficiency states in childhood

Transient defects of T-cell function can occur following a number of common childhood viral infections and as a complication of tuberculosis and leprosy. This is also a feature of autoimmune disorders, malnutrition and burns. Nevertheless, TA-GvHD has not been recognized in these cases and irradiation of blood products is not recommended, even if immunological testing has demonstrated a defect. Despite the profound T-cell defect which develops in infection with HIV, no cases of TA-GvHD have been described in children or adults, perhaps because donor lymphocytes also become infected.

Recommendation: there is no indication for the irradiation of cellular blood components for infants or children who are HIV antibody-positive or who have acquired immune deficiency syndrome (AIDS). However, this should be kept under review.

8 Acute leukaemia and bone-marrow transplantation in children and adults

8.1 Acute leukaemia

There are very few published reports of TA-GvHD in patients receiving intensive chemo(radio)therapy without BMT. A review of the world literature revealed 14 adult cases (nine acute myeloid leukaemia (AML), five acute lymphoblastic leukaemia (ALL)) prior to publication of US guidelines in 1985. Since 1988, there has been only one adult case in AML (Sazama & Holland, 1993). In children, there have been only eight ALL and two AML cases reported in the world literature. In surveys of adult and paediatric practice in the UK, no centres routinely irradiate products for acute leukaemia without transplantation, and no cases of TA-GvHD were reported.

Recommendation: it is not necessary to irradiate red cells or platelets for adults or children with acute leukaemia, except for HLA-matched platelets or donations from first- or second-degree relatives.

8.2 Allogeneic bone-marrow transplantation

It has been common practice to gamma-irradiate blood products given to BMT recipients during the last 20 years. There is no consensus as to the duration of such treatment, current practice in the UK ranging from 2 months to indefinitely, depending on ease of access to irradiation facilities. There are no unequivocal scientific data to indicate when irradiation of blood products can safely be withdrawn after allogeneic BMT. It seems prudent to continue irradiation at least until the immunosuppressive therapy, such as cyclosporin A, is withdrawn (i.e. at least 6 months, in most cases). Since chronic GvHD can also be significantly immunosuppressive, irradiated products should be considered for patients with active chronic GvHD.

Recommendation: all recipients of allogeneic BMT should receive gamma-irradiated blood products from the time of initiation of conditioning chemo/radiotherapy. This should be continued while the patient remains on GvHD prophylaxis, i.e. usually 6 months, or until lymphocytes are $>1 \times 10^9/l$. It may be necessary to irradiate blood products for severe combined immunodeficiency (SCID) patients for considerably longer, up to 2 years, and for patients with chronic GvHD, if there is evidence of immunosuppression.

8.3 Donors of allogeneic bone marrow

There have been two reports of TA-GvHD associated with graft rejection, apparently mediated by third-party lymphocytes, putatively from transfused blood.

Recommendation: to prevent this, blood transfused to bone-marrow donors prior to or during the harvest should be irradiated.

8.4 Autologous bone-marrow/peripheral-blood stem-cell recipients

Virtually all UK centres currently irradiate products for autologous BMT (ABMT) recipients and 30% of centres have a policy of use of irradiated products given to potential ABMT recipients before and during harvesting of marrow or peripheral-blood stem cells (PBSCs). This is to prevent the harvesting of allogeneic T lymphocytes, which might cause TA-GvHD after reinfusion. As with allogeneic transplants, current knowledge does not allow precise guidance on when irradiation can be safely discontinued. Many patients need prolonged periods of red-cell and, particularly, platelet support after ABMT. We would recommend, as a minimum, continuing to use irradiated blood products until there is unequivocal evidence of haemopoietic engraftment and lymphoid reconstitution. In most patients, this would mean at least 3 months of treatment. If, however, the patient has received total body irradiation (TBI), this may take up to 6 months.

Recommendation: patients undergoing bone-marrow or peripheral-blood stem-cell harvesting for future autologous reinfusion should only receive gamma-irradiated cellular blood products during and for 7 days before the bone-marrow/stem-cell harvest to prevent the collection of viable allogeneic T lymphocytes, which could withstand cryopreservation. All patients undergoing ABMT or PBSC transplantation (PBSCT) should then receive gamma-irradiated cellular blood products from the initiation of conditioning chemo/radiotherapy until 3 months post-transplant (6 months if TBI used).

9 Other patient groups

9.1 Lymphoma

Transfusion-associated GvHD has been reported in all forms of lymphoproliferative disease (Spitzer *et al.*, 1990; Anderson *et al.*, 1991). Twenty cases associated with Hodgkin's disease (HD) have been reported, almost certainly an underestimate. Transfusion-associated GvHD has occurred during treatment with chemotherapy alone or with radiotherapy, and the risk of TA-GvHD appears not to be influenced by the stage of the disease.

Transfusion-associated GvHD has also been described in children with HD. There are fewer reports of TA-GvHD in non-Hodgkin's lymphoma (NHL), despite this being a more common disease than HD. The majority have been high-grade and there has been at least one case of TA-GvHD in T-cell NHL. Non-Hodgkin's lymphoma represents a lower risk of TA-GvHD than HD, and it is probably not necessary to use irradiated blood products for NHL patients. With careful surveillance, it may be possible to separate a sub-group at higher risk, e.g. T-cell NHL. Transfusion-associated GvHD has also been reported in children with NHL, and the incidence of TA-GvHD in this situation should be carefully monitored.

The purine antagonists fludarabine, 2-chlorodeoxyadenosine (CdA, cladribine) and 2'-deoxycoformycin (DCF) induce profound lymphopenia, with low CD4 counts, which persist for several years (Cheson, 1995). Case reports have appeared of TA-GvHD following treatment of low-grade B-cell malignancies with fludarabine and cladribine, and several other cases have occurred (Williamson *et al.*, 1996). Considering that these patients do not require intensive transfusion support, this association is considered significant.

Recommendation: we recommend that all adults and children with HD at any stage have irradiated red cells and platelets, but this is not necessary for adults or children with NHL. However, this should be kept under review. Patients treated with purine analogue drugs (fludarabine, CdA and DCF) should have irradiated cellular components.

9.2 Solid tumours

A dozen cases of TA-GvHD have followed treatment of a variety of solid tumours, ranging from rhabdomyosarcoma, Ewing's sarcoma and neuroblastoma in the young to renal carcinoma, cervical carcinoma and glioblastoma in patients in their 60s. In relation to the number of patients with cancer, it is a rare occurrence. However, the effect of dose escalation of chemotherapy regimes in children and young adults is unknown.

9.3 Organ transplantation

Graft-versus-host disease following solid-organ transplantation has been reported after pancreas and spleen, heart, liver and renal transplantation. Considering the immunosuppression used postoperatively, the use of cyclosporin A, which can predispose to GvHD, and the previous use of family-directed transfusion in renal transplants, it must be a rare occurrence. However, it is usually due to the transfer of viable donor lymphocytes within the transplanted organ. No prophylactic treatment of blood products is therefore necessary, but early recognition of GvHD may lead to prompt appropriate treatment. The role of blood components in this context has not been established.

9.4 Acquired immunodeficiency and aplastic anaemia

There are no reports of HIV-infected patients developing TA-GvHD, despite the immunodeficiency. We are unaware of reports in patients with aplastic anaemia or those treated with antilymphocyte globulin or CAMPATH antibodies.

Recommendation: it is not necessary to irradiate blood components for patients with solid tumours, organ transplants, HIV or aplastic anaemia. However, the effects of new regimes of chemo- and immunotherapy must be monitored.

Appendix 14.1: Technical aspects of irradiation of blood components

Choice of blood irradiators

The equipment will contain a long half-life, gamma-emitting source, probably caesium (Cs)-137. The activity must be specified by the manufacturer on an appropriate certificate to ±20%. The source must be double-encapsulated. Its size and shape should be specified, together with the dimensions of the outer housing and details of the thicknesses and nature of all housing materials. This information is necessary to demonstrate adequate containment of the source and may be required for accurate dosimetry.

Adequate shielding must be provided to ensure that dose rates are as low as reasonably achievable at all accessible points in all service modes of operation. Your radiation protection adviser (RPA) will advise on whether this has been achieved.

Because so much lead is used for shielding, the equipment could be top-heavy. Mechanical stability is essential and, possibly, strengthening of the floor. The control panel must be clearly laid out and the function of each control explained fully in the manual. Desirable features include: a safety interlock to ensure the hand cannot get trapped while loading, a means of retrieving samples manually and a means of detecting failure of the turntable mechanism.

Commissioning and dosimetry

The manufacturer, or their agent, should commission the irradiator and provide a calibration certificate, traceable to national standards, for the dose rate at a specified point in the canister. To achieve the minimum recommended dose of 25 Gy in a reasonable time requires a central axis dose rate of at least 3 Gy/min (Leitman, 1993). The timing mechanism for the irradiator should also be checked.

Commissioning would include the provision of generic isodose charts for that type of equipment. However, a thorough survey of the dose distribution throughout the irradiated volume must then be made, as there are literature reports of marked variations with commercial equipment (Masterson & Febo, 1992). The isodose distribution should be determined with the canister full of blood-equivalent material. Appropriate checks can be made on doses and dose distribution, using thermoluminescent dosimeters or commercial dose-mapping systems.

If the minimum dose of 25 Gy results in a maximum in excess of 50 Gy, seek advice on improving the dose uniformity. Spacers may be useful to avoid underdosing the bottom of the pack.

Following calibration/recalibration, a table should be produced which gives irradiation times for specified doses for a set period (e.g. 1 year for Cs-137).

Operation

Both the dose rate and the dose distribution should be checked upon installation, annually and after any source change or mechanical alteration, particularly to the rotating turntable. Results falling outside these guidelines should be discussed with the manufacturer, and usage of the machine should cease pending the outcome of an investigation. In routine use, bags of blood should be packed closely together, with any remaining airspace filled with dummy bags of water. The small residual airspaces will cause only a tiny additional dose (1–2% maximum). Do not allow any bags to protrude above the upper rim of the canister.

Quality control of procedures

All operators must have been adequately trained in the use of the equipment. The names of authorized operators should appear in the local rules (see later) or in a suitable logbook. Standard operating procedures (SOPs) for all laboratory aspects of irradiation must be followed by all staff performing irradiation. There should be a defined person who documents the periodic review of all data relating to the use of the irradiator.

Maintenance

Wipe tests must be carried out at regular intervals to check for leakage of radioactive contamination (every 26 months is statutory in the UK; every 6 months is recommended). The wipe test must be done according to a SOP in the manner specified by the manufacturer and the swabs counted in a low-background area with an appropriate scintillation detector, as recommended by the local RPA.

The maximum permissible activity removed from surfaces likely to be contaminated is 0.18 kBq (0.005 μCi). Action to be taken in the event of a raised count rate must be specified, for example, as follows.

1 If the count rate is above the permissible level, all movements in the vicinity of the irradiator must cease to prevent possible dispersal of radioactivity, and specialist radiation protection advice should be called at once.

2 If the count rate is below the permissible level but consistently above background, the RPA and manufacturer should be informed.

Check weekly that dose rates are below upper limits previously agreed with your RPA on all external surfaces, both when the irradiator is in use and when it is not in use.

Make suitable mechanical and electrical checks, as recommended by the manufacturer and in accordance with the Electricity at Work Regulations (1989). Check operational procedures every 6 months. A list of possible causes of malfunction in the operator's manual is very helpful.

Legislation and official guidance

In addition to general legislation relating to health and safety, e.g. Radiation Safety for Operators of Gamma Irradiation Plants and Approved Code of Practice, the following specific legislation will apply.

1   Radioactive Substances Act (1993) – the radioactive source must be registered with HM Inspectorate of Pollution.

2   Ionizing Radiations Regulations (1985) – these are formulated under the Health and Safety at Work Act. A radiation protection supervisor (RPS) must be appointed in writing and will be responsible to the employer for ensuring that all work is carried on in accordance with the regulations. There must be written local rules and documentation.

3   Transportation and disposal of the radiation source are covered by the Radioactive Substances Act (1993), the Radioactive Substances (Carriage by Road Great Britain Amendment Regulations) (1985) and the Road Traffic Training of Drivers of Vehicles Carrying Dangerous Goods Regulations (1992). New Radioactive Substances (Carriage by Road) regulations are imminent.

4   Electricity at Work Regulations (1989).

This list should be updated annually. If in doubt about any aspect of equipment, dosimetry, maintenance or protection, consult your RPA.

Local rules and documentation

Local rules and documentation for work with a blood-cell irradiator should define the following.

Responsibilities and personnel

These include the employer, head of department, RPS, RPA, staff authorized to operate the irradiator and 'outside workers', e.g. service engineers.

Introduction and code of practice

All persons who intend to use the irradiator must, before starting, read these departmental rules and sign that they have understood and agree to abide by the regulations. The Ionizing Radiations Regulations 1985 and Approved Code of Practice are available for consultation from the RPS and/or RPA.

Any project involving the use of radioactive materials must be discussed with the RPS and head of department.

The location of the irradiator should be a supervised area.

Monitoring

The location and details of a radiation monitoring device must be documented near the irradiator. The monitor should be calibrated annually and the calibration of the meter reading should be available from the RPS.

The gamma-cell irradiator must be monitored weekly as per the instructions in the logbook, drawn up in consultation with the RPA. A record of radiation-monitor readings will be kept in the logbook. If any measurement exceeds a previously agreed level, the RPA must be contacted immediately.

Staff who work frequently with the irradiator will wear whole-body monitors and extremity monitors on the fingers, if either is advised by the RPA.

General operations procedures

This should include manufacturer, contact supplier, source and activity, authorized users and access. A list of named users is located in the irradiator logbook, which must also include a record of the daily usage of the irradiator. Radiation exposure will be reduced if the logbook can be filled in away from the irradiator.

The irradiator must be regularly serviced. This includes leak testing every 6 months.

Contingency plan

1 In the event of sticking of the turntable (or source, depending on the system), the operator must contact the RPS or RPA immediately and prevent access to the area until assistance arrives. A predetermined plan should then be followed.

2 In the event of fire, a member of staff must appraise the fire officers of the presence of the source and assist in checking that the shielding remains intact.

References

Anderson K.C., Goodnough L.T., Sayers M. *et al*. (1991) Variation in blood component irradiation practice: implications for prevention of transfusion-associated graft-vs.-host disease. *Blood* **77**, 2096–2102.

Cheson B.D. (1995) Infectious and immunosuppressive complications of purine analog therapy. *Journal of Clinical Oncology* **13**, 2431–2448.

Commission of the European Communities (1992) *EC Guide to Good Manufacturing Practice*, Vol. IV. *Annex 12, Use of Ionising Radiation in the Manufacture of Medicinal Products*. HMSO, London.

FDA (1993) *Recommendations Regarding License Amendments and Procedures for Gamma Irradiation of Blood Products*. Food and Drug Administration.

Leitman S.F. (1993) Dose, dosimetry and quality improvement of irradiated blood components. *Transfusion* **33**, 447.

Leitman S.F. & Holland P.V. (1985) Irradiation of blood products: indications and guidelines. *Transfusion* **25**, 293–303.

McMilin K.D. & Johnson R.L. (1993) HLA homozygosity and the risk of related-donor transfusion associated graft-vs.-host disease. *Transfusion Medicine Reviews* **7**, 37–41.

Masterson M.E. & Febo R. (1992) Pretransfusion blood irradiation: clinical rationale and dosimetric consideration. *Medical Physics* **19**, 649–657.

NBTS/NIBSC (1993) *Guidelines for the Transfusion Service*. HMSO, London.

Parkman R., Mosier D., Umansky I. *et al*. (1974) Graft-vs.-host disease after intrauterine and exchange transfusions for hemolytic disease of the newborn. *New England Journal of Medicine* **290**, 359–363.

Royal College of Physicians of Edinburgh (1993) *Consensus Conference: Leucocyte Depletion of Blood and Blood Components*.

Sanders M.R. & Graeber J.E. (1990) Posttransfusion graft-vs.-host disease in infancy. *Journal of Pediatrics* **117**, 159–163.

Sazama, K. & Holland, P.V. (1993) Transfusion-induced graft-vs.-host disease. In Garratty, G. (ed.) *Immunobiology of Transfusion Medicine*. Marcel Dekker, New York.

Spitzer T.R., Cahill R., Cottler-Fox M. *et al*. (1990) Transfusion induced graft vs. host disease in patients with malignant lymphoma. *Cancer* **66**, 2346–2349.

Strauss R.G. (1990) Routinely washing irradiated red cells before transfusion seems unwarranted. *Transfusion* **30**, 675–677.

Williamson L.M., Wimperis J.Z., Wood M.E. & Woodcock B. (1996) Fludarabine treatment and transfusion-associated graft-versus-host-disease. *Lancet* **348**, 472–473.

15 Guidelines for Blood Grouping and Red-cell Antibody Testing during Pregnancy and for Performing Red-cell Alloantibody Titrations

Prepared by the Blood Transfusion Task Force

1 Introduction

The typing of red cells for ABO and Rh D and red cell antibody tests on the sera of pregnant women are routinely performed for the protection of the mother and the identification of haemolytic disease of the fetus and of the newborn (HDN) (Judd *et al.*, 1990, 1992; Mollison *et al.*, 1993). These guidelines are primarily addressed to haematology departments undertaking such antenatal testing, although it is strongly recommended that any laboratory undertaking such tests should have a good and close relationship with local obstetricians and paediatricians in the management of this important aspect of antenatal and perinatal care. A large amount of data has now been accumulated about the clinical significance of red-cell antibodies. This should enable more informed decisions to be made regarding the testing frequencies than was possible at the inception of antenatal testing schedules over three decades ago. It is now accepted that samples should be tested only when it is likely that results could influence the clinical management of the pregnancy. In addition, with new financial pressures within the Health Service, together with the shifting emphasis of clinical management from hospitals to primary practitioners and community midwifery care, the need for a rational approach is even more important.

2 Objectives

The objectives of routine serological testing of women are as follows.
1 To identify pregnancies at risk of fetal and neonatal HDN.
2 To identify Rh D-negative women who need anti-D immunoglobulin prophylaxis.
3 To provide compatible blood swiftly for obstetric emergencies.

When red-cell antibodies are present during pregnancy, the purposes of follow-up serological tests are as follows.
1 To identify the fetus that may need treatment before term.
2 To predict infants who are likely to require treatment for HDN in the neonatal period.

Reprinted with permission from *Transfusion Medicine*, 1996, **6**, 71–74.

3   To identify any additional red-cell alloantibodies developing during the course of the current pregnancy. Subjects who develop antibodies may form additional antibodies.

4   To identify additional maternal antibodies induced by intrauterine red-cell transfusions.

3 Testing protocols

3.1 All pregnant women

The first antenatal examination at booking is usually at 10–16 weeks of gestation, at which time maternal samples should be tested for ABO and Rh D groups and the presence of red-cell alloantibodies. When an antibody screen is positive, further testing should be carried out to determine the antibody specificity and significance. Subjects who have the weak Rh D (D^u) blood group are Rh D-positive and do not form immune anti-D. The D^u testing of samples typed as Rh D-negative is wasteful and is not recommended (UK BTS/NIBSC, 1993). All tests should be well established and validated by good laboratory methods according to published guidelines (BCSH, 1991a, b). Because most practitioners do not see many cases of HDN, it is essential that patients with antibodies of clinical significance should be referred for advice to a specialist at the earliest opportunity. Testing for ABO immune antibodies in the maternal serum is not recommended, as their presence neither predicts ABO HDN nor causes problems *in utero*.

3.2 No red-cell antibodies detected at booking

Where no red-cell antibodies are detected at booking, all pregnant women should be retested once during 28–36 weeks' gestation. Some workers believe that Rh D-negative women should have at least two tests performed during this period, one of which should be at 34–36 weeks. In view of the lack of scientific evidence, this requirement is optional, but immunization during late pregnancy is unlikely to result in an antibody that will reach a level sufficiently high to cause HDN requiring treatment.

3.3 Red-cell antibodies present at booking

All women who have previously had an infant affected by HDN should be referred early to a specialist unit for advice before 20 weeks' gestation, for assessment of fetal haemolysis, irrespective of the antibody level. This will enable the need for amniocentesis and/or fetal-blood sampling and intrauterine transfusion to be evaluated. Neither the specificity nor the level of maternal red-cell antibodies can precisely predict the outcome for the infant. When a red-cell antibody (or antibodies) is detected at 10–16 weeks of gestation, subsequent testing of maternal blood should be undertaken to determine the specificity, concentration, origin and level of antibody or antibodies and likelihood of HDN. Anti-D, anti-c̄ and anti-Kell are the antibodies most often implicated in causing moderate to severe HDN (see Section 6).

4 Paternal sample

Where a clinically significant antibody capable of causing HDN is present in a maternal sample, testing the partner's phenotype provides useful information to predict the likelihood of a fetus carrying the relevant red-cell antigens. The possibility of the partner not being the father of the fetus should be borne in mind.

5 Women with anti-D

Blood samples from women with anti-D should be tested at least monthly until 28 weeks' gestation and every 2 weeks thereafter, to monitor the level of anti-D and to identify any additional antibodies that may develop. Each sample should be tested in parallel with the previous sample and the results compared to identify significant changes in antibody level. When intrauterine transfusions are given, the maternal serum should be screened for additional antibodies prior to each transfusion.

Titration of anti-D does not closely correlate with the occurrence of HDN (Bowell *et al.*, 1982). Anti-D quantification (iu/ml) using the national anti-D standard is more reproducible and correlates more closely with the likelihood of HDN.

An increase of the anti-D level by 50% or greater over the previous level indicates a significant rate of increase, irrespective of the period of gestation. This is of special importance when the anti-D level increases to over 10 iu/ml.

Anti-D is the red-cell alloantibody most frequently responsible for serious HDN and generally the significance of the anti-D level during pregnancy is as follows, although exceptions can occur (Nicolaides & Rodeck, 1992):

Anti-D <4 iu/ml   *HDN unlikely*
Anti-D 4–15 iu/ml   *Moderate risk of HDN*
Anti-D >15 iu/ml   *High risk of hydrops fetalis*

6 Women with red-cell alloantibodies other than anti-D

Only immunoglobulin G (IgG) antibodies are capable of entering the fetal circulation. Red-cell antibodies which have a significant IgG component are detectable by the indirect antiglobulin test (IAT) and all non-D antibodies reacting by IAT should be titrated against red cells heterozygous for the corresponding antigen.

Anti-c̄ (Bowell *et al.*, 1986) and antibodies within the Kell blood-group system (Vaughan *et al.*, 1994), with or without other antibodies, are the non-D antibodies most likely to cause haemolytic disease severe enough to warrant antenatal intervention. Women who have these antibodies should therefore be retested with the same frequency as women with anti-D, i.e. at least monthly up to 28 weeks' gestation and every 2 weeks thereafter. For all other antibodies reactive by IAT, retesting once at 28–34 weeks provides sufficient information to determine management of the pregnancy.

Significant titres likely to cause HDN are a titre of 32 or greater, except for Kell-related antibodies, which may affect the fetus regardless of the titre (Vaughan *et al.*, 1994). In general, anti-c̄, -K, -e, -Ce, -Fy^a, -Jk^a and -C^w have the greatest potential to cause HDN.

Anti-Le^a, -Le^b, -Lu^a, -P, -N, -Xg^a and high-titre, low-avidity antibodies (HTLA), such as anti-Kn^a, have not been implicated in HDN.

7 Action at time of delivery

Maternal sample/s and a cord-blood sample should be taken at delivery from RhD-negative women with no immune anti-D. The cord-blood sample should be used to determine the infant's Rh D group, thus identifying women who must receive prophylactic anti-D immunoglolublin. When the infant is Rh D-positive, the direct antiglobulin test (DAT) should be done on cord red blood cells. This enables HDN due to anti-D developing in late pregnancy to be identified. A positive DAT has been shown to be a good predictor of HDN.

A test should be done on the maternal blood sample to establish the size of the feto-maternal bleed, so that additional anti-D immunoglobulin may be given when required.

Whenever the maternal serum contains clinically significant red-cell antibodies, a DAT should be done on cord red cells. Where the DAT is positive, a red-cell eluate may be helpful to identify the red-cell antibody specificity. Wherever possible, the red cells from the cord should be tested for the corresponding red-cell antigens. All infants born to mothers who have clinically significant antibodies in their serum should be closely observed for evidence of HDN during the first 48–72 h of life. They should not be discharged earlier unless subsequent follow-up is arranged.

8 Testing of blood samples from women who have received antenatal prophylaxis with anti-D immunoglobulin

While this is not universal practice in the UK at the present time, antenatal prophylaxis with anti-D IgG is practised in some regions. Passive anti-D may be detectable in the serum by enzyme tests as well as by IAT for up to 12 weeks or more after the administration of anti-D IgG. Testing of maternal serum for anti-D prior to the second prophylactic dose or post-delivery may be confusing and is therefore not recommended, as passive anti-D cannot be differentiated from alloimmune anti-D. When non-D antibodies are present in a woman who received antenatal anti-D IgG prophylaxis, the testing protocol already described for this group of patients should be followed.

9 Simplified action chart

An action chart is shown in Fig. 15.1 for easy reference.

10 Performing red-cell alloantibody titrations

10.1 Introduction
Serial titration of maternal alloantibodies, which have the potential to cause haemolytic disease of the fetus or HDN, is an established non-invasive method of monitoring the pregnancy. Titrations of anti-D and, more recently, anti-c have been replaced by quantitation.

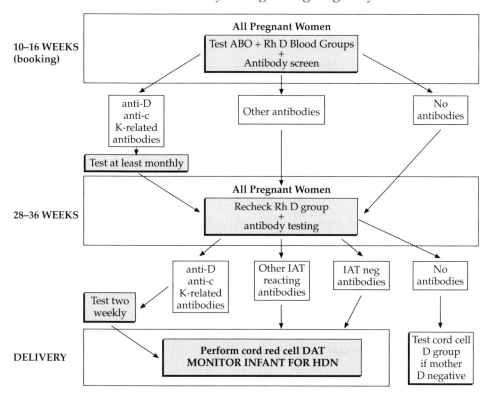

Figure 15.1 Action chart for blood grouping and antibody testing during pregnancy.

The foregoing guidelines for blood grouping and red-cell antibody testing during pregnancy place emphasis on the significance of a rising antibody titre as an indicator of a fetus at risk of haemolytic disease. They also refer to historical-outcome data of pregnancies, demonstrating that significant titres likely to cause haemolysis are 32 or greater, except for Kell-related antibodies which may affect the fetus regardless of titre.

Recent exercises in the National External Quality Assessment Scheme, Blood Group Serology (NEQAS (BGS)) have highlighted the large range of titres reported (titres of 1–128) in a sample containing anti-Fy^a, with a median titre of 8, reflecting the variety of IAT methods used. These exercises have emphasized the limitation of reliance upon a specific titre of 32, and the requirement to improve the reproducibility and comparability of titres.

It is recommended that the National Institute for Biological Standards and Control (NIBSC) anti-D standard should be used to validate the sensitivity of the IAT method employed and that it can serve as an internal control.

10.2 Use of the National Institute for Biological Standards and Control anti-D standard 96/784

Laboratories should validate the sensitivity of their technique by use of the anti-D standard, titrated using the method recommended by NIBSC.

Laboratories should ensure that titres of the anti-D standard are consistent within one doubling dilution, by paying attention to all variables, including cell sources, cell ages and operators. Titres obtained with the anti-D standard can be used as a means of comparing results from different laboratories, using different techniques. Laboratories are also recommended to use this standard as an internal control, to be assured of the consistency and reproducibility of their titration technique.

10.3 Performing titrations

1   Red-cell antigen expression varies with the source and age of the sample. Wherever possible, the same cell sample (heterozygous for the antigen) should be used.

2   All dilutions and titrations should be made using calibrated pipettes and a separate tip for each step. Dilutions should be made in phosphate-buffered saline (PBS).

3   Tube sizes and assay volumes should be chosen to permit thorough mixing of the dilutions.

4   When assaying high-titre samples, an initial dilution should be made to reduce the number of doubling serial transfers to less than 10. A sufficient range of dilutions should be chosen to ensure that two negative results can be observed.

5   The end-point should be macroscopic and well defined. The use of visual comparator aids should be considered, where appropriate.

6   Wherever possible, each sample should be tested in parallel with the previous sample.

7   Titrations should be repeated if there is more than a one-tube difference in the titres obtained from sequential samples.

References

BCSH (1991a) Hospital blood bank documentation and procedures. In Roberts B. (ed.) *Standard Haematology Practice*, pp. 128–138. Blackwell Scientific Publications, Oxford.

BCSH (1991b) Compatibility testing in hospital blood banks. In Roberts B. (ed.) *Standard Haematology Practice*, pp. 150–163. Blackwell Scientific Publications, Oxford.

Bowell P.J., Wainscoat J.S., Peto T.E.A. & Gunson H.H. (1982) Maternal anti-D concentrations and outcome in rhesus haemolytic disease of the newborn. *British Medical Journal* **285**, 327–329.

Bowell P.J., Brown S.E., Dike A.E. & Inskip M.J. (1986) The significance of anti-c̄ alloimmunisation in pregnancy. *British Journal of Obstetrics and Gynaecology* **93**, 1044–1048.

Judd W.J., Luban N.L.C., Ness P.M., Silberstein L.E., Stroup M. & Widmann F.K. (1990) Prenatal and perinatal immunohaematology: recommendations for serological management of the fetus, newborn and obstetric patient. *Transfusion* **30**, 175–183.

Judd W.J., Steiner E.A. & Nugent C.E. (1992) Appropriate serological testing in pregnancy. *Vox Sanguinis* **63**, 293–296.

Mollison P.L., Engelfriet C.P. & Contreras M. (1993) *Blood Transfusion in Clinical Medicine*, 9th edn. Blackwell Scientific Publications, Oxford.

Nicolaides K.H. & Rodeck C.H. (1992) Maternal serum anti-D concentration and assessment of rhesus isoimmunisation. *British Medical Journal* **304**, 1155–1156.

UK BTS/NIBSC Liaison Group (1993) *Guidelines for Blood Transfusion Services in the United Kingdom*, 2nd edn, Section 3, Chapter 3, p. 153. HMSO, London.

Vaughan J.I., Warwick R., Letsky E.A., Nicolini U., Rodeck C.H. & Fisk N.M. (1994) Erythropoiesis suppression in foetal anaemia because of Kell alloimmunisation. *Journal of Obstetrics and Gynaecology* **171**, 247–252.

16 Guidelines for the Clinical Use of Blood-cell Separators
Prepared by the Blood Transfusion Task Force

The following points are recommended.

Clinical management:

1 Clinical decisions regarding the use of cell separators are the responsibility of a medical consultant (or equivalent). Nursing care and responsibilities must adhere to Principles for Adjusting the Scope of Practice (United Kingdom Central Council for Nursing, Midwifery & Health Visiting 1992).

2 Informed consent should be obtained from patients (relatives or guardians) and donors.

3 Selection of patients and donors, and their pre-donation medical and laboratory assessment is the responsibility of a medical officer familiar with the use of cell separators. Particular care must be taken in the selection of volunteer donors (related and unrelated) to ensure that they fulfil the appropriate UK Guidelines for selection of donors and that no undue pressure is put upon them to donate.

4 Paediatric patients require special care and should only be selected and managed in close cooperation with medical and nursing staff strained in the clinical assessment and management of children.

General care and management of complications:

1 Apheresis procedures involve certain risks to donors/patients. All staff responsible for donor/patient care during apheresis must be aware of the more common complications and be trained to identify when they occur.

2 Staff must be trained in how to avoid common complications and also in their management should they occur. Problems with vascular access, reactions to citrate, reactions to replacement fluids and chilling are the commonest complications.

3 Paediatric patients and those with renal disease, liver disease, sickle-cell disease or immunosuppression are more prone to problems, extra care must be taken when treating these patients.

Reprinted with permission from *Clinical and Laboratory Haematology*, 1998, **20**, 265–278.

4 Staff proficiency in the operation of cell separators and the identification and management of patient/donor complications during aphaeresis procedures must be maintained by regular use of equipment.

Post-donation care:
1 Care of the donor/patient must include observation in the immediate post-apheresis period to minimize the occurrence of delayed complications.
2 A record of any post-apheresis complications must be made and of the length of time for which observations were made.

Facilities:
1 Cell separators should be operated in an area reserved exclusively for their use.
2 Adequate space must be provided for routine working and for cardiopulmonary resuscitation.
3 Facilities must comply with Good Manufacturing Practise regulations and with other relevant Guidelines. Appropriate facilities for the management of potentially infective patients must exist.

Staff:
1 Staff responsible for cell-separator procedures must be trained to the highest standards of proficiency in the use of all appropriate equipment. Documentary evidence that training has been undertaken must be kept.
2 Staff involved in patient care must be trained in cardiopulmonary resuscitation to include the use of resuscitation equipment retained on site and they must hold a valid certificate as evidence of appropriate training.

Machine safety:
1 Care should be taken to ensure that cell separators and other associated equipment conform to relevant British and European safety requirements.
2 Regular servicing should be undertaken according to manufacturer's recommendations and service records must be kept.

1 Introduction

These guidelines replace 'Guidelines for the clinical use of blood cell separators' (BCSH, 1991) and supplement the 'Guidelines for automated apheresis of volunteer donors within the UK Blood Transfusion Service' (UK BTS/NIBSC, 1996b).

Since the 1991 'Guidelines for the clinical use of blood cell separators' were published, there has been an increase in the clinical use of cell separators for the treatment of a greater variety of clinical conditions (Rock *et al.*, 1996) and to collect a greater range of therapeutic products. Cell-separator technology has also undergone a considerable evolution, which has permitted the introduction of new procedures, such as photopheresis and immunadsorption. Donors can now donate a variety of therapeutic products during a single procedure. A wide range of patients, including sicker patients, is now being actively treated. It is therefore important that careful consideration is given to the likely clinical conditions to be treated, the most suitable type of equipment to use and the appropriate training of staff when setting up a cell-separator service.

These guidelines for the clinical use of cell separators apply both to patients and to volunteer donors.

Patient procedures include:
- cytapheresis; the removal of white cells (progenitor cells, lymphocytes and granulocytes), platelets and red cells (which may be part of an exchange procedure);
- plasmapheresis (plasma exchange), with or without immunadsorption columns;
- photopheresis.

Donor procedures include:
- cytapheresis; the removal of white cells (progenitor cells, lymphocytes and granulocytes), platelets and red cells;
- plasmapheresis;
- or any combination of the above.

2 Clinical management of a cell-separator service

Clinical decisions regarding the use of cell separators for both patients and volunteer donors are always the responsibility of a medical consultant (or equivalent). In view of the known risks and complications associated with the use of cell separators, appropriate medical/nursing staff must always be in attendance (UK BTS/NIBSC, 1996b). Nursing responsibility must adhere to the Principles for Adjusting the Scope of Practice (UKCC, 1992). The Department of Health (1997) has also issued *Guidance Notes on the Processing, Storage and Issue of Bone Marrow and Blood Stem Cells.*

2.1 Informed consent
The routine of obtaining written informed consent from patients and donors represents good clinical practice and is a requirement of the 'Guidelines for automated apheresis of volunteer donors' (UK BTS/NIBCS, 1996b) (see Appendix 16.2 for suggested consent forms). Clearly written explanatory literature must be available to assist in obtaining informed consent. This should include information about any drugs or replacement fluids that may be used.

2.2 Selection of donors
Donors should be accepted according to the advice given on the selection, medical examination and care of apheresis donors in the 'Guidelines for automated apheresis of volunteer donors' (UK BTS/NIBCS, 1996b). First-time donors should not be under 50 kg

in weight and they should, preferably, have given at least one routine blood donation, without untoward effect, within the last 2 years. Occasionally, truly first-time donors may be accepted if they are specifically motivated – for example, friends, relatives or hospital volunteers – but they must fulfil the remaining criteria for suitability. Normally, donors should be recruited from the UK Blood Transfusion Service (UK BTS) donor panels and requests for such unrelated donors should be made to the local blood centre.

For platelet donations, the donors should not have taken any aspirin or other platelet-active drugs for an appropriate period. For aspirin, this is 5 days, but, for other drugs, this may be shorter.

Care must be taken that undue pressure is not put on persons to donate, particularly if they are related to the patient or are a human leucocyte antigen (HLA)-matched donor. Donors must not be placed in a position where it is difficult for them to discontinue making further donations although they wish to stop.

Patients or related donors may fail to meet the criteria laid down by the UK BTS for acceptance as an apheresis donor (UK BTS/NIBSC, 1996b). The consultant in charge of the unit or his/her deputy must make the final decision regarding an individual's suitability as a donor.

2.3 Medical examination

2.3.1 *Patients*
The doctor in charge of the procedure must ensure that the patient is fit to undergo the procedure and particular account should be taken of pulse and blood pressure, cardiorespiratory status and whether any severe autonomic neuropathy is present. A record must be made in the patient's case notes of all these findings.

Certain laboratory investigations should be performed before and after all procedures. These investigations are to ensure not only the efficacy of the procedure undertaken but also the patient's well-being.

A full blood count should be undertaken to monitor red-cell and platelet loss during apheresis procedures, in order that replacement transfusion can be instituted, as appropriate.

Mandatory microbiological screening tests (UK BTS/NIBSC, 1996a) should be undertaken on a sample collected at the time of donation, or a few days prior to donation if a product is being collected for subsequent transfusion, such as progenitor cells. Currently, informed consent for human immunodeficiency virus (HIV) testing is required.

A coagulation profile (to include, at a minimum, a prothrombin time (PT) and activated partial prothrombin time (APPT)) as a baseline assessment is important for certain groups of patients, particularly those undergoing plasma exchange. This is done to indicate whether a pre-existing coagulopathy is present, as this may influence the choice of replacement fluid.

Baseline biochemistry, to include electrolyte measurement, is of especial importance in renal patients and paediatric patients, who are more prone to electrolyte disturbances during apheresis.

Plasma viscosity, immunoglobulin levels or specific antibody levels may need to be measured regularly, if they are implicated in the patient's pathology, as an important part of assessing the efficacy of apheresis. Similarly, total white-cell count, differential white-cell count and CD 34$^+$ cell count may need to be measured in order to determine the timing of peripheral progenitor-cell collections.

2.3.2 Donors

A medical examination should be carried out, preferably by the medical officer who obtains informed consent. A doctor who does not have primary-care responsibilities for the patient to whom the donation will be given should ideally undertake this examination. This examination is to ensure that the donor meets the required standard of health as laid down by the 'Guidelines for automated apheresis of volunteer donors' (UK BTS/NIBSC, 1996b).

If there is clinical suspicion of cardiorespiratory disease (as indicated by the donor's history and/or the clinical examination), a specialist opinion should be sought.

Mandatory microbiological screening tests (UK BTS/NIBSC, 1996a) must be performed on all volunteer donors. Baseline biochemistry, full blood count, coagulation screen and immunoglobulins may be measured. The results should be within the normal range for the age and sex of the donor. A CD 34$^+$ cell measurement may be required to optimize progenitor-cell collection.

Before white-cell collections (granulocytes, lymphocytes, progenitor cells), ABO/rhesus D (Rh D) typing must be performed and donor/patient compatibility must be assessed. A red-cell cross-match must be performed if major ABO incompatibility is present and, if donor/patient incompatibility is detected, some form of red-cell depletion may be required in order to avoid a haemolytic transfusion reaction.

2.4 Frequency and volume of procedures

2.4.1 Patients

The consequences of multiple apheresis for patients must be considered whenever repeated procedures are required. Few medical conditions require more than 5 consecutive days' apheresis and usually fewer procedures are necessary during the first week of treatment. The volume of plasma removed during a plasma exchange should be related to the patient's estimated plasma volume. Each procedure normally involves a 1–1.5 times plasma-volume exchange, which, in an adult, usually involves a 2–4 litre exchange per procedure.

Peripheral-blood progenitor-cell collections should be timed for individual patients, depending on their peripheral white-count response to growth-factor administration. To harvest sufficient progenitor cells for engraftment, between 10 and 15 litre of blood needs to be processed. Sufficient progenitor cells are often collected from a single procedure but, for some patients, two or more daily collections may be required.

A worksheet should be kept of the details of each procedure. Special note must be made of any adverse patient reactions (see Appendix 16.1).

2.4.2 Donors

Recommendations regarding frequency, volume and duration of donor apheresis procedures are laid down in *Guidelines for the Blood Transfusion Service* (UK BTS/NIBSC, 1996a) and should be adhered to. Donors should not regularly donate plasma more often than once a fortnight. A donor should not generally undergo a total of more than 24 plateletpheresis procedures per annum and not more than 12 leucopheresis procedures per annum. There should normally be a minimum of 48 h between procedures and a donor should not normally undergo more than two procedures within a 7-day period. Not more than 15 litres of plasma should be donated by one donor in a year. For any single donor apheresis procedure, the final collection volume should not exceed 15% of the total blood volume, excluding anticoagulant.

Donors should have a full blood count, total serum proteins and serum albumin measured when they first attend for apheresis and annually thereafter. A system should be in operation for regular review of these results, together with a documented protocol of the action to be taken in the light of any abnormal findings.

2.5 Special considerations for paediatric patients

Advances in cell-separator technology and an increase in the number of clinical indications for apheresis has led to an increase in the applicability of aphaeresis procedures for children, mainly in the field of peripheral-blood progenitor-cell collections.

2.5.1 Informed consent

The nature of the procedure must be explained to the parents/guardian and informed consent obtained on behalf of the child (see consent form, Appendix 16.2).

There may be unusual extenuating circumstances when it may be considered necessary for a child to undergo apheresis as a donor (e.g. for a life-threatening event in a sibling or parent). There are major ethical concerns regarding the role of children as 'volunteered' donors; thus it is highly recommended that advice is sought from a local ethics committee.

2.5.2 Medical examination

Children should be assessed prior to the procedure by medical staff trained in the clinical assessment of children. These staff must be available throughout the procedure.

All apheresis procedures undertaken on children should take place in an area with full paediatric resuscitation equipment, and personnel trained in its use must be available.

2.5.3 Volume and access considerations

It is recommended that only continuous-flow cell separators with minimal extracorporeal volume are used in children. These machines require high flow rates and therefore good venous access. In some children, typically over the age of 10 years, it may be possible to use bilateral antecubital fossae venous access. This may be facilitated by the use of local-anaesthetic creams. However, if repeated procedures are anticipated or in very small children, insertion of a central-venous double-lumen catheter will be required. Hazards associated with the use of these catheters are outlined below (Section 3.1) and raise further ethical problems in 'volunteered' donors.

Children who weigh less than 30 kg will require the apheresis extracorporeal lines to be primed with homologous donor blood, which should have a haematocrit similar to that of the patient. Compatibility testing must be undertaken and cytomegalovirus (CMV) status of the child must be taken into account. Irradiation of this donor blood is required during peripheral progenitor-cell collections for both autologous and allogeneic transplant (BCSH Transfusion Task Force, 1996). For children under 1 year of age, this blood will also require leucodepletion (BCSH Transfusion Task Force, 1997).

During lengthy procedures and particularly when replacement fluids are infused, it is essential that these fluids (cellular or otherwise) are warmed in order to prevent complications, such as central body cooling or sickling in susceptible patients.

In small children (under 30 kg), it is important to be aware that electrolyte disturbances (hypocalcaemia and hyperkalaemia) may occur and that, if repeated procedures are necessary, depletion of plasma proteins, in particular coagulation factors, may also occur.

Recommendation. Clinical decisions regarding the use of cell separators are the responsibility of a medical consultant (or equivalent). Nursing care and responsibilities must adhere to the Principles for Adjusting the Scope of Practice (UKCC, 1992). Informed consent should be obtained from patients (relatives or guardians) and donors. Selection of patients and donors and their predonation medical and laboratory assessment are the responsibility of a medical officer familiar with the use of cell separators. Particular care must be taken in the selection of volunteer donors (related and unrelated) to ensure that they fulfil the appropriate UK guidelines for selection of donors and that no undue pressure is put upon them to donate. Paediatric patients require special care and should only be selected and managed in close cooperation with medical and nursing staff trained in the clinical assessment and management of children.

3 General care during apheresis procedures

Apheresis procedures involve certain risks to donors/patients; these include problems related to anticoagulant use, replacement fluids, fluid and electrolyte imbalance, vascular access, haemolysis, air embolus and infection (Westphal, 1984). There is a mortality rate associated with therapeutic apheresis of three per 10 000 patients (Huestis, 1983). Staff must therefore be trained to the highest standards of proficiency in the operation of apheresis equipment and the care of patients/donors during all procedures. The equipment must be used regularly, so that staff proficiency in its operation and care is maintained.

Patients and donors should never be left in a room without the attendance of an appropriately trained member of staff. Procedures on children should be undertaken in a

designated paediatric area, with appropriately trained medical/nursing staff and with paediatric resuscitation facilities.

3.1 Vascular access

The safest venous access is by repeated venepuncture, most commonly of antecubital fossa
veins. This is the only way currently permitted for venous access in healthy donors. In some
patients, peripheral venous access is not practicable and some form of venous catheter will
need to be inserted. This should only be undertaken in accordance with current 'Guidelines
on the insertion and management of central venous lines' (BCSH Clinical Task Force,
1997; see Chapter 21), the major recommendations of which are included in Appendix 16.3.
Related volunteer donors may also occasionally require a central line to be inserted for harvesting. This should be done in accordance with the above guidelines, and informed consent, specifically for line insertion, should be obtained as part of the procedure.

There are currently a variety of catheters suitable for venous access for apheresis procedures (Table 16.1). Some catheters are only suitable for emergency procedures, as they
are designed to be used only once or for a short period of time, have a single lumen and
are not able to sustain the high flow rates needed for cell-separator use. Dual-lumen
catheters can be left *in situ* for between 5 days (Vascath) and several months (Apheresis
Hickman catheter) and are suitable for progenitor-cell harvesting. Patency of long-term
indwelling catheters can be maintained by instilling heparin (10 u/ml (Hepsal)) after each
use, daily or once or twice weekly, according to manufacturer's instructions, if the line is
not in regular use. This heparin 'lock' must always be discarded when next accessing the
catheter.

3.2 Drugs and infusion fluids

It is recommended that the choice of drugs and other substances given to donors/patients
should be restricted. Anticoagulants used should be citrate-based, acid citrate dextrose
(ACD) and sodium citrate being used most frequently. Heparin is used for some procedures. Replacement fluids that may be used include dextran, hydroxyethyl starch, modified
fluid gelatin, and crystalloids. Human albumin solutions (HAS), fresh-frozen plasma (FFP)
and human red cells are also sometimes used, usually as part of an exchange procedure.
Predosage of donors with corticosteroids to enhance the yield during granulocyte collections is sometimes undertaken. Records of the cumulative dose of corticosteroids should be
kept for each donor. Recombinant growth factors (granulocyte colony-stimulating factor
(G-CSF)) are not currently licensed for stimulating granulocytes prior to collection from
donors but have been used for this purpose in ethically approved clinical trials.

The use of all drugs and replacement fluids should conform with recommendations
outlined in the appropriate data sheet (ABPI, 1999–2000).

Staff working in cell-separator units with responsibility for patient care must have
knowledge of the side-effects of the constituents of the fluids and drugs they are using and
also any drugs patients may be already taking which may affect the apheresis procedure,
e.g. angiotensin converting enzyme (ACE) inhibitors.

Table 16.1 Examples of catheters used for venous access. This list is not comprehensive – other catheters are available. Mention of specific trade-mark names does not represent an endorsement of any given catheter

Maker	Gauge	Lumen	Wall	Duration of use	Position	Indication
BARD	Vascath 10.8Fg	Double	Thick	5 days	IVC, SVC, femoral veins	PBSCH, PEX, RBCEX
	Hickman 13.5Fg	Double	Thick	Months	Tunnelled into SVC	PBSCH, PEX, RBCEX
Terumo Medical Corp.	16Fg	Single back-eye needle	Thin	Single use	Antecubital fossa	Single-use emergency
Cooke	12Fg	Double Hickman	Thick	Months	Tunnelled into SVC	PBSCH, PEX, RBCEX
Vygon Dualyse catheter	12Fg	Double	Thin	5 days	IVC, SVC, femoral veins	PBSCH, PEX, RBCEX
Kimal	8Fg, 12.5Fg, 15Fg	Double	Medium	Years	SVC	PBSCH, PEX, RBCEX
Ohmeda Venflon	16Fg, 14Fg	Single	Thin	Single use	Antecubital fossa	Single-use emergency

IVC, inferior vena cava; PBSCH, peripheral-blood stem (progenitor)-cell harvest; PEX, plasma exchange; RBCEX, red blood-cell exchange; SVC, superior vena cava.

The use of FFP should conform to current guidelines (BCSH Transfusion Task Force, 1992).

Recombinant growth factors (G-CSF) are routinely used for patients to stimulate peripheral progenitor-cell release and improve collection efficiency. They should be used in accordance with local guidelines and manufacturer's recommendations. Growth factors have also been used for related donors, with local ethical-committee approvals, to stimulate peripheral progenitor-cell release prior to collection and use for allogeneic transplant. Currently, these growth factors cannot be used for unrelated volunteer donors, although this is under review.

3.3 Management of complications

Any complications that develop during apheresis procedures (Table 16.2) should be treated appropriately. The consultant in charge of apheresis must make recommendations for appropriate treatment, with clear indications as to what action must be taken by medical and/or nursing staff.

3.3.1 *Anticoagulants* (Table 16.2)

Citrate toxicity
This has been recorded in up to 15% of procedures and can lead to cardiac arrhythmias (Sutton *et al.*, 1989). The development of toxicity depends on a variety of factors, including the concentration of citrate anticoagulant used, the concentration of citrate in the replacement fluid, the rate of citrate infusion and patient susceptibility. Citrate acts by chelating calcium ions, and symptoms are due to hypocalcaemia and include circumoral paraesthesiae, muscle twitching, nausea and/or vomiting, chills, syncope and tetany (rare). Chilling of the patient/donor exacerbates the symptoms of citrate toxicity.

Severe hypocalcaemia can occur without any of the above warning symptoms.

Avoidance
• The patient/donor should be warned about symptoms and asked to report any immediately. Oral calcium supplements before/during the procedure may prevent the development of hypocalcaemia.
• Use the manufacturer's recommended anticoagulant at the correct ratio to comply with *Guidelines for the Blood Transfusion Service* (UK BTS/NIBSC, 1996a).
• If different citrate formulations are to be used, it is essential to monitor the citrate levels in the return line to the patient/donor and to monitor ionized calcium levels in the patient/donor to ensure the maximum citrate dose rate is not exceeded. Advice on the need to undertake such monitoring should be sought from the manufacturer of the cell separator to be used.
• If patient susceptibility is suspected – for example, impaired renal or liver function – reinfuse at a slow rate and monitor for signs of hypocalcaemia.

Treatment. It is safer to correct hypocalcaemia by stopping or slowing the reinfusion rate than by infusing concentrated calcium solutions – hypercalcaemia induced in this

Table 16.2 Patient/donor complications associated with use of cell separators

Subject	Sign/symptom	Possible cause	Possible management
Vascular access	High return pressure	Haematoma	Check tubing for kinks
	Low access pressure	Kink in tubing	Check position of valves
		Valves in closed position	Adjust or resite access or return line
		Vascular inadequacy	Reduce inlet flow
			Stop procedure
Delivery of anticoagulant	Significant tingling/numbness	Citrate toxicity	Decrease citrate infusion rate
	Hypotension		Pause/stop procedure
	Nausea/vomiting		Consider administration of
	Fasciculation/carpopedal spasm/tetany		calcium (oral/i.v.)
	Unstable interface during PBSCH	Underanticoagulation	Check tubing for kinks
			Increase AC : inlet ratio
	Gross clotting evident		Stop procedure
Fluid balance	Increased blood pressure	Fluid overload	Operate at a negative fluid balance
	Dyspnoea, feeling faint	Vasovagal	Stop procedure
	Hypotension	Hypovolaemia	Operate at a positive fluid balance
			Increase colloid : crystalloid ratio
Chilling	Decrease in donor/patient temperature	Cold environment	Increase room temperature
	Decrease in access pressure		
	Patient/donor complains of cold	Cold replacement fluids	Use blood warmer
Transfusion reaction	Urticaria	Plasma products	Administer antihistamine and/or hydrocortisone
			Stop procedure
	Increased patient/donor temperature	Incompatible transfusion	Stop procedure
	Shock	Septicaemia	
	Bronchospasm	Anaphylaxis	
	Rigor		

i.v. intravenous; PBSCH, peripheral-blood stem-cell harvest; AC, anticoagulant.

way can be as dangerous as hypocalcaemia. Calcium gluconate, 5 ml of 10% given slowly intravenously, can be used for the treatment of serious citrate reactions where clinical and electrocardiographic evidence of hypocalcaemia exists, and then only under medical supervision (BCSH Transfusion Task Force, 1994).

Inadequate citration

If inadequate levels of citrate are achieved, this may lead to clotting in the extracorporeal cell-separator circuit. This may either result in the reinfusion of material with procoagulant activity and potentially precipitate disseminated intravascular coagulation (DIC), or cause haemolysis in the cell separator, leading to reinfusion of haemolysed blood.

Avoidance
- Use the manufacturer's recommended anticoagulant at the correct ratio.
- Monitor the anticoagulant pump, the rate of delivery via the drip chamber and the volume of anticoagulant used throughout the procedure to ensure constant correct delivery of anticoagulant.
- Monitor the separation chamber of the return-line filter for evidence of clotting. Also monitor the return line for evidence of negative pressure, which can be an early indicator of clotting within the circuit.
- Monitor the colour of the separated plasma for evidence of haemolysis.

Adverse reactions to heparin
These include bleeding, allergy/anaphylaxis, thrombocytopenia, dyspnoea and abdominal pain.

If protamine is used to reverse heparin, the following adverse reactions can occur: chills and light-headedness, allergy and/or anaphylaxis, dyspnoea and/or chest pain, and flushing. Because of these adverse reactions and the prolonged effect of heparin, citrate is recommended as the anticoagulant of choice for most cell-separator procedures and the use of heparin in normal donors should be avoided.

3.3.2 Replacement fluids
The following materials have been used alone or in combination for fluid replacement in therapeutic exchange procedures.
- HAS 4.5%.
- FFP.
- Whole blood and/or packed cells.
- Volume expanders, e.g. modified fluid gelatin (MFG), hydroxyethyl starch (HES).
- Dextran, crystalloids, e.g. saline, Hartmann's solution.

No therapeutic materials should be added to HAS, blood or other blood products.

For plasma-exchange procedures, the choice of replacement fluid depends on the frequency and volume of the exchange procedure and the underlying disorder. However, in all patients, it is important to maintain adequate levels of protein during the procedure, as inadequate protein replacement can rapidly lead to hypovolaemia and hypotension.

Procedures can be done safely for most patients with a mixture of crystalloid, colloid and albumin, depending on the patient's condition. If plasma exchange is to be performed more than once a week, the volume of the exchange is $1.5 \times$ plasma volume and replacement fluid is part crystalloid and part albumin, the patient's albumin levels, as well as levels of other plasma proteins, progressively fall.

If replacement fluid is albumin solution only, the patient's albumin levels will be maintained, but there will be a progressive fall in levels of coagulation factors (including fibrinogen and antithrombin III), immunoglobulins, complement and cholinesterase. Reduction in coagulation factors can lead to bleeding episodes, particularly if there is a potential bleeding point – for example, recent renal biopsy. This will be enhanced if heparin is used as the anticoagulant. Reduction in antithrombin III levels may predispose to thromboembolic episodes postexchange and also reduces the effectiveness of heparin. Reduction in cholinesterase levels can lead to prolonged periods of apnoea in response to the muscle relaxant suxamethonium used in general anaesthesia or precipitate a myasthenic crisis.

If volume expanders are used as part replacement, certain problems should be recognized.

1 Fluid overload precipitating congestive cardiac failure in the susceptible patient.

2 Allergic reaction, particularly with dextrans.

3 Haemaccel has a high concentration of calcium and should not be mixed with citrated blood, as this could produce clotting in the reinfusion blood line.

Fresh-frozen plasma should not be used as a replacement fluid, except in the management of thrombotic thrombocytopenic purpura (TTP). Intensive plasma exchange, using coagulation-factor-free replacement fluids, results in progressive reduction in plasma coagulation factors, but FFP should only be used to correct these abnormalities when abnormal bleeding occurs. There are certain adverse effects associated with the use of FFP, which may prove hazardous if used inappropriately for plasma exchange (see also Table 16.2).

1 Allergic reactions: urticaria has been reported in 1–3% of patients. Life-threatening anaphylaxis is reported as occurring in one in 20 000 transfusion episodes (Bjerrum & Jersild, 1971).

2 Transfusion-transmitted infection: the risk of infection by HIV, hepatitis B and C and parvovirus following a transfusion of FFP is similar to that following the transfusion of red cells. Two forms of virally inactivated FFP (solvent detergent, Octaplas, Octapharma, Vienna, and methylene-blue-treated FFP, UK BTS) are expected to become available during 1999 and may be used as a replacement fluid to reduce these risks. Fresh-frozen plasma has not been implicated in CMV transmission (Bowden & Sayers, 1990) or in transfusion-acquired graft-versus-host disease.

3 Haemolysis: ABO-incompatible plasma may contain potent anti-A or anti-B, which can cause lysis of recipient cells. Fresh-frozen plasma of the same ABO group as the recipient should be used whenever possible and, if group O FFP has to be used for non-O recipients, it must have been screened to exclude donations from high-titre anti-A and anti-B group O donors.

4 Transfusion-related acute lung injury (TRALI) may result from potent donor antibodies to patient granulocytes (Nordhagen *et al.*, 1986).

5 Immune suppression resulting from plasma infusion has also been reported (Blumberg & Heal, 1988).

Adverse effects can be minimized by adhering to current 'Guidelines for the use of fresh frozen plasma' (BCSH Transfusion Task Force, 1992). Major reactions to FFP, such as TRALI, must be reported to the Serious Hazards of Transfusion Office (SHOT Office, Manchester Blood Centre, Plymouth Grove, Manchester M13 9LL).

3.3.3 Fluid- and electrolyte-balance problems (Table 16.2)

Selection of the type and amount of replacement fluid is an important consideration when undertaking therapeutic plasma exchange (Sutton *et al.*, 1989). Cytapheresis procedures do not usually require replacement fluids and are therefore not usually complicated by problems associated with their use.

Hypervolaemia

This is most commonly seen in renal patients and can be controlled by maintaining the albumin level and finishing the exchange with the patient in a negative fluid balance. Any plasma exchange, however, must always aim to replace a minimum of 75% of the patient's total calculated plasma volume. Patients with hyperviscosity are often already hypervolaemic and care must be taken in performing plasma exchange on these patients, especially when they are anaemic, as changes in their haematocrit can acutely change the total blood viscosity and precipitate a hyperviscosity crisis (Beck *et al.*, 1982).

Hypovolaemia

This is avoided by using protein-containing solutions for replacement. In paediatric patients where the extracorporeal volume of the circuit exceeds 12% of the total blood volume, a whole-blood prime should be used to avoid hypovolaemia (see Section 2.5).

Electrolytes

Problems resulting from abnormalities of calcium homeostasis are the most frequently encountered electrolyte disturbance associated with the use of cell separators. They result primarily from the use of citrate-containing anticoagulants. The resulting hypocalcaemia is most commonly seen in patients who have severe liver dysfunction, in those receiving citrated FFP and during procedures such as T-lymphocyte collection, where there is a high citrate : blood ratio (Silberstein *et al.*, 1986). Management of this problem is discussed in Section 3.3.1.

Other electrolyte abnormalities are uncommon, apart from in patients with renal disease who have pre-existing abnormalities. In these cases, it is possible to alter the electrolyte composition of the exchange fluid as appropriate.

Children are particularly prone to electrolyte disturbances (see Section 2.5).

3.3.4 *Chilling* (Table 16.2)

Rapid reinfusion without using a blood warmer can cause chilling and rigors. Chilling also increases the problems of hypocalcaemia. Certain groups of patients are more prone to complications associated with chilling, including patients with:

- sickle-cell disease;
- paraproteinaemia;
- cold-haemagglutinin disease;
- cryoglobulinaemia;

and

- paediatric patients.

Haemolysis, gelling or agglutination may occur in the extracorporeal circuit in these conditions. It is therefore important in these groups of patients to use a blood warmer to:

- warm all solutions used for priming;
- warm all replacement fluids;
- warm any reinfused blood;

and also to increase the temperature of the working environment.

Blood warmers are mechanical devices for warming fluids being returned to the donor/patient to minimize chilling. A variety of different commercially produced blood warmers are available. Such devices must comply with British Standard (BS) 5724 Part 1. Safety of Electrical Equipment (1979, 1989) and BS EN 60601–1–(1993). They must be operated and maintained according to manufacturer's instructions.

3.3.5 *Complications of vascular access* (Table 16.2)

Peripheral venous access
Peripheral access may be associated with haematoma formation, bruising and occasionally nerve damage. Poor vascular access may require resiting of the venepuncture or abandonment of a procedure. Careful explanations must be given to the donor/patient when these complications occur and appropriate medical management must be undertaken.

Central venous access
The use of central venous catheters can be associated with well-described complications, and these complications lead to the majority of fatalities associated with apheresis (Sutton *et al.*, 1989). Subclavian/superior vena-caval catheters can be associated with vessel perforation, haemothorax, pneumothorax, infection and thrombosis. The use of femoral catheters can be associated with the occurrence of haemorrhage, thrombosis and infection.

3.3.6 *Haemolysis* (Table 16.2)
Forcing blood by pump through a narrow orifice, particularly when blood is concentrated to a high haematocrit, may result in haemolysis. Inadequate anticoagulation is also associated with haemolysis.

Avoidance
- All the software must be carefully examined prior to setting up the machine to ensure there are no kinks or twists in the tubing.
- Constant observation of the colour of the plasma to detect the presence of haemolysis.
- When using filtration machines, constant monitoring of the transmembrane pressure is essential and particular care must be taken if frequent episodes of low flow occur as, in this situation, haemolysis is more likely to occur.

If haemolysis is suspected the procedure must be terminated, as the return of damaged red cells to the patient/donor could precipitate DIC and mimic a haemolytic transfusion reaction.

3.3.7 *Air embolus*

Most cell separators incorporate air-detector devices in the reinfusion line. However, with the use of blood warmers and other software beyond the machine's air detectors, there is a risk of air embolism if all the lines are not fully primed.

Never rely totally on fail-safe alarm systems. Occasionally they can break down and constant monitoring of all reinfusion lines is necessary to prevent air embolism from occurring.

3.3.8 *Infection*

Equipment contamination
Do not leave cell separators and associated equipment primed for longer than necessary and not for more than 1 hour prior to use.

Bacterial infection
If bacterial contamination has occurred during the set-up and priming procedure, there is a risk of causing a severe bacteraemia, which could be fatal in an immunosuppressed patient. Plasma exchange using crystalloid, colloid or albumen as replacement fluid depletes the patient's immunoglobulin level. The combination of low immunoglobulins and immunosupressive therapy predisposes the patient to infection. Prophylactic administration of intravenous immunoglobulin to patients particularly at risk should only be considered under special circumstances.

Recommendation. Apheresis procedures involve certain risks to donors/patients. All staff involved in donor/patient care during apheresis must be aware of the more common complications and be trained to identify them when they occur. Staff must also be trained in how to avoid common complications and also in their management should they occur. Problems with vascular access, reactions to citrate and to replacement fluids and chilling are the commonest complications. Paediatric patients and those with renal disease, liver disease, sickle-cell disease or immunosuppression are more prone to problems; extra care must be taken when treating these patients. Staff proficiency in the operation of cell separators and the identification and management of patient/donor complications during apheresis procedures must be maintained by regular use of equipment.

4 Postdonation care

It is important to ensure as far as possible that all donors/patients take the required amount of rest and drink at least one cup of fluid before leaving the apheresis venue and, if no adverse reactions have occurred, this information is noted in the relevant notes.

Any adverse reaction must be dealt with promptly, appropriately and sympathetically and must be documented. The patient/donor must have recovered as fully as possible before being allowed to leave the venue.

The nurse/doctor in charge must remain on the unit until the last donor/patient has left the premises.

Recommendation. Care of the donor/patient must include observation in the immediate postapheresis period to minimize the occurrence of delayed complications. A record of any postapheresis complications must be made and of the length of time for which observations were made.

5 Facilities

5.1 Accommodation

Ideally, cell separators should be operated in an area reserved exclusively for this work, although patients and donors can be managed in the same area. This area should be adequate to allow a cardiac-arrest team to operate. There should be sufficient space to allow for staff to operate all equipment without danger to themselves, patients and donors. All cell-separator units where products for subsequent transfusion are collected, such as platelets, peripheral-blood progenitor cells, lymphocytes or granulocytes, must comply with guidelines for good manufacturing practice (Medicine Control Agency, 1997). Collection and storage of progenitor cells must comply with current guidelines (BCSH Transfusion Task Force, 1994) and with Department of Health (1997) recommendations. Each cell-separator unit must have adequate space for patients/donors to rest and be monitored following a procedure, particularly if there have been any adverse reactions.

All procedures must be undertaken with resuscitation facilities available, as agreed by a consultant in charge of a hospital cardiac-arrest team. Staff must be trained in cardiopulmonary resuscitation (CPR) and in the use of the available equipment.

Patients categorized as high-risk from the point of view of infection should be managed in collaboration with a local control-of-infection officer. Local guidelines must be observed to minimize risk of transmission of infection. Advice from manufacturers may need to be obtained regarding appropriate decontamination procedures for apheresis equipment used for such patients.

Recommendation. Cell separators should be operated in an area reserved exclusively for their use. Adequate space must be provided for routine working and for CPR. Facilities must comply with good manufacturing practice regulations and with other relevant guideline recommendations. Appropriate facilities for the management of potentially infective patients must exist.

6 Staff

6.1 Training

The consultant in charge of the unit has responsibility for establishing a programme for initial and continued training of the apheresis staff to ensure an appropriate level of proficiency. Training may take place at a site other than an apheresis unit and may be supervised by a trainer qualified in assessment, but the consultant in charge of the unit and his/her nurse manager/sister must be satisfied that the content of the training is appropriate.

The consultant in charge of the apheresis unit, in consultation with the nurse manager or sister in charge of the unit, must be satisfied that the appropriate training has been completed before allowing staff to carry out apheresis procedures.

In the absence of a nationally recognized training programme, a suitable comprehensive training programme (3–6 months) should be devised, in conjunction with the appropriate machine manufacturers, and opportunities provided for regular updating (e.g. study days, conferences, etc.). Training should be done in accordance with standard operating procedures (SOPs) and cover aspects of donor/patient care, operation of machines and troubleshooting, and recognition and management of adverse effects. Training in CPR must be undertaken on a regular basis, using recognized trainers; a valid CPR certificate must be held by staff who perform patient apheresis procedures.

A suitable assessment designed to determine the level of competence of such staff must be performed and documentation of knowledge and technical ability (training records) must be kept and updated annually.

Recommendation. Staff responsible for cell-separator procedures must be trained to the highest standards of proficiency in the use of all appropriate equipment. Documentary evidence that training has been undertaken must be kept. Staff involved in patient care must be trained in CPR, including the use of resuscitation equipment retained on site, and they must hold a valid certificate as evidence of appropriate training.

7 Machine safety

Numerous types of cell separators are now available, but all operate on either a continuous- or an intermittent-flow principle, allowing rapid return of citrated blood.

These systems consist of a device that will carry out whole-blood separation, normally using a disposable apheresis set and a citrate and/or heparin anticoagulant solution. Such an integrated system withdraws blood from the donor/patient, mixes it with anticoagulant in the required ratio and separates and collects the component selected, safely returning the remaining blood components to the donor/patient.

The machine must comply with the relevant aspects of the Health and Safety at Work Act. Additionally, such machines must comply with the requirements of BS 5724: Part I: Safety of Medical Electrical Equipment (1979) and BS EN 60601–1–(1993).

7.1 Machine maintenance

Cell-separator machines should be serviced in accordance with manufacturers' instructions. A planned maintenance scheme should be followed.

Machine maintenance and servicing must be in accordance with procedures outlined in Equipment information HEI.98 Management of Medical Equipment, Devices (1990).

Apheresis machines should be routinely cleaned with a suitable decontaminating agent. A standard procedure for dealing with blood spillage must be in operation.

In the event of a mechanical failure of the machine, a service engineer should be able to be contacted by telephone during normal working hours.

Recommendation. Care should be taken to ensure that cell separators and other associated equipment conform to relevant British and European safety requirements. Regular servicing should be undertaken according to manufacturers' recommendations and service records must be kept.

Appendix 16.1: Guidelines for operators outlining standards of care for patients and donors undergoing blood-cell separation

A consultant fully experienced in the operation of cell separators has overall responsibility for the health and welfare of patients/donors and for the observance of the codes of practice.

Registered general nurses are responsible for nursing-care aspects and for preparation and operation of the cell separator.

The nurse in charge has responsibility for:

- the physical and psychological needs of the patient/donor;
- making sure that support facilities are available and functioning;
- completing a comprehensive record/worksheet;
- making sure there is instruction on postprocedural care and subsequent follow-up of patient/donor.

Standards and monitoring required to prevent complications

The clinical hazards associated with procedures and the avoidance of such complications are clearly outlined in this chapter.

To minimize operational errors, the following should apply.

1 Information required with reference to specific patient/donor management.
   (a) The physical and psychological condition of the patient/donor.
   (b) Any associated nursing care required.
   (c) The basic parameters required to establish the total blood and plasma volume: height, weight and haematocrit (relevant to the volume to be removed or exchanged and the anticoagulant ratio to be used).
   (d) The details of current drug therapy, particularly anticonvulsants, antiarrhythmics and steroids. It may be necessary to modify drug regimens or to give supplemental doses to maintain the desired drug concentration in the blood, especially when large quantities of plasma are to be removed.
   (e) If there is a history of cardiac valvular diseases, specialist advice about antibiotic prophylaxis should be sought.

2 A SOP must be available for the machine in use. It should include a detailed description of all procedures likely to be undertaken.

The SOP must clearly lay out details of the following.

- Maintenance of donor/patient records and care plans.
- Checking and prescribing required for drugs, anticoagulants and intravenous solutions, also recording all batch numbers of harnesses, packs, intravenous solutions and local anaesthetic (if used).

- A description of the complications which may arise during the procedure and the corrective and preventive action to be taken. This should include details of the following.
    (a) Procedures to be undertaken in the event of a respiratory or cardiac arrest and application of the techniques involved and the equipment in use.
    (b) Procedures following accident or untoward incident.
    (c) Action in the event of fire or a bomb alert.
- A list of appropriate laboratory tests for the procedure concerned, so that advice concerning intervention or adjustment to treatment can be sought.

Appendix 16.2: Donor and patient consent forms (cell separators)

Donor consent form

---

1 I .... (full name)

of .... (full address)
hereby acknowledge that I have volunteered to donate blood by means of a cell separator. The nature and purpose of the donation of blood by this means and the risks involved to the donor have been explained to me by:

Dr ....*

I hereby consent to the donation of ....
by means of a cell separator and I agree to undergo medical assessment which will also involve giving a sample of my blood for tests including a test for HIV/AIDS. I consent to such further or alternative operative measures or treatment as may be found necessary during the course of the donation.

Signature of volunteer donor ....

Date ....

2 I confirm that I have explained the nature and purpose of this procedure to the person who signed the above form of consent.

Signature of doctor ....

Date ....

* The explanation must be given by a medical practitioner.

Patient consent form

Please check and complete the following personal details.

SURNAME
FORENAME
ADDRESS

POSTCODE
DATE OF BIRTH

CASE SHEET NUMBER ....

To be completed by patient/guardian/parent/next of kin

I am the patient/guardian/parent/next of kin (delete where appropriate). I understand the procedure .... which has been explained by Dr .... I understand that this will involve the use of a cell-separator machine and the infusion of anticoagulant solution while blood is being processed. Any other procedure, in addition to that named above, will be performed if it is necessary and in the best interests of myself/my child/my next of kin (delete where appropriate).

I agree to the administration of local anaesthetic or to sedation if required.

I agree to the procedure named on this form.

Signature: .... **Date:** ....

NAME (block caps): ....

To be completed by the medical practitioner
I have fully explained to the patient/parent/guardian/next of kin:
1   The procedure named on the consent form.
2   Alternatives which are available.
3   The significant side-effects of this form of therapy.

Signature: .... **Date:** ....

NAME (block caps): ....

Appendix 16.3: Guidelines on the insertion and management of central venous lines (BCSH Clinical Task Force, 1998)

Major recommendations

1   Tunnelled central venous lines (catheters) are indicated for the repeated administration of chemotherapy, antibiotics, parenteral feeding and blood products, and for frequent blood sampling.

2   Single-lumen catheters can be used, but additional peripheral access will usually also be required.

3   Fully implantable catheters (ports) are more suitable for children and for less frequent but long-term use, while non-fully implantable lines are better for short-term use and intensive access.

4   Insertion should be performed by experienced operators, regardless of speciality. Lines should be inserted in children by paediatric specialists.

5   Imaging facilities (fluoroscopy, intravenous contrast studies and standard radiography) must be available.

6   Line insertion should take place in an operating theatre or similar clean environment.

7   Skin cleansing is of utmost importance.

8   Routine antibiotic prophylaxis should not be used.

9   Dressings are not required in the long term, but regular flushing (by protocol, according to the type of line) is essential to avoid thrombosis.

10   Pre-existing haemorrhagic, thrombotic or infective problems must be effectively managed before line insertion.

11   Thrombosis and infection must be promptly diagnosed and vigorously treated. Both complications may require removal of the line.

12   Catheters should only be removed by experienced personnel. Catheter breakage requires expert radiological intervention.

13   Patients should receive clear and comprehensive verbal and written information and be encouraged to look after their own lines.

14   Units should audit complications associated with central lines and should use the data to develop preventive measures.

References

ABPI (1999–2000) *Compendium of Data Sheets and Summaries of Product Characteristics.* Datapharm Publications, London.

BCSH (1991) Guidelines for the clinical use of blood cell separators. In Roberts B. (ed.) *Standard Haematology Practice*, pp. 231–251. Blackwell Science, Oxford.

BCSH Clinical Task Force (1997) Guidelines on the insertion and management of central venous lines. *British Journal of Haematology* **98**, 1041–1047.

BCSH Transfusion Task Force (1992) Guidelines for the use of fresh frozen plasma. *Transfusion Medicine* **2**, 57–63.

BCSH Transfusion Task Force (1994) Guidelines for collection, processing and storage of human bone marrow and peripheral stem cells for transplantation. *Transfusion Medicine* **4**, 165–172.

BCSH Transfusion Task Force (1996) Guidelines on gamma irradiation of blood components for the prevention of transfusion associated graft-versus-host disease. *Transfusion Medicine* **6**, 261–271.

BCSH Transfusion Task Force (1997) British Committee for Standards in Haematology guidelines for the administration of blood products: transfusion of infants and neonates. *Transfusion Medicine* **7**, 248.

Beck J.R., Quinn B.M., Meier R.A. & Rawnsley H.M. (1982) Hyperviscosity syndrome in paraproteinaemia. *Transfusion* **22**, 51–53.

Bjerrum O.S. & Jersild C. (1971) Class specific anti IgA associated with severe anaphylactic transfusion reactions in a patient with pernicious anaemia. *Vox Sanguinis* **21**, 411.

Blumberg N. & Heal J.M. (1988) Evidence for plasma mediated immunomodulation transfusions of plasma rich blood components are associated with a greater risk of acquired immunodeficiency. *Transplantation Proceedings* **206**, 1138–1142.

Bowden R. & Sayers M. (1990) The risk of transmitting cytomegalovirus by fresh frozen plasma. *Transfusion* **30**, 762–763.

Department of Health (1997) *Guidance Notes on the Processing, Storage and Issue of Bone Marrow and Blood Stem Cells*. Department of Health.

Huestis D. (1983) Mortality in therapeutic haemapheresis. *Lancet* **i**, 1043.

Management of Medical Equipment, Devices (1990) *Equipment Information HEI.98*. Health and Safety Executive, London.

Medicine Control Agency (1997) *Rules and Guidance for Pharmaceutical Manufacturers and Distributors*. HMSO, London.

Nordhagen R., Conradi M. & Demtorp S.M. (1986) Pulmonary reaction associated with transfusion of plasma containing anti-5b. *Vox Sanguinis* **51**, 102–108.

Rock G.A., Guillerin L., Dau P.C. *et al.* (1996) Application of plasma exchange in autoimmune disorders. *Transfusion Science* **17**, 207–282.

Silberstein L.E., Navyshkins Haddad J.J. & Strauss J.F. (1986) Calcium homeostasis during therapeutic plasma exchange. *Transfusion* **26**, 151–155.

Sutton D.M.C., Nair R.C. & Rock G. (1989) The Canadian Apheresis Study Group. Complications of plasma exchange. *Transfusion* **29**, 4–7.

UK BTS/NIBSC (1996a) *Guidelines for the Blood Transfusion Service*, 3rd edn. HMSO, London.

UK BTS/NIBSC (1996b) Guidelines for automated apheresis of volunteer donors within the UK Blood Transfusion Service. In *Guidelines for the Blood Transfusion Service*, 3rd edn, pp. 37–52. HMSO, London.

UK Central Council (UKCC) for Nursing, Midwifery and Health Visiting (1992) *The Scope of Professional Practice*. UKCC, Portland Place, London.

Westphal R.G. (1984) Health risks to cytapheresis donors. *Clinics in Haematology* **13**, 289–301.

17 Guidelines for the Estimation of Fetomaternal Haemorrhage

Prepared by the Blood Transfusion Task Force

1 Introduction

Transplacental haemorrhage (TPH) may occur following a sensitizing event during pregnancy or at delivery and can lead to Rh D immunization. Assessment of TPH is an important element in determining the amount of anti-D to be administered to an Rh D-negative mother following a sensitizing event or after delivery of an Rh D-positive infant. The joint Consensus Conference of the Royal College of Physicians of Edinburgh/Royal College of Obstetricians and Gynaecologists on anti-D prophylaxis stated that one to two of every 100 Rh D-negative pregnant women at risk still become sensitized.

The guidelines for the use of anti-D immunoglobulin for Rh prophylaxis (UK Blood Transfusion Service, Immunoglobulin Working Party, 1991) stated that at least 500 iu of anti-D must be given to every Rh D-negative woman with no preformed anti-D within 72 h of delivery of an Rh D-positive infant. This dose will be sufficient to prevent sensitization from a 4-ml fetal red blood cell (r.b.c.) bleed. However, 0.4% of women have a TPH of greater than 4 ml and up to 0.3% greater than 15 ml and will not be protected by the standard 500 iu dose of anti-D. It is therefore important that the size of any fetomaternal bleed is accurately estimated so that, if necessary, a supplementary dose of anti-D can be administered and maternal alloimmunization prevented.

2 Purpose of the guidelines

Despite earlier publications describing methods for assessing fetomaternal haemorrhage (FMH) (Wagstaff, 1978; UK Blood Transfusion Service, Immunoglobulin Working Party, 1991), it is recognized that there is little standardization of techniques (Milkins *et al.*, 1997), and this can lead to inaccuracies in determining the size of any FMH.

These guidelines set out recommendations for best practice, including: (i) quality assurance; (ii) sample requirements; (iii) serological testing; (iv) criteria for the assessment of FMH; (v) techniques for assessing FMH; (vi) examination of the blood film; (vii) calculation of the FMH; and (viii) follow-up and confirmation of the result.

Reprinted with permission from *Transfusion Medicine*, 1999, **9**, 87–92.

3 Quality assurance

The recommendations are as follows.

1 All laboratories carrying out FMH assessment participate in an external quality assurance scheme, e.g. UK NEQAS.

2 Standard operating procedures are available for the technique in use.

3 Training protocols are available.

4 There is a mechanism in place for ongoing assessment of staff proficiency for the technique in use.

4 Sample requirements

4.1 Women from whom blood samples are required

Blood samples are required from all Rh D-negative women at delivery and Rh D-negative women following a potentially sensitizing event after 20 weeks' gestation. A sensitizing event may be defined as therapeutic termination of pregnancy, spontaneous complete or incomplete abortion, amniocentesis, chorionic villus sampling, fetal blood sampling, insertion of shunts, embryo reduction, ante-partum haemorrhage, external cephalic version, closed abdominal injury, ectopic pregnancy, intrauterine death or stillbirth (Lee *et al.*, 1999). Sensitizing events before 20 weeks do not require an FMH assessment.

4.2 Type of samples

4.2.1 At delivery

1 Mother: an ethylenediaminetetra-acetic acid (EDTA) sample for FMH assessment and a clotted or EDTA sample for blood grouping and antibody screening.

2 From the cord: an EDTA or clotted sample, as locally required, taken with a syringe and needle from a cord vessel for blood grouping.

4.2.2 Following a sensitizing event between 20 weeks and delivery

An EDTA sample from the mother.

4.3 Sample labelling

The samples should be labelled in accordance with the British Committee for Standards in Haematology (BCSH) guidelines on pretransfusion compatibility testing (BCSH, 1996). The samples should also be clearly marked 'Cord' and 'Maternal', as appropriate. The request form should contain the full patient's details, including location, and relevant clinical details, including the date and time of delivery or sensitizing event.

4.4 Timing of samples

The maternal sample should be taken within 2 h of a normal delivery, manual removal of placenta or sensitizing event. The sample should be processed and results reported in sufficient time to ensure that, if necessary, a supplementary dose of anti-D can be given within 72 h of the delivery or sensitizing event.

5 Serological techniques

Rhesus D and ABO typing must be carried out on both the maternal and cord samples. The maternal sample should also be screened for clinically significant red-cell antibodies. Techniques used should be in accordance with the BCSH guidelines on pretransfusion compatibility testing (BCSH, 1996).

Anti-D detected in the maternal plasma/serum may be immune in origin or due to the administration of prophylactic anti-D. Where it is not certain that the anti-D present is immune in origin, a standard dose of anti-D should be administered.

6 Criteria for performing a fetomaternal haemorrhage estimation

An FMH estimation should be performed if a Rh D-negative woman has delivered a Rh D-positive baby or if a fetal blood group is not available. This will allow an appropriate supplementary dose of anti-D immunoglobulin (Ig) to be given to the woman within the correct time period, when necessary.

An FMH estimation should also be performed following a potentially sensitizing event after 20 weeks' gestation in a Rh D-negative woman (see Section 4.2).

Fetomaternal haemorrhage assessment is not indicated if preformed immune anti-D is present in the mother's plasma/serum.

7 Methods of assessment for fetomaternal haemorrhage

Techniques used for FMH assessment include acid elution (Mollison, 1972), rosetting (Jones & Silver, 1958) and flow cytometry (Johnson *et al.*, 1995). The techniques recommended for the screening and quantitation of FMH in this chapter are as follows.
1   Acid elution.
2   Flow cytometry.
Flow cytometry for the estimation of FMH is an evolving technique and offers the advantage that if an anti-D reagent is used to relabel the fetal cells Rh D-positive cells only are detected. It is recognized that not all laboratories have access to a flow cytometer and that in many laboratories only the acid-elution technique is available.

8 Acid-elution technique

It is very important that particular attention is paid to detail. Two recommended methods can be found in Appendix 17.1. All other methods (including commercial kits) should be standardized against one of these two recommended methods.

Care must be taken to exclude false-positive results. Increased levels of fetal haemoglobin (HbF) are seen in various genetic disorders, including β- and αβ-thalassaemias and hereditary persistence of HbF.

8.1 Slide preparation

Thin blood films are freshly made on clean, dry slides, previously degreased, if necessary. The thickness of the blood film is important for accurate results and it is recommended that the maternal whole-blood sample is diluted 1 : 2 or 1 : 3 with saline before making the film. It is important to ensure that the diluted sample is well mixed immediately before the film is made. Each slide must be spread evenly and, when examined under the microscope, should show red cells touching but not overlapping.

8.2 Controls

Controls must be performed with each batch of slides stained and should be treated in exactly the same way as the maternal sample.

1 Positive control: fresh EDTA cord blood diluted 1 : 100 in adult EDTA male blood. The sample should be well mixed before film preparation.

2 Negative control: adult male blood.

8.3 Staining

The effectiveness of the staining is dependent upon a number of factors, including temperature, age, quality and pH of the stain. All these factors must be standardized.

8.4 Examination of the stained films

It is recommended that this is divided into screening and quantitation.

Controls must be examined first to ensure that the staining and preparation are satisfactory. If the controls are not to the required standard, the whole process must be repeated.

8.4.1 Screening

A minimum of 25 fields should be examined using a ×10 objective. If no fetal red cells are seen, the FMH can be reported as <4 ml fetal red cells and no further anti-D is needed. If any fetal red cells are seen, a full quantitation must be performed.

8.4.2 Quantitation

Slides giving a positive screening result must be examined further to estimate the number of fetal cells present. It is recommended that fetal cells are expressed as a proportion of adult cells, with a minimum of 6000 cells being counted, using a ×40 objective. Lowering the condenser may make it easier to count ghosts.

This method is aided by the use of a Miller Square disc or an Indexed Square. Their use is described in Appendix 17.2.

8.5 Calculation of the fetomaternal haemorrhage

This is calculated using the formula described by Mollison (1972). This assumes that the maternal red cell volume is 1800mL, fetal cells are 22% larger than maternal cells and only

92% of fetal cells stain darkly. The fetal bleed should be calculated thus: uncorrected volume of bleed $= 1800 \times$ fetal cells counted (F)/adult cells counted (A) corrected for fetal volume $(1.22) = (1800 \times F/A) \times 1.22 = J$ and corrected for staining efficiency $(1.09) = J \times 1.09 =$ fetal bleed. An example is given in Appendix 17.2. When the fetomaternal bleed has been determined, a supplementary dose of anti-D is given, in accordance with recommendations, i.e. 125 iu/ml fetal red cells. A minimum of 500 iu must be given. When there is an FMH of more than 15 ml, it is preferable to use the larger anti-D Ig intramuscular (i.m.) preparation (2500 iu or 5000 iu) (Lee *et al.*, 1999).

8.6 Women with high levels of fetal haemoglobin

A standard dose of anti-D should be given. If free anti-D is present in the plasma no further anti-D Ig is necessary. However, if no free anti-D is present, a supplementary dose should be given and the original and a new sample should be sent to an appropriate centre for flow-cytometry analysis.

9 Flow cytometry

The flow-cytometry method is evolving and therefore only general guidance is given and a detailed method is not included.

9.1 Sample

1   Anticoagulated blood must be used.
2   The washing procedure must be validated to ensure that:
    (a)   all cells are sedimented by the centrifugation procedure;
    (b)   all cells are thoroughly resuspended before staining.

9.2 Staining

Indirect and direct methods of staining are available for identifying Rh D-positive fetal red cells.

9.2.1 Indirect staining

1   A polyclonal antiserum or a monoclonal antibody that gives clear discrimination between Rh D-positive and Rh D-negative cells must be used.
2   It is recommended that a fluorescent isothyocyanate (FITC)- or phycoerythrin (PE)-labelled Fab anti-human IgG reagent is used to prevent agglutination of fetal Rh D-positive red cells.
3   The anti-D and fluorescent anti-IgG reagent should be tested in a checkerboard assay to determine the optimum combination that gives maximum discrimination between negative and positive populations.

9.2.2 Direct staining

FITC or PE-labelled monoclonal anti-D antibodies are commercially available. The antibodies must be validated against mixtures of D-positive and negative cells to ensure that a clear discrimination between negative and positive populations can be made. The direct test should always be done on a maternal sample prior to the administration of anit-D.

Where the mother has received a dose of prophylactic anti-D it is possible that the Rh D-positive fetal cells will be sensitised to such an extent that binding of the fluorescent-labelled anti-D will be inhibited. This may falsely indicate that no Rh D-positive cells are present. It is recommended that where it is known that the mother has received anti-D an indirect and direct flow cytometric test should be undertaken.

9.3 Quantitation

Red blood cells should be selected for analysis by using forward- and side-scatter parameters. A gate setting should be selected such that >99% of red cells will be analysed for fluorescent staining. Validation of the gate settings may be accomplished by back-gating with r.b.c.s stained, for example, with an anti-glycophorin-FITC reagent. The use of the following in-house standards is recommended which use ABO-compatible Rh D-negative and Rh D-positive donors:

- 100% D-negative cells;
- 99% D-negative and 1% D-positive (approximating an 22 ml bleed);
- 99.75% D-negative and 0.25% D-positive (approximating a 5.5 ml bleed).

It is recommended that, as a minimum, duplicate test samples be analysed.

To minimize the coefficient of variation obtainable, no less than 500 000 events should be collected. Where the flow cytometer does not allow this, samples should be continuously reanalysed until an analysis of a sufficient number of cells (through summation by simple addition of the results from several individual counts) has been obtained.

The gain setting on FL1 or FL2 should be set so that <5% of negative events fall below the first log decade. Regions must be set on FL1 or FL2 to separate negative and positive cells; less than 0.05% of negative events should fall in the positive region. Background positive events obtained with 100% D-negative cells must be subtracted from the test positive events.

9.4 Calculation of fetomaternal haemorrhage

The percentage of Rh D-positive events (i.e. presumed red cells) is used to calculate the volume of fetal blood from the presumed maternal blood volume. The maternal blood volume is assumed to be 1800 ml of packed red cells; no account is taken of either maternal haematocrit, maternal body mass or the occurrence of maternal haemodilution just prior to delivery.

Cord red-cell volume is assumed to be 22% greater than that of adult red cells; hence the volume of fetal cells calculated as a percentage of the maternal red-cell number found to be Rh D-positive should be proportionately increased in order to take this difference into account. Thus, if 0.5% of the maternal blood is D-positive, then the fetal bleed will be calculated to be:

Uncorrected for fetal r.b.c. volume: $1800 \times 5/1000 = 9$
Corrected for fetal r.b.c. volume: $= 9 + (9 \times 22/100) = 10.98$

Table 17.1 Protocol for follow-up and confirmation

Acid elution/flow cytometry	Serum/plasma	Action
No fetal cells present	No free anti-D	Give further dose of anti-D Retest the serum/plasma for presence of free anti-D in 48 h
No fetal cells present	Free anti-D	No further action
Fetal cells present	No free anti-D	Quantitate and give appropriate further dose of anti-D Repeat FMH assessment in 48 h
Fetal cells present	Free anti-D	Repeat FMH assessment in 48 h

10 Confirmation

For any FMH greater than 4 ml, an appropriate supplementary dose of anti-D Ig must be given immediately. A repeat estimation of the FMH should be carried out 48 h following the initial anti-D injection. The serum/plasma should be screened for anti-D. The protocol given in Table 17.1 for follow-up and confirmation must be followed.

It is recommended that, wherever possible, a transplacental haemorrhage of greater than 4 ml should be confirmed by flow-cytometric analysis. If this method is not available, then a separate operator should confirm the FMH by the Kleihauer technique or, if this is not possible, e.g. out of routine working hours, a new film should be examined.

11 Follow-up

Where a large FMH (>4 ml) has been identified, a sample should be taken from the mother 6 months after the sensitizing event and the serum or plasma tested for the presence of anti-D.

Acknowledgments

The writing group wish to acknowledge the help of Dr Eric Austin and Dr Anatole Lubenko in writing the section on flow cytometry.

Appendix 17.1: Demonstration of fetal haemoglobin in individual red cells: acid-elution technique

Principle

Fetal haemoglobin (HbF) is more resistant than adult haemoglobin (HbA) to both alkali denaturation and acid elution. When dry blood films are fixed and then immersed in an acid-buffer solution, HbA is denatured and eluted, leaving red-cell ghosts. Red cells containing HbF are resistant and the haemoglobin can be stained; these cells stand out in a sea of ghost maternal cells. There are many factors which influence the quality of the results.

Two techniques will be described. The first is based on the classical Kleihauer method and the second is a shorter modification, on which commercially available kits are based. For both, strict timing is essential.

Method 1
Reagents
Fixative. Solution A: Citric acid monohydrate 0.1 m ($C_6H_8O_7.H_2O$, mol.wt 210.14) 21.01 g to 1 l distilled water.
Solution B: Disodium hydrogen phosphate 0.2 m ($Na_2HPO_4.2H_2O$, mol.wt 177.99)
           35.60 g to 1 l distilled water.
Working buffer: pH 3.3 Solution A: 73.4 ml.
                        Solution B: 26.6 ml.
Check pH and adjust if necessary; pH is critical.

Stains
Ehrlich's acid haematoxylin.
Eosin Y 10 g/l in distilled water.

Method
1   The making of the films is described above.
2   Fill a Coplin jar with the working citrate–phosphate buffer (pH 3.3) and allow to warm to 37°C. Allow air bubbles to escape.
3   Fix slides in 80% ethanol for 5 min. Rinse in tap water and air-dry.
4   Immerse slides in citrate–phosphate buffer at 37°C for 5 min. Agitate slides at 1 and 3 min to ensure even exposure to the buffer.
5   Rinse slides in tap water and air-dry.
6   Stain slides in Ehrlich's acid haemotoxylin for 3 min. Rinse slides in tap water.
7   Counterstain with eosin for 3 min. Rinse in tap water and dry.

Results
Haemoglobin F-containing cells are stained densely red and are refractile. The cells that contained HbA are ghosts. White cells stain grey/blue.

Method 2: rapid technique
Reagents
Solution A: Haemotoxylin 7.5 g in 100% ethanol to 1 l.
Solution B: Ferric chloride 24 g.
              Hydrochloric acid (2.5 mol/l) 20 ml.
              Distilled water to 1 l.
Eluting solution (pH 1.5) Solution A: 2 parts.
                            Solution B: 1 part.
                            80% Ethanol 1 part.
Counterstain: Eosin Y 10 g/l in distilled water.
Solutions A and B can be stored at room temperature. If stored in a refrigerator, the eluting

solution must be allowed to reach room temperature before use. The eluting solution should be made up freshly each time.

Method
1   Make films as described above.
2   Fix in 80% ethanol for 5 min. Air-dry.
3   Flood slides with the eluting solution at room temperature for 20 s. Rinse in distilled water and air-dry.
4   Stain with 1% eosin for 2 min.
5   Rinse in tap water and air-dry.

The staining characteristics are identical to those describe above. Examination and reporting are described elsewhere in the chapter.

Appendix 17.2: Quantification of fetomaternal haemorrhage using visual counting

Using a Miller square (Fig. 17.1)
1   Using a ×40 objective, select an area of the film where cells are touching but not over-lapping appreciably.
2   Count adult cells (A) in the small square, including all cells which overlap the left-hand or upper edges but not those overlapping the right-hand or lower edges.
3   Count fetal cells (F) in the large square, treating cells overlapping the edges as above.
4   Move across the slide so that the next area to fall within the counting grid is contiguous with the preceding one and repeat the procedure.
5   Continue until the proportion of fetal cells among a minimum of 6000 adult cells has been counted.
6   Assume the total adult cells scanned (A × 9) = 6003 and total fetal cells counted = 18.
7   Calculate the FMH using the formula of Mollison:

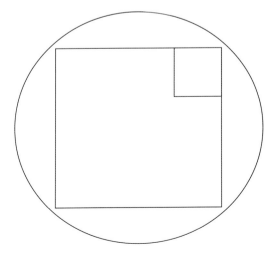

Fig. 17.1 Miller square.

Volume of fetal cells (in ml) = 2400/ratio of adult to fetal cells

For example, if the total adult cells scanned (A × 9) was 6003 and the total fetal cells counted (F) was 18, then the ratio of A/F is 6000/18 = 333.5. The fetal haemorrhage is therefore 2400/333 = 7.2 ml.

Note. It is essential to survey a minimum of 6000 cells to achieve reasonable precision. In the above example, the 95% confidence limits of an estimate of 7.2 ml would be 6.36–8.03 ml, allowing for the fact that only 667 adult cells are actually counted (this number being multiplied by 9 to estimate the number of adult cells actually scanned). If 6000 cells were actually counted, the 95% confidence limits would be narrower – 6.91–7.49 ml.

Using an indexed square

The procedure is as above, except that adult cells are counted in 10 of 100 squares in a 10 × 10 grid and the ratio of adult to fetal cells is then A/(F × 10).

Suppliers of both graticules

Graticules Ltd., Morley Road, Tonbridge, Kent TN9 1RN.
- Miller Square E57 16 mm order no. 01A16032, 19 mm 01A19032, 21 mm 01A21032, price on 17.8.99 £35.70.
- Indexed Square E35 16 mm order no. 01B16221, 19 mm 01B19221, 21 mm 01B121221, price on 17.8.99 £35.70.
- Use of either graticule requires a Kellner × 10 (F10) eyepiece, order no. 5E 02081, price on 17.8.99 £59.

References

BCSH (1996) Guidelines for pre-transfusion compatibility procedures in blood transfusion laboratories. *Transfusion Medicine* **6**, 273–283.

Johnson P.R.E., Tait R.C., Austen E.B., Shwe K.H. & Lee D. (1995) The use of flow cytometry in the quantitation and management of large feto-maternal haemorrhage. *Journal of Clinical Pathology* **48**, 1005–1008.

Jones A.R. & Silver S. (1958) The detection of minor erythrocyte populations by mixed agglutinates. *Blood* **13**, 763.

Lee D., Contreras M., Robson S.C., Rodeck C.H. & Whittle M.J. (1999) Recommendations for the use of anti-D immunoglobulin for Rh prophylaxis. *Transfusion Medicine* **9**, 93–97.

Milkins C.E., Wardle J., O'Hagan J. *et al.* (1997) Measurement of feto-maternal haemorrhage (FMH) – a report of the first two surveys from the UK National External Quality Assessment pilot scheme for FMH. *Transfusion Medicine* **7** (Suppl. 1), 52.

Mollison P.L. (1972) Quantitation of transplacental haemorrhage. *British Medical Journal* **3**, 31–34.

UK Blood Transfusion Services Immunoglobulin Working Party (1991) Recommendations for the use of anti-D immunoglobulin. *Prescribers Journal* **31**, 137–145.

Wagstaff W. (1978) *Practical Aspects of Anti-D Prophylaxis of Haemolytic Disease of the Newborn.* Broadsheet 90, Association of Clinical Pathologists, 189 Dyke Road, Hove BN3 1TL.

18 Guidelines Addendum for the Administration of Blood Products: Transfusion of Infants and Neonates

Prepared by the Blood Transfusion Task Force

Following discussions at the Ministerial Advisory Committee on the Microbiological Safety of Blood and Tissues for Transplants (MSBT), new recommendations have been agreed regarding the selection of blood products for neonates and infants less than 1 year of age. These have been drawn up in order to reduce transfusion risks to this vulnerable group to a minimum. The recommendations endorse earlier advice contained in British Committee for Standards in Haematology (BCSH, 1994), but go further in several significant ways. The information has been circulated to consultant haematologists within blood services of the UK, with the expectation that it will be disseminated to clinical colleagues. The key features of the new recommendations include the following.

- Donations from first-time donors should not be used. Components should only be prepared from donors who have been tested on a previous occasion and found negative for all current required microbiological markers.
- One donation should be dedicated to cover the needs of any infant likely to require several red-cell transfusions over a short period of time. This can be achieved by the use of multiple satellite packs containing sterile dispensed aliquots.
- Red-cell and platelet components should be leucocyte-depleted to reduce the possibility of cell-associated virus transmission and to minimize possible long-term immunomodulatory effects. Where appropriate (e.g. where leucodepletion is not possible), cytomegalovirus (CMV)-seronegative donations should be used.
- For transfusions involving a significant volume of plasma, it may also be necessary to minimize the effects of ABO incompatibility by the use of donors screened to exclude high-titre anti-A and anti-B.

Reference

BCSH (1994) Guidelines for administration of blood products: transfusion of infants and neonates. *Transfusion Medicine* **4**, 63–69.

Reprinted with permission from *Transfusion Medicine*, 1997, **7**, 248.

19 Guidelines on the Provision of Facilities for the Care of Adult Patients with Haematological Malignancies (including Leukaemia and Lymphoma and Severe Bone Marrow Failure)

Prepared by the Clinical Haematology Task Force

1 Introduction

The British Committee for Standards in Haematology (BCSH) Clinical Haematology Task Force produced its first 'Guidelines on the care of adult patients with leukaemia and lymphoma' in 1986. That report recommended the establishment of leukaemia centres for the specialist care of these patients, and its publication generated much debate within the profession. Since that time, significant changes in the management of leukaemia have taken place, particularly the extension of high-dose chemotherapy and bone-marrow transplantation (BMT) to older patients and the use of unrelated donors for transplants. The intervening 7 years have failed to see the establishment of specific leukaemia centres, either regionally or nationally, other than those already in place before 1986 in the special health authorities. In addition, the change in the operating environment of the National Health Service (NHS) to one of purchaser and provider has made the concept of leukaemia centres less valid.

This chapter has been prepared with a view to advising providers, and reminds NHS purchasers of the facilities and expertise they should be seeking when planning to place contracts for leukaemia and lymphoma care for adults, including BMT. Purchasers are keen to see the best value for their money, and leukaemia care, especially involving BMT, is relatively expensive. While accepting that efficiency savings are always to be welcomed, the cheapest option may not always provide a sufficient quality of care. Another manifestation of the purchaser/provider relationship and the establishment of NHS trust hospitals has been the desire of many trusts to expand the range of services offered to their (neighbouring) purchasers. One such service has been BMT, especially autografting. Evidence from allogeneic BMT (Horowitz et al., 1992) suggests that, in these conditions, the number of cases treated each year affects outcome, i.e. the greater the experience of the unit, the better the results. If standards are to be maintained in an environment of increasing pressure to reduce costs, it is important to address those aspects of care that are considered essential, or minimal, for the safe treatment of groups of patients (ASCO/ASH, 1990).

Because the concept of leukaemia centres has not been developed, this chapter does not presume to suggest how services for these disorders should be provided for the patients of

Reprinted with permission from *Clinical and Laboratory Haematology*, 1995, **17**, 3–10.

any purchasing authority. Rather, it is subdivided so that the different levels of facilities required for carrying out specific treatment procedures or treatment for particular groups of patients are clearly identified. These treatments or procedures have been divided into four levels of care, as described below. The appropriate level of treatment should be determined by the complexity of care and support services for patient management; this may be independent of the age of the patient. Shared care between larger and smaller centres is highly desirable and should not be discouraged by financial considerations.

1.1 Level 1 care – general haematology patients

This includes general haematology patients, such as those with chronic lymphocytic leukaemia, low-grade non-Hodgkin's lymphoma (NHL), chronic myeloid leukaemia and other myeloproliferative disorders, multiple myeloma (older patients receiving non-intensive treatment) and myelodysplasia, being diagnosed and managed using conventional doses of chemotherapy, which would not normally be planned to produce prolonged neutropenia. The numbers of patients in these categories significantly exceed those with acute leukaemia and high-grade lymphoma. The workload for haematologists is steadily rising, because of an increased incidence of myelodysplasia in an ageing population, increasing incidence of lymphoma and expanding use of chemotherapy, both in haematology and by other specialities.

Hospitals providing general haematology care at this level should be capable of the safe management of a patient with transient severe neutropenia, prior to transfer to a centre providing care at a higher level, including that of patients with severe aplastic anaemia. Some hospitals at this level will wish to use combined chemotherapy regimens for lymphomas, such as CHOP and ChlVPP.

1.2 Level 2 care – remission induction

This will cover facilities required for remission induction in acute myeloid or acute lymphoblastic leukaemia, using current standard intensive chemotherapy regimes, such as those used in Medical Research Council (MRC) trials, Acute Myeloid Leukaemia (AML) 10 and UK Acute Lymphoblastic Leukaemia (UKALL) 12. Such facilities will also be required for managing patients with Hodgkin's lymphoma or NHL, using pulses of chemotherapy, such as CHOP, MOPP, EVAP, DHAP and VAPEC-B. Early aftercare of patients receiving autologous transplants elsewhere is also appropriate at this level.

1.3 Level 3 care – autologous transplants

Level 3 facilities will be capable of carrying out autologous transplants, using either bone marrow or peripheral-blood stem cells (PBSCs), and conditioning regimens, such as high-dose melphalan or BEAM.

1.4 Level 4 care – related allogeneic bone-marrow transplants

At this level, related allogeneic BMTs and autologous transplants using total body irradiation (TBI) or busulphan/cyclophosphamide (Bu/Cy) would be included. The reason for including autologous transplants using these regimens at level 4, rather than level 3, is that evidence is emerging from MRC trials of continuing morbidity and mortality over 1 year post-transplant in patients receiving TBI + Bu/Cy conditioning.

Centres of level 4 standard will already have a proven record in autologous transplantation and be registered with the MRC and EBMT. In order to maintain expertise, there should be agreement between the centre and the prime purchaser(s) for at least 10 sibling donor allografts in addition to 10 autografts annually. In some geographical locations, a centre functioning at this level may be viable, despite being unable to meet the target of 10 allografts, while performing more than 10 autografts annually. The programme should not commence with patients rejected by other more established allograft centres. New centres should achieve the target number of cases within 2 years.

A small number of centres at level 4 will be capable of carrying out transplants using techniques for patients without a sibling donor. This may involve allogeneic BMT from a matched unrelated donor (MUD transplantation) or a number of other techniques, including autologous transplantation after long-term bone-marrow culture, etc. The unit should normally be transplanting at least 10 allogeneic (related) cases per year, estimated from the average for the previous 3 years (Executive Committee of WMDA, 1992). There must be agreement between physicians, senior nurses and managers for a programme of unrelated volunteer transplants, with the aim being at least three per year in addition to the minimum of 10 related transplants. The programme should not commence with patients rejected by more established centres.

As most districts are too small to provide sufficient patients to maintain local expertise, centres of level 3 and 4 standard will be dealing with a significant proportion of tertiary referrals. Contracts should secure access to comprehensive care on a planned basis. In view of the unpredictability of need and the potentially large cost involved, simple block contracts and ECRs may not be appropriate. Purchasers may wish to move towards more sophisticated block or threshold contracts and to increase their use of cost and volume and cost-per-case contracts (similar to those required in haemophilia care) (NHSME, 1993b). Further guidance on contracting for specialized services has recently been provided by the NHS Management Executive (NHSME, 1993a). A number of 'multiple purchaser' models are described in this handbook and the concept of 'lead purchasing' is developed.

Important issues that must be considered by purchasers are summarized in the following sections.

1.5 Capital requirements
- Beds: number of single rooms, number of beds overall and their location.
- Isolation facilities: single rooms, positive-pressure ventilation, laminar air flow.
- Equipment: availability on haematology ward of intravenous pumps, ambulatory pumps, pulse-oximetry.
- Hospital infrastructure: capability of providing urgent respiratory/bronchoscopy service, central venous access (e.g. Hickman line) insertion service, renal dialysis, intensive care unit, nutrition team, central pharmacy drug preparation.

- Laboratory: range of general and special haematology investigations provided, transfusion services and whether on site or remote, ease of access to microbiological diagnosis and advice, participation in external quality assessment schemes and laboratory accreditation (e.g. with Clinical Pathology Accreditation (CPA) (UK) Ltd.).
- Availability of cytopheresis, plasmapheresis, cell sorting and cell storage. Access to molecular biology, histopathology, cytogenetics and a research background should all be taken into account in determining the level of care that can be delivered.
- Radiotherapy: ready access to a department possessing suitable equipment and staff with relevant skills.

1.6 Staffing

- Medical staff: availability of resident doctors at or above junior house officer (JHO); consultant and intermediate-grade cover. Ability to provide 24 h cover with experienced staff (see British Society for Haematology (BSH) document on haematology staffing (BSH, 1992)). Ward rounds with consultant microbiologists, virologists and other interested specialists. Skills in palliative care and pain relief at consultant level.
- Nursing: numbers and skill mix over a 24 h period. Availability of expert advice and support from nurse specialists in haematology/oncology and related areas, e.g. palliative care. Extent of the role undertaken by ward staff, e.g. inclusion of intravenous (i.v.) administration, phlebotomy, venous cannulation, etc. Staff education.
- Existence of guidelines and protocols. Extent to which admission to designated haematology beds can be guaranteed.
- Pharmacy: central drug make-up and particular input from a specific pharmacist (Allwood & Wright, 1993).
- Support services: other issues of importance in determining the type of patients that can be dealt with would include support from social work, chaplaincy, psychiatry, other staff support, physiotherapy, occupational therapy.
- Centres treating patients with lymphoma secondary to human immunodeficiency virus (HIV) infection will require staffing and facilities appropriate to patients with acquired immune deficiency syndrome (AIDS).

1.7 Blood transfusion

Improvements in blood transfusion support have been partly responsible for the increasing success in the treatment of patients with leukaemia, lymphoma and severe bone marrow failure and have allowed the use of intensive treatment regimens, causing prolonged bone marrow suppression.

The blood transfusion support of such patients requires close collaboration between the clinical service and the hospital blood transfusion laboratory. In hospitals providing level 3 care and above, one of the consultant haematologists may have specialist training and experience in blood transfusion and be responsible for the clinical and laboratory transfusion services (Royal College of Pathologists, 1989). Alternatively, this may be the responsibility of one of the regional transfusion-centre consultants, who may have sessions on the unit or at least be in regular and specific contact with the consultant staff of the unit.

The blood transfusion laboratory, in turn, needs to liaise closely with the regional transfusion centre and other suppliers of blood components and blood products. Blood transfusion support must be available 24 h a day and should be able to provide the necessary blood components and blood products on demand.

2 Requirements for treatment and care of patients at level 1

2.1 General
Treatment at this level requires all the usual facilities of a district general hospital (DGH), including access to radiotherapy services.

2.2 Capital requirements
• Beds: a flexible number of specific haematology beds should be available on a general medical ward and patients admitted under the care of a consultant haematologist.
• Isolation facilities: one room for neutropenic patients awaiting transfer is desirable.
• Equipment: no special equipment over and above that found on an acute general medical ward.
• Hospital infrastructure: the environment of the average DGH is adequate for this level of care.
• Laboratory: there must be a full haematology and blood transfusion laboratory on site with rapid availability of blood counts, blood and blood products. Medical laboratory scientific officers (MLSOs) and scientific staff should be familiar with cytochemical techniques and there must be easy access to chromosome analysis and immunophenotyping. Routine biochemistry and microbiology must be immediately available.
• Radiotherapy: must be readily available but not necessarily on site.

2.3 Staffing
• Medical staff: there must be 24 h availability of dedicated or shared juniors at senior house officer (SHO) or registrar level. A consultant haematologist must be available for advice at all times. Agreed protocols for common medical problems should be available (neutropenic fever, hypercalcaemia, etc.).
• Nursing: the patient's named nurse should have 6 months' experience in haematology (or oncology). There should be access to the advice of a clinical nurse specialist (CNS) in haematology/oncology. On wards with a high proportion of haematology beds, this role may be incorporated with that of a suitably qualified and experienced ward sister. In the case of wards with a smaller haematology workload, the CNS may be peripatetic and cover more than one hospital.

By day and night, there should be sufficient i.v. skilled nurses to ensure that all i.v. therapy is given at the prescribed times (or within the range 5–7 h for 6-hourly drugs and 10–14 h for 12-hourly drugs).

Where there is no specific haematology out patient department, nursing support to clinics should include the CNS and/or nurses from haematology ward areas.

• There should be clear and practicable written guidelines/protocols on: i.v. drug administration; care of i.v. access devices; cytotoxic drug handling and administration; blood transfusion; infection control; management of pyrexia.

• Pharmacy: there must be a proper cytotoxic drug-handling facility, with a pharmacist experienced in the field available for advice (see national guidelines (Allwood & Wright, 1993)). There must also be access to haemopoietic growth factors and all appropriate antimicrobial agents and antiemetics.

• Support services: the provision of care should include access to a named social worker, psychological and emotional support facilities, a terminal care/palliative medicine service and spiritual advisers of all faiths.

• Audit/research: data collection should be an integral part of the service, permitting audit and outcome review and facilitating collaboration with other centres in trials and other studies. Purchasers should enquire about the extent to which patients are entered on therapeutic trials.

2.4 Blood transfusion

The following transfusion services should be available:

1 Platelet concentrates. Depending on the distance from the regional transfusion centre, a number of platelet concentrates may have to be stored under appropriate conditions (BCSH, 1992) in the blood transfusion laboratory, so that they are available for the treatment of thrombocytopenic bleeding.

2 Red cell and platelet concentrates from donors seronegative for cytomegalovirus (CMV) infection. These concentrates should be available for patients who are potential BMT recipients to prevent primary CMV infection.

3 Leucocyte-depleted red cell and platelet concentrates for certain groups of patients (Royal College of Physicians, Edinburgh, 1993) – for example:

(a) young patients with aplastic anaemia requiring transfusion before onward referral, to minimize the risk of sensitization to transplantation antigens;

(b) potential BMT recipients, as an alternative to CMV-seronegative red-cell and platelet concentrates, to prevent CMV infection;

(c) older patients with bone-marrow failure receiving regular red-cell transfusions, to prevent recurrent non-haemolytic transfusion reactions.

The BCSH has established a working party to develop formal guidelines on leucocyte-depleted blood products (BCSH, 1998; see Chapter 12).

4 Human leucocyte antigen (HLA)-matched platelet concentrates for patients refractory to platelet transfusions from random donors because of HLA alloimmunisation (BCSH, 1992).

5 Coagulation factor replacement, e.g. fresh-frozen plasma (FFP), cryoprecipitate and coagulation factor concentrates.

6   Gamma-irradiated cellular blood components to prevent transfusion-associated graft-versus-host disease (GvHD) in susceptible recipients (Anderson *et al.*, 1991; BCSH, 1996; see Chapter 14).

7   Cell separator facilities for plasma exchange and leucaphaeresis, either on site or elsewhere. The BCSH guidelines for the clinical use of cell separators have already been published (Roberts, 1991) and the BCSH Blood Transfusion Task Force has prepared 'Guidelines for the collection, storage and processing of human bone marrow and peripheral stem cells prior to transplantation' (BCSH, 1994).

8   Reference laboratory services for red cell serology, platelet serology and HLA class I and II antigen typing and matching.

3 Requirements for treatment and care of patients at level 2

3.1 General
Care at this level requires all the facilities available at level 1, with some refinements. There should be provision for direct admission of patients to the haematology ward, to encourage self-referral of existing patients.

3.2 Capital requirements
• Beds: specific haematology beds must be available on a single general medical ward.
• Isolation facilities: a number of single rooms with en suite facilities must be available.
• Equipment: central venous catheters and pumps (portable and static) must be available.
• Hospital infrastructure: there should be ready access to bronchoscopy, dialysis and intensive care facilities. Central venous (Hickman) or Portacath insertion must be available from a committed specialist experienced in this work.
• Laboratory: similar facilities are required to those for level 1.
• Radiotherapy: must be readily available but not necessarily on site.

3.3 Staffing
• Medical: as for level 1, but junior doctors should be part of the firm looking after the patient and must be familiar with unit protocols. Consultant haematological and microbiological advice must be available at all times. In the case of haematology, this requires two consultants, both of whom must be clinically committed, experienced in the management of such patients and aware of recent advances.
• Nursing: senior ward nursing staff (F grade and above) should hold a recognized certificate in haematology or oncology nursing (e.g. English National Board ENB 237, ENB A27 or one of the recognized short courses in haematology and BMT nursing) or possess demonstrably equivalent experience and knowledge. All staff allocated to care for these patients should have a range of i.v. skills.
• Pharmacy: cytotoxic drug reconstitution must be centralized in the pharmacy and there should ideally be a specific pharmacist allocated to the unit.

• Support services: as for level 1, but involvement in trials will necessitate a data handling capability that exceeds that of level 1. A data manager should be available, although this member of staff may be shared with other centres.

3.4 Blood transfusion

All the transfusion facilities should be available as for level 1 care. However, a greater requirement for CMV-seronegative and gamma-irradiated blood components can be anticipated, particularly for BMT patients receiving shared care with a larger centre.

4 Requirements for treatment and care of patients at level 3

4.1 Capital requirements

• Beds: at least four rooms should be available and form part of a larger haematology unit. The case for positive pressure ventilation and/or air filtration at this level has not been proved. When necessary, patients may be nursed on the open ward, but patients selected for this should be those whose blood counts are recovering or who have received less intensive chemotherapy regimens. In order to maintain expertise, the unit should perform at least 10 autologous BMT (ABMT) or PBSC procedures per year.

• Isolation facilities: as for level 2.

• Equipment: substantial numbers of intravenous pumps are required and special equipment, such as pulse-oximeters and resuscitation facilities, should be available on the ward.

• Hospital infrastructure: a rapid facility for central venous line insertion must be available and there should ideally be on site bronchoscopy, dialysis and intensive care facilities and a nutrition team.

• Laboratory: the haematology department requires the full range of facilities as for level 2 and also access to cell culture facilities and cryobiology. The provision of immunophenotyping services, molecular biology, histopathology, cytogenetics and research facilities should either be on site or immediately available. There must be a bacteriology laboratory on site and ready access to special virology investigations and advice. An automated blood-culture system should be available.

• Radiotherapy: ready access to a department with experienced staff should be available, preferably on site, with a named radiotherapist being associated with the clinical service.

4.2 Staffing

• Medical staff:
  (a) at least two consultant haematologists to provide cross cover;
  (b) at least three other haematology medical staff (above JHO), who may be either trainee or staff grades;
  (c) on call from a limited pool of doctors, with clear protocols and 24 h consultant advice available.

The total number of medical staff must be sufficient for keeping up to date and to cover general haematological services.

• Nursing: the named nurse should have at least 6 months' experience of autograft/PBSC transplantation. At least 25% of all staff should have completed a recognized course in haematology or oncology. All unit/ward nursing staff should have the full range of i.v. therapy skills. The unit should possess nursing staff with counselling skills and there should be access to hospital-based MacMillan nurses.

• Pharmacy: central cytotoxic drug reconstitution and a specific unit pharmacist are essential. There must be access to the fullest range of haemopoietic growth factors, antimicrobial agents and antiemetics.

• Support services: cell separation. There must be ready access to a cell separator for the preparation of PBSC. If at unit level, this will require staffing by at least one experienced staff nurse who will be in attendance throughout all procedures and capable of dealing with emergency situations (see Chapter 16). There must be access to social workers and skilled counsellors.

4.3 Blood transfusion

All the transfusion facilities should be available as for level 1 and 2 care. In addition, the following should be available.

1 Facilities for the collection, processing and storage of bone-marrow cells and PBSCs. Individuals concerned with this procedure must be aware of the need to conform to good manufacturing practice (GMP) (BCSH, 1994).

2 Immediate access to a local source for gamma-irradiation of blood components.

5 Requirements for treatment and care of patients at level 4

5.1 Capital requirements

• Beds: a specific area or unit containing at least four single rooms with en suite facilities. Rooms should not be used by patients other than those receiving treatment directly related to autologous or allogeneic transplantation. Ideally, the ward should have a designated kitchen area. Provision for separate relatives' overnight accommodation should be available adjacent to the unit. Readmissions after allogeneic transplant should be to the same unit for the first year.

• Isolation facilities: rooms should preferably have laminar air flow or positive air handling with high efficiency particulate air (HEPA) filtration.

• Equipment: as for level 3. Rooms must contain piped oxygen and suction facilities. Resuscitation equipment should be immediately available within the unit. Beds should tilt at both ends.

• Hospital infrastructure: as for level 3. There should be on site anaesthetic, surgical, respiratory, dialysis, intensive therapy unit (ITU), dermatological, pharmacological, microbiological, psychological and computer assisted tomography (CT) scanning facilities;

magnetic resonance imaging (MRI) is of value in the diagnosis of central nervous system (CNS) complications. Such colleagues should have experience in the particular problems encountered in BMT patients.

- Laboratory: as for level 3, but in addition the laboratory must be capable of aseptic bulk manipulation of donor marrow, e.g. T-cell adjustment. Centres performing MUD transplants will have greater need for these techniques and for long term bone marrow culture.

Quality control measures must be in place to ensure the clonogenic capacity and sterility of the resulting donor stem cells. Ideally, such work should be performed by specific clinical scientists or MLSO staff, following standard operating procedures (SOPs). For research and other purposes, data on stem cell yield, efficacy of T-cell adjustment and CMV status should be stored on database to permit retrieval at a later date. Such centres will be actively involved in research at a national or international level, especially if performing MUD transplants.

Biochemistry services must be able to provide same-day cyclosporin levels and liver function tests.

- Radiotherapy: level 4 requires the availability of TBI facilities. If not on site, common protocols should be followed. There must be an identified radiotherapist member of the BMT team and a physicist experienced in the planning and administration of TBI. The department should have the capacity to permit no more than a 2–3-week wait for TBI.

5.2 Staffing

- Medical.

    (a)   There should be at least two consultant haematologists/transplant physicians with experience and training in BMT and able to provide 24 h cover. In centres performing MUD transplants, consultant staff should have at least 5 years' experience of allogeneic BMT. Such consultants should be available to return to the unit at short notice.

    (b)   There must be at least three junior haematological medical staff (SHO grade or above) providing daytime and on-site night-time cover in rota with junior medical colleagues who are familiar with transplant patients on the unit. One of these staff (probably a higher specialist trainee or staff grade) will act as a transplant coordinator to liaise with patients, relatives, nursing and medical staff and other professional groups (MLSOs, scientists).

- Nursing: the named nurse should have at least 6 months' experience of allogeneic BMT work. Staff at F grade and above and at least 25% of all staff should hold a recognized certificate in haematology (or oncology) which includes the specific care of patients undergoing allogeneic BMT. A senior member of nursing staff should have specific responsibility and time for the coordination of non-medical aspects of pre-BMT work.

Staff support provision should reflect the stresses inherent in providing an allogeneic BMT service.

Nurses in centres performing MUD transplants must have prolonged experience of allogeneic BMT and the care of patients with GvHD.

- Pharmacy: as for level 3.
- Support services: an identified BMT coordinator is essential to facilitate cooperation with donor registries.

5.3 Blood transfusion

As for level 3, but with comprehensive facilities for molecular as well as serological techniques of tissue typing and matching.

Appendix 19.1 Glossary for purchasers

Bone-marrow transplant:
Autologous (ABMT): in this procedure marrow is aspirated from the patient and returned (with or without manipulation) following high dose chemo/radiotherapy.
Allogeneic (BMT): marrow from a normal donor (usually a fully matched sibling) is given to the patient after high dose chemo/radiotherapy.
Matched unrelated donor (MUD): marrow from a normal volunteer donor identified from a computer database is used where a sibling donor is unavailable.
Cytochemistry: The use of special stains to identify the lineage of leukaemic cells.
Cytogenetics: The study of chromosomes by light microscopy.
Haematological malignancy: 'Cancer' affecting the blood, bone marrow or lymphatic system.
Hickman line: A long term indwelling catheter placed into a large central vein to facilitate investigation and treatment of patients with haematological malignancies.
Human leucocyte antigen (HLA) matching: Comparing the HLAs (tissue type) of patients and prospective donors.
Immunophenotyping: The use of immunological methods (usually employing monoclonal antibodies) to identify the precise type of leukaemia or lymphoma cells.
Leukaemia:
Acute: a disorder of haematological precursors (myeloid or lymphoid) in which normal maturation is blocked. May be rapidly fatal if untreated but potentially curable.
Chronic: an accumulation of mature white blood cells (myeloid or lymphoid) causing impaired bone marrow function and/or antibody production. Controllable with treatment but not curable (with the exception of BMT for young patients with chronic myeloid leukaemia).
Lymphoma:
Hodgkin's: a tumour of lymph nodes of variable cell type, distinguished by the presence of Reed–Sternberg cells. Frequently curable with standard chemo/radiotherapy.
Non-Hodgkin's (NHL): A tumour of lymph nodes with different clinical features and microscopic appearance from Hodgkin's disease.
High-grade NHL: acute onset, aggressive course but potentially curable.
Low-grade NHL: insidious onset and course, controllable but usually not curable.
Molecular biology: The study of genes and their abnormalities at the nucleic acid level, using a variety of techniques, including the polymerase chain reaction (PCR).

Myelodysplasia: A group of morphological and functional bone marrow disorders, which may develop into acute myeloid leukaemia.

Myeloma: A tumour of plasma cells which may cause anaemia, renal failure, hyper-calcaemia and bone destruction. Controllable but very rarely curable with treatment.

Myeloproliferative disorder: Increased activity of all cell types in the bone marrow, leading to overproduction of circulating red cells, granulocytes, platelets or combinations of these. Usually controllable with simple therapy.

Morphology: The study of cell and tissue structure.

Neutropenia: A reduction in polymorphonuclear granulocytes, leading to an increased tendency to bacterial and fungal infection.

Peripheral blood stem cells (PBSC): Cells found in the peripheral blood (similar to those in bone marrow) which are capable of division and maturation to mature blood cells while maintaining their own numbers.

Remission: A state of apparent absence of disease (morphological, cytogenetic or molecular).

References

Allwood M. & Wright P. (eds) (1993) *The Cytotoxic Handbook*, 2nd edition. Radcliffe Medical Press Ltd., Oxford, p. 315.

Anderson, K.C., Goodnough, L.T., Sayers, M. *et al.* (1991) Variation in blood component irradiation practice: implications for prevention of transfusion-associated graft-versus-host disease. *Blood* **77**, 2096–2102.

ASCO/ASH (1990) Recommended criteria for the performance of bone marrow transplantation. *Blood* **75**, 1209.

BCSH (1992) Guidelines for platelet transfusions. *Transfusion Medicine*, **2**, 311–331.

BCSH (1994) Guidelines for the collection, storage and processing of human bone marrow and peripheral stem cells prior to transplantation. *Transfusion Medicine* **4**, 165–172.

BCSH (1996) Guidelines on gamma-irradiation of blood components for the prevention of transfusion-associated graft-versus-host disease. *Transfusion Medicine* **6**, 261–271.

BCSH (1998) Guidelines on the clinical use of leucocyte-depleted blood components. *Transfusion Medicine* **8**, 59–71.

British Society for Haematology (BSH) (1992) Report of a Presidential Working Party to consider Consultant Haematology Staffing Requirements in UK Hospitals (unpublished but circulated to BSH members).

Executive Committee of WMDA (1992) Bone marrow transplants using volunteer donors – recommendations and requirements for a standardized practice throughout the world. *Bone Marrow Transplantation* **10**, 287–291.

Horowitz M.M., Przepiorka D., Champlin R.E. *et al.* (1992) Should HLA-identical sibling bone marrow transplants for leukemia be restricted to large centers? *Blood* **79**, 2771–2774.

NHS Management Executive (NHSME) (1993a) *Contracting for Specialised Services – a practical guide.* NHSME, EL(93)98, p. 63.

NHS Management Executive (NHSME) (1993b) Provision of haemophilia treatment and care. Health Service Guidelines, HSG **93**, 30.

Roberts B. (ed.) (1991) Clinical use of blood cell separators. In *Standard Haematology Practice*, pp. 231–251. Blackwell Science, Oxford.

Royal College of Pathologists (1989) Recommendations for training for a haematologist who has a special interest in blood transfusion within the hospital service. Bulletin of the Royal College of Pathologists **68**, 9–10.

Royal College of Physicians, Edinburgh (1993) Consensus Conference on leucocyte depletion of blood and blood components (1993). Royal College of Physicians, Edinburgh.

20 Guidelines for the Prevention and Treatment of Infection in Patients with an Absent or Dysfunctional Spleen
Prepared by the Clinical Haematology Task Force

1 Introduction

Overwhelming postsplenectomy infection should be preventable if simple precautions are taken. An ad hoc working party of the British Committee for Standards in Haematology has reviewed recommendations for patients without a spleen and drawn up a consensus. Members of the working party were selected for their personal expertise and to represent relevant professional bodies. The guidelines, which are set out below, include and extend the Chief Medical Officer's 1994 update.

Fulminant, potentially life-threatening infection is a major long-term risk after splenectomy (King & Shumacker, 1952; Cullingford *et al.*, 1991). Splenic macrophages have an important filtering and phagocytic role in removing bacteria and parasitized red blood cells from the circulation (Rosse, 1987). Although the liver can perform this function in the absence of a spleen, higher levels of specific antibody (Hosea *et al.*, 1981) and an intact complement system are probably required. The ability of an asplenic patient to mount an adequate protective antibody response may relate more to the indication for or age at splenectomy and to the presence of underlying immune suppression than to the absence of the spleen.

This chapter presents the conclusions of an ad hoc working party of the British Committee for Standards in Haematology on procedures for managing patients without a spleen. In accordance with guidance on best practice (Effective Health Care Bulletin, 1994; Clinical Guidelines Working Group, 1995), the guidelines are based on an assessment of published evidence and the expert opinion of the working party.

2 Methods

2.1 Assessment of published evidence
The CD-ROM databases Silver Platter Medline (1966–95) and Excerpta Medica (1974–95) were searched by using the keywords infection, splenectomy, asplenia and hyposplenism. Abstracts in English (of English and non-English articles) were reviewed. In addition, bibliographies of previous reviews and papers describing original research were cross-checked.

Reprinted with permission from *British Medical Journal*, 1996, **312**, 430–434.

2.2 Guideline development group

In view of the potential bias in guideline development by small groups (Newton *et al.*, 1992), a national working group representative of key disciplines was convened under the auspices of the British Committee for Standards in Haematology. The working-group members were from general practice, haematology, immunology, microbiology, paediatrics, surgery and public-health medicine. The formal consensus of the guideline development group was integrated with the findings of systematic review of published evidence to formulate the ensuing recommendations.

3 Background

3.1 Infecting microorganisms

Most instances of serious infection are due to encapsulated bacteria, such as *Streptococcus pneumoniae* (pneumococcus), *Haemophilus influenzae* type b and *Neisseria meningitidis* (meningococcus) (Traub *et al.*, 1987). Pneumococcal infection is most common and carries a mortality of up to 60% (Ellison & Fabri, 1983; Holdsworth *et al.*, 1991). Infection with *H. influenzae* type b is much less common, but none the less significant, particularly in children (Teare & O'Riordan, 1992). The meningococcus may also be associated with serious infection (McMullin & Johnston, 1993). Other infections include *Escherichia coli* (Edwards & Digiola, 1976), malaria (Oster *et al.*, 1980), babesiosis (Rosner *et al.*, 1984) and *Capnocytophaga canimorsus* (DF-2 bacillus), which is associated with dog bites (McCarthy & Zumla, 1988).

3.2 Patient categories

3.2.1 Operative splenectomy

Surgical removal of the spleen is performed for severe splenic trauma, for splenic cysts or as part of a resective procedure for tumours of the spleen or adjacent organs (Jackson, 1983). Partial splenectomy with retention of some splenic tissue is increasingly practised (Buyukunal *et al.*, 1987). However, in view of the uncertainty of the level of splenic function achieved by partial splenectomy or autotransplantation of splenic tissue, it is prudent to institute similar measures to prevent infection in these patients to those for asplenic subjects.

Although there has been a reduction in the use of splenectomy for staging haematological malignancies, such as Hodgkin's disease, the procedure may still be used in hereditary spherocytosis, immune thrombocytopenic purpura and autoimmune haemolytic anaemia. Patients receiving immunosuppressive chemotherapy or radiotherapy or both are at greatest risk of serious infection after splenectomy (Siber *et al.*, 1978).

3.2.2 Functional hyposplenism

Functional hyposplenism may be detected on a blood film as red cells containing Heinz and Howell–Jolly bodies, thrombocytosis and monocytosis (Hoffbrand & Lewis, 1989).

Splenic dysfunction may occur secondary to sickle-cell anaemia (haemoglobin SS (HbSS), HbSC), thalassaemia major, essential thrombocythaemia and lymphoproliferative diseases (Hodgkin's disease, non-Hodgkin's lymphoma and chronic lymphocytic leukaemia). Functional hyposplenism may also occur in coeliac disease (Marsh & Stewart, 1970), inflammatory bowel disease (Jewell, 1987) and dermatitis herpetiformis (Losowsky, 1987).

Bone-marrow transplantation is a further cause of functional hyposplenism, leading to an increased incidence of pneumococcal bacteraemia and *H. influenzae* type b pneumonia (Winston *et al.*, 1979). Although most studies have shown an association of infections with chronic graft-versus-host disease (Aucouturier *et al.*, 1987), in some patients there is also impaired splenic function, with Howell–Jolly bodies (Aucouturier *et al.*, 1987; Kalhs *et al.*, 1988). Infections occur 6 months after bone-marrow transplantation, after co-trimoxazole prophylaxis against pneumocystis pneumonia has been stopped (Kalhs *et al.*, 1988). More detailed recommendations for managing patients receiving bone-marrow transplantation have been given by Fielding (1994). All patients having bone-marrow transplantation should be immunized against pneumococcal infection 9–12 months after transplantation, and those with chronic graft-versus-host disease should receive appropriate long-term prophylactic antibiotics, especially if the spleen has been removed or irradiated before transplantation.

3.2.3 Congenital asplenia
Congenital asplenia is associated with cardiac abnormalities and biliary atresia (Dyke *et al.*, 1991).

3.2.4 Effect of age
Asplenic children under 5 – and especially infants splenectomized for trauma – have an infection rate of over 10%, much higher than in adults (<1%) (Robinette & Fraumeni, 1977). Children with sickle-cell anaemia (HbSS, HbSC) are at especially high risk of overwhelming infection (Cummins *et al.*, 1991).

Other groups of patients may for other reasons be considered at risk of infection with encapsulated organisms – for example, patients with chronic lymphocytic leukaemia or myeloma (Gowda *et al.*, 1995) and patients with human immunodeficiency virus (HIV)-related disease or other immunodeficiency states. Local or national guidelines for the prevention of infection in these groups should be consulted (Gibb & Walters, 1993).

3.3 Duration of risk
Although most infections occur within the first 2 years after splenectomy, up to a third may be manifested at least 5 years later. Cases of fulminating infection have been reported more than 20 years after splenectomy (Evans, 1985). The risk of dying of serious infection, though unquantifiable (Shaw & Print, 1989), is clinically significant and almost certainly lifelong.

Patients falling into all the above categories, once identified, should receive appropriate vaccination and advice about lifelong antibiotic prophylaxis.

Table 20.1 Key guidelines

- All splenectomized patients and those with functional hyposplenism should receive pneumococcal immunization (A, B)
- Documentation, communication and reimmunization require attention (A, B)
- Patients not previously immunized should receive *Haemophilus influenzae* type b vaccine (A, B)
- Meningococcal immunization is not routinely recommended (B)
- Influenza immunization may be beneficial (B)
- Lifelong prophylactic antibiotics are recommended (oral phenoxymethylpenicillin or an alternative) (A, B)
- Asplenic patients are at risk of severe malaria (A)
- Animal and tick bites may be dangerous (A)
- Patients should be given a leaflet and a card to alert health professionals to their risk of overwhelming infection (A, B)
- Patients developing infection despite measures must be given a systemic antibiotic and urgently admitted to hospital (A, B)

N.B. There are no randomized controlled trials or case-controlled studies on this issue.
A, based on published evidence; B, expert opinion.

4 Guidelines (Table 20.1)

The Chief Medical Officer has highlighted the importance of preventive measures for post-splenectomy sepsis (Chief Medical Officer, 1994).

4.1 Immunizations

Asplenia in itself is not a contraindication to routine immunization. Normal inoculations, including live vaccines, can be given safely to children and adults with absent or dysfunctional spleens.

4.1.1 Pneumococcal immunization

Current vaccine

The currently available polyvalent pneumococcal vaccine contains purified capsular polysaccharide from the 23 most prevalent serotypes (Health and Public Policy Committee, 1986). The vaccine is more than 90% effective in healthy adults under the age of 55 (Shapiro *et al.*, 1991). Once vaccinated, failure of protection may relate to waning specific antibody levels or be due to infection with serotypes not represented in the vaccine. Children under 2 years of age have inherently reduced ability to mount an antibody response to polysaccharide antigens. However, pneumococcal vaccine may have some (if reduced) efficacy for particular serotypes. The same considerations apply to other patients who have functional hyposplenism because of an underlying disorder (Grimfors *et al.*, 1989). The vaccine is best avoided in pregnancy (Walker, 1995).

Timing

The vaccine should be given a minimum of 2 weeks before elective splenectomy, in order to ensure an optimal antibody response. If this is not practicable, the patient should be immunized as soon as possible after recovery from the operation and before discharge from hospital. The general practitioner should be notified of the splenectomy and vaccinations given, in order to avoid potential reactions due to premature reimmunization. Unimmunized patients splenectomized some time earlier should be immunized at the first opportunity. Immunization, however, should be delayed at least 6 months after immunosuppressive chemotherapy or radiotherapy, during which time prophylactic antibiotics should be given. Hyposplenic patients should be immunized as soon as the diagnosis is made, although, because of the reduced efficacy in young children (Department of Health, 1992), it may be better to rely initially on prophylactic antibiotics and immunize after the second birthday.

Reimmunization of asplenic patients is currently recommended every 5–10 years (Department of Health, 1992). It may be necessary to revaccinate more frequently, particularly if there is an underlying disease causing immunosuppression. Antibody levels may decline more rapidly than expected in asplenic patients (Giebink *et al.*, 1981) and reimmunization may be required as early as 3 years after the first dose, especially in lymphoproliferative disorders or sickle-cell anaemia (Weintrub *et al.*, 1984).

Adverse reactions
Side-effects of immunization are usually self-limiting hypersensitivity, with pain and swelling at the site of the injection after 24 h. Much less commonly, fever, malaise and generalized aches, disappearing after 48–72 h, may occur. Occasional patients with chronic immune thrombocytopenic purpura may have a relapse of their thrombocytopenia after immunization (Kelton, 1981).

4.1.2 Haemophilus influenzae *type b immunization*
Most children in Britain up to 4 years of age will have received *H. influenzae* type b vaccine. When over 18 years, most patients will have acquired some immunity through natural exposure, but this may not provide adequate protection in the context of an absent or dysfunctional spleen. The vaccine has been shown to be immunogenic in patients with impaired splenic function associated with sickle-cell anaemia (Rubin *et al.*, 1992). The level of antibodies to *H. influenzae* type b required for protection is known for people with an intact spleen. There is evidence that a higher specific antibody level is required in patients lacking a spleen (Rubin *et al.*, 1992). The need for reimmunization is unclear.

4.1.3 Meningococcal immunization
In Britain, meningococcal infection is most commonly due to a group B strain (Jones & Karczmarski, 1995). The present meningococcal vaccine covers groups A and C, which occur more commonly abroad. As the protection conferred with the current vaccine is of short duration, meningococcal immunization is not routinely recommended for asplenic patients, except when travelling to areas where there is an increased risk of group A infection. Otherwise, the vaccine should be restricted to groups for whom it is already specifically recommended – that is, close contacts of cases due to group A or C disease and outbreaks in closed or semiclosed institutions (Walker, 1995). Reimmunization should

be considered after 2 years in those remaining at risk, especially children. A forthcoming conjugated vaccine should provide longer-lasting immunity.

4.1.4 Influenza immunization

Influenza vaccine is recommended yearly for patients with 'immunosuppression due to disease or treatment' (Chief Medical Officer, 1993), and may be of value to asplenic patients by reducing the risk of secondary bacterial infection.

4.2 Antibiotic prophylaxis

Prophylactic oral phenoxymethylpenicillin has been used effectively for years in children with sickle-cell anaemia (Gaston *et al.*, 1986). Although amoxycillin has been recommended more recently (Waghorn, 1993), this drug may be less well tolerated in young children and is more expensive. The advantages of amoxycillin over penicillin in adults are that it is better absorbed as an oral preparation and it has a broader spectrum and a longer shelf-life (Chattopadhay, 1989). Patients who are allergic to penicillin should be offered erythromycin (see Appendix 20.1).

Lifelong prophylactic antibiotics should be offered in all cases, especially in the first 2 years after splenectomy, for all children aged up to 16 (Cummins *et al.*, 1991) and when there is underlying impaired immune function (Scopes, 1991). In addition, for patients not allergic to penicillin, a supply of amoxycillin should be kept at home (and taken on holiday) and used immediately should infective symptoms of raised temperature, malaise or shivering develop. In such a situation, the patient should seek immediate medical help. In the event of a feverish illness, patients taking erythromycin as prophylaxis should increase the dose to a therapeutic level or change to an alternative broader-spectrum preparation and seek medical advice immediately.

Antibiotic prophylaxis may not prevent sepsis. Indeed, phenoxymethylpenicillin does not cover *H. influenzae* and neither does amoxycillin reliably. The emergence of antibiotic-resistant bacterial strains (Klugman & Koornhof, 1989) must be considered if empirical treatment of sick patients is to be used. Local resistance patterns may dictate the need to use other antibiotics.

4.3 Recommendations for travellers

Asplenic patients should be strongly advised of the increased risk of severe falciparum malaria. Scrupulous adherence to antimalarial prophylaxis cannot be overemphasized, and specialist advice from an infectious-disease or tropical-disease unit or the local consultant in communicable-disease control should be sought. Meningococcal A plus C vaccine is recommended for all those travelling to sub-Saharan Africa, India and Nepal (Fielding, 1994).

Patients who are not otherwise taking antibiotic prophylaxis should do so during periods of travel (Conlon, 1993) and should keep a therapeutic course of antibiotics with them for the duration of the holiday, taking into account resistance patterns, such as the high incidence of penicillin-resistant pneumococci in Spain and some other European countries.

4.4 Other measures

It is essential to educate patients regarding the risk and the importance of prompt recognition and treatment of infections. Asplenic patients should be encouraged to wear a Medic-Alert disc (Medic-Alert Foundation (a registered charity), 156 Caledonian Road, London N1 9UU) and carry a card with information about their lack of a spleen, other clinical details and contact telephone numbers. In an emergency, this information may be life-saving. An information leaflet and patient card about splenectomy are available from the Department of Health (HMSO, Oldham Broadway Business Park, Broadgate, Chadderton, Oldham OL9 0JA).

4.4.1 Environmental

Protective clothing and washing after potential exposure in endemic areas for histoplasmosis, babesiosis and malaria may be beneficial.

4.4.2 Animal bites

Ensure adequate antibiotic cover after dog (and other animal) bites, as asplenic patients are particularly susceptible to infection by *C. canimorsus* (DF-2 bacillus) and should receive a 5-day course of co-amoxiclav (erythromycin in allergic patients).

4.4.3 Tick bites

Babesiosis is a rare tick-borne infection, and patients (especially those in contact with animals) should be warned of the danger of tick bites transmitting the disease. Clinical presentation is with fever, fatigue and haemolytic anaemia. Diagnosis is made by identifying parasites within red cells on blood films and by specific serology. Quinine (with or without clindamycin) is usually effective treatment (Shute, 1975).

4.4.4 Mosquito bites

Travel to areas where malaria is endemic should be discouraged. Patients should be made aware of their increased risk and advised about chemoprophylaxis relevant to local patterns of resistance and measures to reduce exposure to malaria parasites.

4.5 Treatment of acute infection

In suspected pneumococcal, meningococcal or other serious infection, immediate medical attention is required. Primary-care physicians attending a known asplenic patient with clinically significant infection should (provided there is no history of penicillin allergy) give an immediate dose of intramuscular or intravenous benzylpenicillin before transfer to hospital. The intravenous route is preferable. For adults and children over 10, 1200 mg (2 million units (MU)) benzylpenicillin should be dissolved in 10 ml water for injection and injected over 3–4 min. A blood sample can be taken for culture immediately before giving the penicillin, but the injection should not be delayed if facilities are not immediately to hand.

Once the patient has been admitted to hospital, blood samples should be taken and intravenous benzylpenicillin continued – but, for patients who have been receiving antibiotic prophylaxis, patients allergic to penicillin, patients with possibly resistant organisms and children under 5, cefotaxime or ceftriaxone should be given instead. Patients allergic to penicillin who are also allergic to cephalosporins may be given chloramphenicol after taking expert advice (see Appendix 20.1).

Appendix 20.1: Dosing regimens for antibiotic prophylaxis and treatment

Antibiotic	Oral prophylaxis	Treatment for suspected infection*
Penicillin		
Adult	250–500 mg 12-hourly†‡	1.2 g 4–6-hourly§
Child aged 5–14 years	250 mg 12-hourly‡	200–300 mg/kg/day in six divided doses
Child under 5 years‖	125 mg 12-hourly‡	(maximum 6 g)§
Erythromycin (base)		
Adult + child over 8 years	250–500 mg daily	0.5–1.0 g 6-hourly by mouth or intravenously
Child aged 2–8 years	250 mg daily	250 mg 6-hourly by mouth
		12.5 mg/kg/day intravenously by infusion in four divided doses
Child under 2 years	125 mg daily	12.5 mg/kg/day by mouth or intravenously by infusion in four divided doses
Amoxycillin/co-amoxiclav (doses according to amoxycillin content)		
Adult	250–500 mg daily	0.5–1.0 g 8-hourly by mouth or intravenously
Child aged 5–14 years	125 mg daily	250 mg 8-hourly by mouth
		90 mg/kg/day intravenously in three divided doses
Child aged 1–5 years	10 mg/kg/day	125 mg 8-hourly by mouth
		90 mg/kg/day intravenously in three divided doses
Child under 1 year	10 mg/kg/day	62.5 mg 8-hourly by mouth
		90 mg/kg/day intravenously in three divided doses
Cefotaxime		
Adult	Not suitable	2 g 8-hourly intravenously
Child under 14 years	Not suitable	100 mg/kg/day intravenously in three divided doses (maximum 12 g)
Ceftriaxone		
Adult	Not suitable	1–2 g once daily intravenously
Child under 14 years	Not suitable	80 mg/kg/day intravenously in a single dose (maximum 4 g)
Chloramphenicol (only patients allergic to penicillins and cephalosporins)		
All patients	Not suitable	Expert advice

* Established infection may require much higher doses given in hospital.
† If compliance is a problem, 500 mg once daily is acceptable.
‡ Phenoxymethylpenicillin (oral).
§ Benzylpenicillin (intravenous).
‖ Seek expert advice for neonatal doses.

References

Aucouturier P., Barra A., Intrator L. *et al.* (1987) Long lasting IgG subclass and antibacterial polysaccharide antibody deficiency after allogeneic bone marrow transplantation. *Blood* **70**, 779–785.

Buyukunal C., Danismend N. & Yeker D. (1987) Spleen saving procedures in paediatric splenic trauma. *British Journal of Surgery* **74**, 350–352.

Chattopadhay B. (1989) Splenectomy, pneumococcal vaccination and antibiotic prophylaxis. *British Journal of Hospital Medicine* **41**, 172–174.

Chief Medical Officer (1993) *Influenza Immunisation*. PL/CMO (93)13, HMSO, London.

Chief Medical Officer (1994) *Asplenic Patients and Immunisation: Update 1*, p. 3. HMSO, London.

Clinical Guidelines Working Group (1995) *The Development and Implementation of Clinical Guidelines*. Report No. 26, Royal College of General Practitioners, London.

Conlon C.P. (1993) The immunocompromised traveller. *British Medical Bulletin* **49**, 412–422.

Cullingford G.L., Watkins D.N., Watts A.D.J. & Mallon D.F. (1991) Severe late postsplenectomy infection. *British Journal of Surgery* **78**, 716–721.

Cummins D., Heuschkel R. & Davies S.C. (1991) Penicillin prophylaxis in children with sickle cell disease in Brent. *British Medical Journal* **302**, 989–990.

Department of Health (1992) *Immunisation against Infectious Disease*, p. 102. HMSO, London.

Dyke M.P., Martin R.P. & Berry P.J. (1991) Septicaemia and adrenal haemorrhage in congenital asplenia. *Archive of Diseases in Children* **66**, 636–637.

Edwards L.D. & Digiola R. (1976) Infections in splenectomised patients: a study of 131 patients. *Scandinavian Journal of Infectious Diseases* **8**, 255–261.

Effective Health Care Bulletin (1994) *Implementing Clinical Practice Guidelines: Can Guidelines be Used to Improve Clinical Practice?* Effective Health Care Bulletin No. 8.

Ellison E. & Fabri P.J. (1983) Complications of splenectomy: etiology, prevention and management. *Surgery Clinics of North America* **63**, 1313–1330.

Evans D. (1985) Post-splenectomy sepsis 10 years or more after operation. *Journal of Clinical Pathology* **38**, 309–311.

Fielding A.K. (1994) Prophylaxis against late infection following splenectomy and bone marrow transplant. *Blood Review* **8**, 179–191.

Gaston M.H., Verter J.I., Woods G. *et al.* (1986) Prophylaxis with oral penicillin in children with sickle cell anaemia: a randomised trial. *New England Journal of Medicine* **314**, 1593–1599.

Gibb D. & Walters S. (1993) *Guidance for Management of Children with HIV Infection*, 2nd edn, 29 pp. AVERT, Horsham.

Giebink G.S., Le C.T., Cosio F.G., Spika J.S. & Schiffmann G. (1981) Serum antibody responses of high-risk children and adults to vaccination with capsular polysaccharides of *Streptococcus pneumoniae*. *Review of Infectious Diseases* **3** (Suppl.), 168–178.

Gowda R., Razvi F.M. & Summerfield G.P. (1995) Risk of pneumococcal septicaemia in patients with chronic lymphoproliferative malignancies. *British Medical Journal* **311**, 26–27.

Grimfors G., Bjorkholm M., Hammarstrom L., Askergren J., Smith C.I.E. & Holm G. (1989) Type-specific anti-pneumococcal antibody subclass response to vaccination after splenectomy with special reference to lymphoma patients. *European Journal of Haematology* **43**, 404–410.

Health and Public Policy Committee, American College of Physicians (1986) Pneumococcal vaccine. *Annals of Internal Medicine* **104**, 118–120.

Hoffbrand A.V. & Lewis S.M. (1989) *Postgraduate Haematology*, 3rd edn, p. 20. Blackwell Scientific, Oxford.

Holdsworth R.J., Irving A.D. & Cuschieri A. (1991) Post-splenectomy sepsis and its mortality rate: actual versus perceived risks. *British Journal of Surgery* **78**, 1031–1038.

Hosea S.W., Brown E.J., Hamburger M.I. & Frank M.M. (1981) Opsonic requirements for intravascular clearance after splenectomy. *New England Journal of Medicine* **304**, 246–250.

Jackson J.W. (1983) Operations for carcinoma of the thoracic oesophagus and cardia. In Dudley H., Pories W. & Carter D. (eds) *Rob and Smith's Operative Surgery: Alimentary Tract and Abdominal Wall*, 4th edn, Vol. 1, p. 177. Butterworths, London.

Jewell D.P. (1987) Crohn's disease. In Weatherall D.J., Ledingham J.G.G. & Warrell D.A. (eds) *The Oxford Textbook of Medicine*, 2nd edn, Vol. 12, pp. 122–123. Oxford University Press, Oxford.

Jones D.M. & Karczmarski E.B. (1995) Meningococcal infections in England and Wales: 1994. *Community Disease Report Weekly* 5, 125–129.

Kalhs P., Panzer S., Kletter K. *et al.* (1988) Functional asplenia after bone marrow transplantation. *Annals of Internal Medicine* 109, 461–464.

Kelton J.G. (1981) Vaccination-associated relapse of immune thrombocytopenia. *Journal of the American Medical Association* 245, 369–371.

King H. & Shumacker H.B., Jr (1952) Splenic studies: susceptibility to infection after splenectomy performed in infancy. *Annals of Surgery* 136, 239–242.

Klugman K.P. & Koornhof H.J. (1989) Worldwide increase in pneumococcal antibiotic resistance. *Lancet* ii, 444.

Losowsky M.S. (1987) Malabsorption. In Weatherall D.J., Ledingham J.G.G. & Warrell D.A. (eds) *The Oxford Textbook of Medicine*, 2nd edn, Vol. 12, p. 106. Oxford University Press, Oxford.

McCarthy M. & Zumla A. (1988) DF-2 infection. *British Medical Journal* 297, 135–136.

McMullin M. & Johnston G. (1993) Long term management of patients after splenectomy. *British Medical Journal* 307, 1372–1373.

Marsh G.W. & Stewart J.S. (1970) Splenic function in adult coeliac disease. *British Journal of Haematology* 19, 445–447.

Newton J.C., Hutchinson A., Steen I.N., Russell I. & Haines E. (1992) Educational potential of medical audit: observations from a study of small groups setting standards. *Quality in Health Care* 1, 256–259.

Oster C.N., Koontz L.C. & Wyler C.J. (1980) Malaria in asplenic mice: effects of splenectomy, congenital asplenia and splenic reconstitution on the course of infection. *American Journal of Tropical Medicine and Hygiene* 29, 1138–1142.

Robinette C.D. & Fraumeni J.F., Jr (1977) Splenectomy and subsequent mortality in veterans of the 1939–1945 war. *Lancet* ii, 127–129.

Rosner F., Zarrabi M.H., Benach J.L. & Habicht G.S. (1984) Babesiosis in splenectomized adults. *American Journal of Medicine* 76, 696–701.

Rosse W.F. (1987) The spleen as a filter. *New England Journal of Medicine* 317, 704–706.

Rubin L.G., Voulalas D. & Carmody L. (1992) Immunogenicity of *Haemophilus influenzae* type b conjugate vaccine in children with sickle cell disease. *American Journal of Diseases in Children* 146, 340–342.

Scopes J.W. (1991) Continued need for pneumococcal prophylaxis after splenectomy. *Archive of Diseases in Children* 66, 750.

Shapiro E.D., Berg A.T., Austrian R. *et al.* (1991) The protective efficacy of polyvalent pneumococcal polysaccharide vaccine. *New England Journal of Medicine* 325, 1453–1460.

Shaw J.H. & Print C.G. (1989) Postsplenectomy sepsis. *British Journal of Surgery* 76, 1074–1081.

Shute P.G. (1975) Splenectomy and susceptibility to malaria and babesia infection. *British Medical Journal* i, 516.

Siber G.R., Weitzman S.A., Aisenberg A.C., Weinstein H.J. & Schiffman G. (1978) Impaired antibody response to pneumococcal vaccine after treatment for Hodgkin's disease. *New England Journal of Medicine* 299, 442–448.

Teare L. & O'Riordan S. (1992) Is splenectomy another indication for *Haemophilus influenzae* type b vaccination? *Lancet* 340, 1362.

Traub A., Giebink G.S., Smith C. *et al.* (1987) Splenic reticuloendothelial function after splenectomy, spleen repair and spleen autotransplantation. *New England Journal of Medicine* 317, 1559–1564.

Waghorn D.J. (1993) Prevention of post-splenectomy sepsis. *Lancet* 341, 248.

Walker G. (1995) *ABPI Data Sheet Compendium 1994–95*, p. 986. ABPI, London.

Weintrub P.S., Schiffman G., Addiego J.E. *et al.* (1984) Long-term follow-up and booster immunisation with polyvalent polysaccharide in patients with sickle cell anaemia. *Journal of Pediatrics* 105, 261–263.

Winston D.J., Schiffman G., Wang D.C. *et al.* (1979) Pneumococcal infections after human bone marrow transplantation. *Annals of Internal Medicine* 91, 835–841.

21 Guidelines on the Insertion and Management of Central Venous Lines

Prepared by the Clinical Haematology Task Force

1 Introduction

These guidelines are a review of basic principles and relevant research for nursing and medical staff involved in the care of patients with skin-tunnelled catheters. They complement existing guidelines for nursing staff (Royal College of Nursing, 1995). The guidelines are not intended as a substitute for local policies and protocols but should provide a useful source of reference for those writing such documents. Non-tunnelled lines and dialysis lines are not discussed, but some reference is made to peripherally inserted central catheters (PICC lines).

Major recommendations

1   Tunnelled central venous lines (catheters) are indicated for the repeated administration of chemotherapy, antibiotics, parenteral feeding and blood products, and for frequent blood sampling.

2   Single-lumen catheters are to be preferred as they cause fewer problems, but multiple-lumen catheters have specific indications.

3   Fully implantable catheters (ports) are more suitable for children and for less frequent but long-term use, whereas non-fully-implantable lines are better for short-term use and intensive access.

4   Insertion should be performed by experienced operators, regardless of speciality. Lines should be inserted in children by paediatric specialists.

5   Imaging facilities (fluoroscopy, intravenous contrast studies and standard radiography) must be available.

6   Line insertion should take place in an operating theatre or similar clean environment.

7   Skin cleansing is of the utmost importance.

8   Routine antibiotic prophylaxis should not be used.

9   Dressings are not required in the long term, but regular flushing (by protocol, according to the type of line) is essential to prevent thrombosis.

Reprinted with permission from *British Journal of Haematology*, 1997, **98**, 1041–1047.

10   Pre-existing haemorrhagic, thrombotic or infective problems must be effectively managed before line insertion.

11   Thrombosis and infection must be promptly diagnosed and vigorously treated. Both complications may require removal of the line.

12   Catheters should be removed only by experienced personnel. Catheter breakage requires expert radiological intervention.

13   Patients should receive clear and comprehensive verbal and written information and be encouraged to look after their own lines.

14   Units should audit complications associated with central lines and use the data to develop preventive measures.

2 Indications for catheter insertion

These catheters are indicated: (i) when venous access is poor; (ii) when embarking on prolonged intravenous chemotherapy and/or total parenteral nutrition (TPN) or for repeated administration of blood products, etc.; (iii) when intravenous therapy involves drugs known to be venous sclerosants; and (iv) when ambulatory chemotherapy is to be given as an out-patient.

3 Choice of catheter

Catheters are divided into: (i) tunnelled fully implantable devices; and (ii) non-fully implantable devices. They may have single or multiple lumina. Multiple-lumen catheters are advantageous in patients undergoing bone-marrow transplantation or high-dose chemotherapy where a number of agents and blood products are required to be infused simultaneously. Multiple-lumen catheters are more expensive and associated with increased morbidity (Henriques *et al.*, 1993), so they should be used only when indicated.

Catheters are made of either silicon rubber or polyurethane, the former being associated with a lower risk of thrombosis and the latter providing a larger lumen for the same outer diameter of the line. Non-fully implantable lines have a Dacron cuff, which induces an inflammatory reaction, leading to fibrosis. Fixation of the catheter usually occurs within 3–4 weeks of insertion. The Dacron cuff does not prevent infection, but lines with additional antimicrobial cuffs are available.

The four commercially available types of catheter are summarized in Table 21.1. It is important to choose the appropriate luminal size of catheter for the patient and the proposed application.

4 Insertion of catheter

We recommend that catheters are inserted only by experienced personnel. The procedure should be performed in a clean area, e.g. X-ray department, operating theatre or cardiac catheterization suite, where a high standard of asepsis is practised. Units which currently

Table 21.1 Tunnelled central venous lines: catheters available

Catheter	Type	Advantages	Disadvantages	Cost of catheter	Cost of maintenance
Hickman (Bard) and Hickman-like (e.g. Cook, Vygon)	End hole, not fully implantable (NFI)	Readily available Widespread experience of use	Need regular flushing using heparin Interference with activities Higher risk of infection	Low	High
Groshong	Side hole, with valve, NFI	Radio-opaque tip Less frequent flushing without need for heparin Valve makes bleeding or air embolism less likely Smaller than Hickman lines for same flow rate Easier to insert percutaneously (dedicated insertion kit)	As for Hickman Unsuitable for collection of PBSC	Medium	High
Apheresis	End or side hole, large bore, NFI	Permits high blood flows, e.g. for PBSC collection	As for Hickman Limited line survival Requires high doses of heparin Uncomfortable for patient	Medium	High, but usually short-term
Subcutaneous port	Fully implantable	Less risk of displacement Less interference with activities Reduced risk of infection Infrequent flushing More suitable for long-term use	Not suitable for frequent repeated access Requires special needles Infection worse if it occurs	High	Low

PBSC, peripheral-blood stem cells.

insert central venous lines on the wards should audit their infection rates in order to support continuation of this practice. Published evidence shows, however, that the risk of infection depends mainly on the presence of bacteria on the skin (Campbell *et al.*, 1994).

In the operating theatre, a mobile image intensifier can be used to provide imaging guidance; the appropriate radiological safety precautions must be taken, including the wearing of lead aprons. Normally, a line is inserted under local anaesthesia with sedation, such as intravenous midazolam. This is not appropriate for children, who will require a general anaesthetic. Open insertion in adults is also better performed under general anaesthesia, first attempting to insert the catheter into the external jugular and then, if unsuccessful, into the main jugular vein.

There are two general types of tunnelled central venous catheter: antegrade and retrograde. Antegrade tunnelled catheters must be measured and cut to the correct length, leaving as smooth a tip as possible. This is best done using fluoroscopic guidance and works well in most patients. With retrograde tunnelling, the tip of the catheter is positioned under fluoroscopy and should be above the right atrium. The catheter is then tunnelled retrogradely before the hub is fixed on to its proximal end. Tunnelling may not reduce the rate of infection but minimizes the risk of accidental displacement.

Lines are increasingly inserted percutaneously and the optimum method is by the use of imaging guidance under local anaesthesia and sedation. Anatomical surface markings can be unreliable for the initial puncture, and both ultrasound and venography via the antecubital vein may be helpful. These techniques also establish the patency of the veins. A lateral insertion site reduces the risk of pneumothorax and avoids 'pinch-off' of the catheter between the clavicle and the first rib (Robertson *et al.*, 1989). An alternative is to use the jugular vein; this is a rapid, straightforward procedure, which is particularly useful in patients with abnormal coagulation, as it minimizes the risk of inadvertent arterial puncture (Lameris *et al.*, 1990). In patients in whom the internal jugular and both subclavian veins are occluded or otherwise unavailable for puncture, catheters may be inserted into the femoral veins, into the hepatic veins or directly into the inferior vena cava (IVC), using an interventional radiological technique. These techniques must only be performed by experienced radiologists, and electrocardiogram (ECG) monitoring is required when lines are advanced into the IVC, as there is a significant incidence of dysrhythmia.

A variety of catheter puncture kits can be used. It is recommended that a coaxial catheter introduction system is used, with a 20- or 21-gauge needle for the initial puncture. There are also 25-gauge micropuncture sets available and these are useful for children, minimizing the risk of bleeding in patients with abnormal coagulation and the need for intervention if the pleura is punctured.

With subcutaneous ports, subclavian venous access is achieved under aseptic conditions, in the same way as for externalized tunnelled lines (Sherry *et al.*, 1992). A suitable site for the port is chosen in the chest wall, in a position in which it may be accessed by the patient. It is important to provide a bony support for the port during access, allow for a short but gently curved path from the reservoir to the site of venous access and avoiding mammary tissue.

Peripherally inserted central catheters require less in the way of facilities or operator experience and may be inserted in a side room on the ward by nursing staff (Roundtree, 1991). Tip placement should be checked by X-ray and often requires adjustment. The role of these lines in the UK remains to be established. The subject has been reviewed by Braun (1994).

5 Patient care prior to catheter insertion

Skin cleansing is the most important part of care before line insertion. Chlorhexidine is the most effective agent (Maki *et al.*, 1991). If povidone iodine is to be used (assuming the patient is not allergic), the skin should be cleaned for 3 min and the iodine allowed to dry. Depilation may be necessary but shaving of the chest wall should not be performed. Patients should ideally shower with Hibiscrub prior to line insertion and wash their hair with chlorhexidine to reduce staphylococcal burden.

6 Antibiotic prophylaxis

Various published studies have produced conflicting results as to the value of prophylaxis in non-neutropenic cancer and non-cancer patients requiring a central venous catheter for intravenous treatments. There are a number of prospective randomized trials examining the use of either vancomycin or teicoplanin in adults and children undergoing treatment for haematological and non-haematological malignancies (Ranson *et al.*, 1990; Schwartz *et al.*, 1990; Schaison & Decroly, 1991; Lim *et al.*, 1993; Vassilomanolakis *et al.*, 1995).

The majority of Gram-positive infections preventable by glycopeptide prophylaxis are due to coagulase-negative staphylococci. Although these cause a considerable amount of morbidity, they are rarely associated with mortality and are amenable to therapy. The inexorable spread of vancomycin-resistant enterococci, which cause significant infections in cancer patients (Montecalvo *et al.*, 1994; Edmond *et al.*, 1995; Noskin *et al.*, 1995) and which are being increasingly isolated in the UK (Anon., 1995), are causing many to rethink their use of glycopeptides. The Centers for Disease Control and Prevention (1994) have issued guidelines for limiting the use of vancomycin, stating that the agent should not be used for routine prophylaxis, i.v. colonization, catheter-related infections with β-lactam-sensitive organisms or empirical therapy of febrile neutropenic patients.

The overall balance is therefore against the routine use of a glycopeptide as prophylaxis for catheter insertion, certainly in non-neutropenic patients. The data on patients neutropenic at the time of catheter insertion are clinically of greater importance but, inevitably, more scanty. If the patient is severely neutropenic (white blood-cell count (WBC) $<0.5 \times 10^9/1$) and likely to bleed during the procedure, then anecdotal evidence suggests a high risk of infection. Studies of the benefits of prophylaxis in this setting are urgently needed. Recent work suggests that loading of catheters with a silver–teicoplanin complex during manufacture may reduce adherence of microorganisms and prevent colonization (Jansen *et al.*, 1994).

7 Immediate patient care postcatheter insertion

After the procedure, the wounds should be dressed; once bloodstained, dressings should be changed immediately. Because of the 1–2% incidence of traumatic pneumothorax post-operatively (Ray *et al.*, 1996), a chest X-ray is required if the patient becomes dyspnoeic. The incidence of pneumothorax relates to the site used for line insertion into the subclavian vein. Most pneumothoraces do not require treatment but should be monitored. Needle evacuation is often sufficient when treatment is required, and formal chest drainage is rarely indicated.

Occlusive dressings should be avoided, and it is better to use a porous adhesive dressing, such as Tegaderm (3M Healthcare Products, USA) or a semi-occlusive dressing such as OpSite IV 3000 (Smith & Nephew, UK). The latter should be changed weekly. Other dressings should be changed daily until the wound is healed, after which no dressing is required but the catheter should be looped and fixed to the skin.

The upper suture over the insertion site into the subclavian vein may be removed at 7–10 days and the lower one at the exit point may be removed after 3 weeks. This, however, may remain long-term if there is any concern regarding the line falling out spontaneously. Subcuticular proline does not need to be removed and ensures that the line remains in place. Sutures over a Portacath insertion site are removed at 7–10 days.

With the Groshong catheter, the line may be glued to a retaining cassette sutured to the skin. The glue takes 24 h to set.

8 Long-term catheter care

This subject has been audited by Morris *et al.* (1995). Once the wound has healed, there is no need for any dressing. For non-fully implantable devices, it is necessary to loop the tails and fix them to the chest. When required, the tails are taken down to avoid twisting at the exit site. The patient should be advised to keep the catheter exit site dry for 10 days and subsequently to use a short-term occlusive dressing while bathing, showering or swimming in order to prevent colonization by Gram-negative organisms, especially *Pseudomonas* spp.

Flushing protocols for the four main types of catheter are shown in Table 21.2. Care must always be taken to maintain positive pressure while clamping the line at the end of flushing, in order to avoid reflux of blood.

9 Patient information

A patient's guide should include the following sections.
1   What is a central venous (e.g. Hickman) line?
2   Uses of the line.
3   Caring for the line.
4   Keeping the line clean:
    (a)   before exit site healed;
    (b)   after site healed.
5   Flushing the line.
6   Changing the bung.

A suitable leaflet may be generated locally or may be obtained from Bard Ltd. (Forest House, Brighton Road, Crawley, West Sussex, RH11 9BP). Examples of guidance are given in Table 21.3.

Table 21.2 Catheter-flushing protocols

Catheter	Solutions	Frequency	Cautions
Hickman (Bard) and Hickman-like (e.g. Cook, Vygon)	Heparin 50 u/ml	After access or at least weekly	Maintain positive pressure until catheter clamped
Groshong	Saline	After access or at least weekly	
Apheresis	Heparin 1000 u/ml or 5000 u/ml according to risk of thrombosis	After access or at least twice weekly	Maintain positive pressure Calculate 'dead space' and avoid systemic heparinization
Subcutaneous port	Heparin 100 u/ml If attached to Groshong lines, heparin not required	Before and after access or at least monthly	Maintain positive pressure until needle removed
Heparin solutions	10 u/ml, e.g. Heplok, Hepsal 100 u/ml, e.g. Hep-Flush, Canusal 1000–5000 u/ml, e.g. heparin injection (unfractionated)		

Table 21.3 Examples of patient guidance

Do contact your nurse or doctor if your central line is red, sore or oozing pus or if you have a temperature >38°C

Do contact your nurse or doctor if your line becomes damaged or leaks – after placing an extra clamp above the damaged area

Do contact your nurse or doctor if your arm becomes swollen or you notice any enlarged veins on your chest or neck

Do not leave the clamp open unless you are using the line

Do not allow anyone to handle the line if they are not sure what to do

10 Patient care of own catheter, access and training issues

Prior to discharge, the clinical staff should ensure that the patient or his/her carer is educated in the use of the catheter. It is more desirable that the patient/carer looks after the line rather than a district nurse inexperienced in its usage. After insertion, initial support in catheter care should come from the parent unit in the form of flushing, dressing and clinical review. Access to the line by different personnel should be kept to a minimum, as the more people using the line the greater the risk of infection. This should be undertaken only by trained staff or the patient him/herself, particularly in the domiciliary setting. Careful hand-washing is essential and gloves should be worn when opening or replacing bungs.

A blood-sampling protocol should be developed locally, but ideally would require the removal of the heparinized dead space (approximately 5 ml) prior to sampling. The volume to be removed before coagulation studies are performed is uncertain with central venous lines, but for activated partial thromboplastin time (APTT) studies from arterial lines it is recommended that six times the dead space volume is removed (Laxson & Titler, 1994). This recommendation is not appropriate for the paediatric patient with a Broviac catheter or in those patients with an apheresis line whose luminal space contains greater than 5000 units of heparin. Coagulation studies in such circumstances produce erroneous results, and the sample should be taken from a peripheral vein. In the bone-marrow transplant setting, the lumen for cyclosporin A and other drug levels should be identified and the drugs administered through a different lumen.

11 Management of problem patients

11.1 Thrombocytopenic

If the patient is thrombocytopenic, the catheter should be inserted by a jugular approach, with care to avoid puncturing the carotid artery. A subclavian approach is associated with tunnelling through muscle and it is also possible inadvertently to breach the subclavian artery. If the platelet count is $<50 \times 10^9/l$ the patient should be transfused with platelet concentrate, ideally to a count $>100 \times 10^9/l$. If there is evidence of bleeding postcatheter insertion, the patient should receive further platelet transfusion(s) to maintain the count in excess of $50 \times 10^9/l$ for the next 48 h. Problems may arise in patients refractory to random-donor platelets (Pheeko *et al.*, 1996).

11.2 Disseminated intravascular coagulation

In those patients with disseminated intravascular coagulation, e.g. in association with acute promyelocytic leukaemia, there should be vigorous correction of any abnormality of coagulation. The prothrombin time should be <1.3 times normal and fibrinogen >1.0 g/l. If fibrin degradation products (FDPs) are very high, this will have an additional adverse effect on coagulation.

Patients on oral anticoagulants should stop their tablets to achieve an International Normalized Ratio (INR) <1.3 before line insertion. If time is limited, fresh-frozen plasma (FFP), factor concentrates or vitamin K may be required, but the latter may interfere with subsequent anticoagulation (BCSH, 1990). Intravenous heparin should be stopped 3 h before insertion and restarted when haemostasis is secured.

11.3 Haemophilia

Haemophiliac patients (with haemophilia A, B or C) will require appropriate factor replacement. Correction should be maintained for >48 h. Clinicians caring for these patients should seek advice from their local haemophilia reference centre.

11.4 Infection

Infection at the time of line insertion represents a relative contraindication to proceeding, and consideration should be given to temporary line placement. If the patient has a unilateral skin infection on the anterior upper chest wall, the unaffected side should be used.

11.5 Radiotherapy

A patient who has received previous radiotherapy to one side of the chest should have the catheter inserted on the opposite side, although patients with breast cancer may prefer a line inserted under their prosthesis.

11.6 Venous insufficiency

If there are symptoms and signs of venous insufficiency, subclavian venous stenosis may be reliably diagnosed by injecting contrast medium through the ipsilateral anterior cubital fossa or, more rapidly but less reliably, by ultrasound. This represents a further contraindication to catheter insertion on that side.

12 Prevention and management of catheter complications

The main complications are: (i) thrombosis; and (ii) infection.

12.1 Thrombosis

Partial and complete catheter blockage is evidenced by difficulty in aspirating blood or infusing fluid. Forcible introduction of fluid down an obstructed lumen may cause catheter rupture. Catheter blockage may be due to kinking of the catheter in the subclavian vein, occlusion of the catheter tip on the vessel wall or luminal thrombus. Plain X-ray or a catheter contrast study may be helpful in confirming the diagnosis.

Catheter kinking can sometimes be relieved by a change in the position of the patient and is less common with lateral insertion of the catheter under fluoroscopic control. Occlusion of the catheter tip against the vessel wall can be rectified by tilting the patient head down.

Catheter thrombosis may be spontaneous or may result from a prothrombotic state associated with either underlying malignancy or treatment, particularly with L-asparaginase. Thrombosis may be prevented by adhering to appropriate flushing protocols (see Table 21.2). The use of low-dose warfarin may also be effective and may be particularly indicated in patients who have had a previous catheter thrombosis (Bern *et al.*, 1990). However, this study excluded patients with platelet counts $<125 \times 10^9/l$ or any coagulopathy, and the use of low-dose warfarin in patients with abnormal haemostasis should be approached with caution.

In catheter occlusion due to thrombus but without symptomatic thrombosis, instillation of a fibrinolytic solution, such as 2 ml urokinase 4000 u/ml, should be tried. The solution should be injected gently into the catheter with a push–pull action to maximize mixing within the lumen. The lumen should then be clamped and left for at least 2–3 h. The catheter should then be unclamped and the solution with disaggregated clot aspirated.

If this procedure fails or there is symptomatic upper-limb thrombosis and the catheter needs to be left *in situ* for further use, a prolonged urokinase infusion through the catheter may be employed (Haire *et al.*, 1990). Anticoagulation is indicated following urokinase infusion, but, if rethrombosis occurs, a further urokinase infusion may clear the catheter. There are no data on the level of anticoagulation required posturokinase infusion to prevent thrombosis. There are similarly no data on ideal levels of anticoagulation in thrombocytopenic patients or on the duration of anticoagulant therapy in catheter-related thrombosis.

If the catheter is to be removed, some authorities advise urokinase infusion prior to catheter removal, either through a peripheral vein or through the catheter itself. After catheter removal, the patient should be anticoagulated. In non-thrombocytopenic patients, standard heparin and warfarin are reasonable. In thrombocytopenic patients, low-molecular-weight heparin may be used. One published regimen utilizes enoxaparin 40 mg subcutaneously twice daily for 14 days, followed by 40 mg daily for at least 8 weeks (Drakos *et al.*, 1992).

12.2 Catheter infection

Recommendations for good practice regarding prevention, diagnosis and treatment of infections (and other aspects of central venous catheterization) have been published by Elliott *et al.* (1994).

There are three categories.

1 A catheter-related bacteraemia is defined as at least two blood cultures positive with the same organism obtained from at least two separate sites at different times, in association with evidence of colonization of the catheter with the same organism. The latter part of the definition can only be strictly fulfilled by removing the catheter. Attempts to incriminate the catheter as the source of bacteraemia (without removing it) by using quantitative blood cultures, such as the Isolator system (Oxoid), have met with mixed success and the method is labour-intensive. Simple sensitive diagnostic techniques are still awaited (Reimer, 1994).

2 An exit-site infection presents with erythema, tenderness and occasionally a discharge at the insertion site.

3 A tunnel infection is characterized by pain and induration along the track of the catheter.

The incidence of these infections varies in different centres with different groups of patients and different practices. In a series of 690 Hickman-catheter insertions, followed up for a mean of 195 days at a single centre between 1978 and 1987, the incidences of catheter-related bacteraemias, exit-site infections and tunnel infections were 57%, 23% and 7%, respectively (Newman *et al.*, 1993).

The management of catheter infections remains controversial. Attempts should be made to make a microbiological diagnosis by culturing blood from all catheter lumina, a peripheral sample of blood and the exit site before commencing antibiotics. Table 21.4 summarizes current recommendations, based upon consensus and the literature. Recent evidence suggests that *in situ* use of glycopeptides may be highly effective and infusion is better than bolus injection (McCarthy *et al.*, 1995; Ley *et al.*, 1996). The 'antibiotic lock' technique, however, may be less effective with subcutaneous ports (Longuet *et al.*, 1995).

Table 21.4 Recommendations for the management of catheter-related infections

Category of infection	Neutropenic patient	Non-neutropenic patient
Presumed catheter-related bacteraemia/fungaemia	Initial empirical antibiotic therapy; modify according to isolates Treat for at least 10–14 days (consider longer if still neutropenic) Remove catheter if cultures remain positive after 48 h of therapy or if proven catheter-related infection with *Staphylococcus aureus, Bacillus* spp., pseudomonads, *Mycobacterium* spp. or fungi	Remove catheter if no longer needed Treat with antibiotics targeted against isolates

Exit-site infection	Initial empirical therapy, including glycopeptide
	Treat for at least 10–14 days or longer until infection resolved
	   Modify according to isolates. Remove catheter if evidence of progression or if blood cultures positive for *Staphylococcus aureus, Bacillus* spp., pseudomonads, *Mycobacterium* spp. or fungi
	   Line may be salvaged by surgical incision and drainage
		Remove catheter if no longer needed
		Treat empirically with flucloxacillin

Tunnel infection	Remove catheter and drain pus Initial empirical therapy, including glycopeptide Treat for at least 10–14 days or until resolution of soft-tissue infection Modify according to isolates	Treat empirically with flucloxacillin

13 Technique of catheter removal

Indications for catheter removal include: (i) sepsis; (ii) irremediable blockage; (iii) axillary or other venous thrombosis attributable to the line; (iv) exteriorization of the cuff; (v) irreparable damage to the catheter, including that caused by 'pinch-off' syndrome; and (vi) the end of treatment.

Patients should be adequately sedated and receive good local anaesthesia, although a brief general anaesthetic may be required.

1   Simple traction on the catheter may be effective.

2   It may be necessary to dissect the Dacron cuff.

3   If difficulty is encountered, insertion of a guide-wire is recommended, followed by dissection of the Dacron cuff. Bard catheters are designed such that the cuff can remain behind. This is not desirable for neutropenic patients and, if the catheter is removed for infection, the cuff should always be removed.

It is important to remove the catheter in the direction of the tunnel. The line should be inspected carefully after removal to ensure that it is complete and the tip sent to the microbiology department for culture. After removal, the patient should sit up and pressure applied to the exit point, tunnel and venotomy site.

14 Repair of damaged catheters and tip retrieval

Only trained personnel should be allowed to undertake these tasks. If the catheter tip is sheared off during removal, it is likely to travel into the pulmonary artery. Either a 'basket' or a 'lassoo' technique is used to retrieve the tip under fluoroscopic guidance. Repair kits should be available to rectify catheter damage and a variety must be stocked if different lines are in use. Further details are beyond the scope of these guidelines.

15 Recommendations for audit

A locally based audit should include patient-identification data, diagnosis, date of line insertion, number of previous lines, operator and department where line inserted, complications associated with the line and date of and reason for removal.

16 Acknowledgement

We gratefully acknowledge the assistance of Miss Alison Hammond in preparing multiple drafts of these guidelines.

References

Anon. (1995) Vancomycin-resistant enterococci in hospitals in the United Kingdom. *Communicable Disease Report Weekly* **5**, 281.

BCSH (1990) Guidelines on oral anticoagulation. *Journal of Clinical Pathology* **43**, 177–183.

Bern M.M., Lokich J.J., Wallach S.R. *et al.* (1990) Very low doses of warfarin can prevent thrombosis in central venous catheters. *Annals of Internal Medicine* **112**, 423–428.

Braun M.A. (1994) Image-guided peripheral venous access catheters and implantable ports. *Seminars in Interventional Radiology* **11**, 358–365.

Campbell W.E., Mauro M.A. & Jacques P.F. (1994) Radiological insertion of long-term venous access devices. *Seminars in Interventional Radiology* **11**, 366–376.

Centers for Disease Control and Prevention (1994) Preventing the spread of vancomycin resistance: report from the Hospital Infection Control Practices Advisory Committee. *Federal Register* **59**, 25757–25763.

Drakos P.E., Nagler A., Or R., Gillis S., Slavin S. & Eldor A. (1992) Low molecular weight heparin for Hickman catheter-induced thrombosis in thrombocytopenic patients undergoing bone marrow transplantation. *Cancer* **70**, 1895–1898.

Edmond M.B., Ober J.F., Weinbaum D.L., Pfaller M.A., Hwang T. & Sanford M.D. (1995) Vancomycin-resistant *Enterococcus faecium* bacteremia: risk factors for infection. *Clinical Infectious Diseases* **20**, 1126–1133.

Elliott T.S.J., Faroqui M.H., Armstrong R.F. & Hanson G.C. (1994) Guidelines for good practice in central venous catheterization. *Journal of Hospital Infection* **28**, 163–176.

Haire W.D., Lieberman R.P., Lund G.B., Edney J. & Wieczorek B.M. (1990) Obstructed central venous catheters: restoring function with a 12-hour infusion of urokinase. *Cancer* **66**, 2279–2285.

Henriques H.F., Kanny-Jones R., Knoll S.M., Copes W.S. & Giordano J.M. (1993) Avoid complications of long-term venous access. *American Surgery* **9**, 555–558.

Jansen B., Ruiten D. & Pulverer G. (1994) A central venous catheter loaded with silver–teicoplanin is able to prevent catheter colonization. In *94th General Meeting, American Society for Microbiology, Las Vegas, 23–27 May 1994, Abstracts*, p. 615.

Lameris J.S., Post P.J.M., Zonderland H.M., Gerritsen P.G., Kappers-Klunne M.C. & Schutte H.E. (1990) Percutaneous placement of Hickman catheters: comparison of sonographically guided and blind techniques. *American Journal of Radiology* **155**, 1097–1099.

Laxson C.J. & Titler M.G. (1994) Drawing coagulation studies from arterial lines: an integrative literature review. *American Journal of Critical Care* **3**, 16–22.

Ley B.E., Jalil N., McIntosh J. *et al.* (1996) Bolus or infusion teicoplanin for intravascular catheter associated infections in immunocompromised patients? *Journal of Antimicrobial Chemotherapy* **38**, 1091–1095.

Lim S.H., Smith M.P., Machin S.J. & Goldstone A.H. (1993) A prospective randomized study of prophylactic teicoplanin to prevent early Hickman catheter-related sepsis in patients receiving intensive chemotherapy for haematological malignancies. *European Journal of Haematology* **54** (Suppl.), 10–13.

Longuet P., Douard M.C., Maslo C., Benoit C., Arlet G. & Leport C. (1995) Limited efficacy of antibiotic lock technique in catheter related bacteraemia of totally implanted ports in HIV infected and oncologic patients. In *15th Interdisciplinary Meeting on Anti-Infectious Chemotherapy, Paris, 7–8 December 1995, Abstracts*, p. 135.

McCarthy A., Byrne M., Breathnach F. & O'Meara A. (1995) 'In-situ' teicoplanin for central venous catheter infection. *Irish Journal of Medical Science* **164**, 125–127.

Maki D., Ringer M. & Alvarado C.J. (1991) Prospective randomised trial of povidone iodine, alcohol and chlorhexidine for prevention of infection associated with central venous and arterial catheters. *Lancet* **338**, 339–343.

Montecalvo M.A., Horowitz H., Gedris C. *et al.* (1994) Outbreak of vancomycin, ampicillin and aminoglycoside-resistant *Enterococcus faecium* bacteremia in an adult oncology unit. *Antimicrobial Agents and Chemotherapy* **38**, 1363–1367.

Morris P., Grace S., Glackin V. *et al.* (1995) Audit of skin tunnelled catheters in neutropenic patients. *Bone Marrow Transplantation* **15** (Suppl. 2), 168 (abstract).

Newman K.A., Reed W.P., Schimpff S.C., Bustamante C.I. & Wade J.C. (1993) Hickman catheters in association with intensive cancer chemotherapy. *Supportive Care in Cancer* **1**, 92–97.

Noskin G.A., Cooper I. & Peterson L.R. (1995) Vancomycin-resistant *Enterococcus faecium* sepsis following persistent colonization. *Archives of Internal Medicine* **155**, 1445–1447.

Pheeko K., Hambley H., Win N., Murphy M., Carr R. & Schey S. (1996) *South Thames Haematology Specialist Committee; Audit of Practice in Platelet Refractoriness.*

Ranson M.R., Oppenheim B.A., Jackson A., Kamthan A.G. & Scarffe J.H. (1990) Double-blind placebo controlled study of vancomycin prophylaxis for central venous catheter insertion in cancer patients. *Journal of Hospital Infection* **15**, 5–102.

Ray S., Stacey R., Imrie M. & Filshie J. (1996) A review of 560 Hickman catheter insertions. *Anaesthesia* **51**, 981–985.

Reimer L.G. (1994) Catheter-related infections and blood cultures. *Clinics in Laboratory Medicine* **14**, 51–58.

Robertson L.J., Mauro M.A. & Jacques P.F. (1989) Radiologic placement of Hickman catheters. *Radiology* **170**, 1007–1009.

Roundtree D. (1991) The PIC catheter: a different approach. *American Journal of Nursing* **91** (8), 22–26.

Royal College of Nursing of the United Kingdom Leukaemia and Bone Marrow Transplant Nursing Forum (1995) *Skin Tunnelled Catheters: Guidelines for Care*, 2nd edn. Scutari Projects, Viking House, 17/19 Peterborough Road, Harrow, Middlesex HA1 2AX.

Schaison G.S. & Decroly F.C. (1991) Prophylaxis, cost and effectiveness of therapy of infections caused by Gram-positive organisms in neutropenic children. *Journal of Antimicrobial Chemotherapy* **27** (Suppl. B), 61–67.

Schwartz C., Henrickson K.J., Roghmann J. & Powell K. (1990) Prevention of bacteraemia attributed to luminal colonization of tunnelled central venous catheters with vancomycin-susceptible organisms. *Journal of Clinical Oncology* **8**, 1591–1597.

Sherry L., Morris M.D., Paul F., Jacques M.D., Matthew A. & Mauro M.D. (1992) Radiology assisted placement of implantable subcutaneous infusion ports for long-term venous access. *Radiology* **184**, 149–151.

Vassilomanolakis M., Plataniotis G., Koumakis G., Hajichristou H., Dova H. & Efremidis A.P. (1995) Central venous catheter-related infections after bone marrow transplantation in patients with malignancies: a prospective study with short-course vancomycin prophylaxis. *Bone Marrow Transplantation* **15**, 77–80.

Index

Page numbers in **bold** refer to tables